Childhood Onset of "Adult" Psychopathology

Clinical and Research Advances

Childhood Onset of "Adult" Psychopathology

Clinical and Research Advances

EDITED BY

Judith L. Rapoport, M.D.

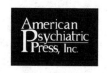

Washington, DC
London, England

Copyright © 2000 American Psychiatric Press, Inc.
ALL RIGHTS RESERVED
Manufactured in the United States of America on acid-free paper
03 02 01 00   4 3 2 1
First Edition

American Psychiatric Press, Inc.
1400 K Street, N.W., Washington, DC20005
www.appi.org

Library of Congress Cataloging-in-Publication Data
Childhood onset of "adult" psychopathology: clinical and research advances/
  edited by Judith L. Rapoport. — 1st ed.
        p.   cm.   —(American Psychopathological Association series)
    Includes bibliographical references and index.
    ISBN 0-88048-821-2
    1. Child psychopathology Congresses. 2. Mental illness
Longitudinal studies Congresses. 3. Psychology, Pathological Congresses.
I. Series.
    [DNLM: 1. Psychopathology—Child Congresses.
2. Psychopathology—Infant Congresses. 3. Developmental
Disabilities—prevention and control—Child Congresses.
4. Developmental Disabilities—prevention and control—Infant
Congresses. 5. Mental Disorders—Child Congresses. 6. Mental
Disorders—Infant Congresses. WS 350 C5362 1999]
RJ499.C4878 1999
618.92′ 89—dc21
DNLM/DLC
for Library of Congress   99-26039
                                                                         CIP

British Library Cataloguing in Publication Data
A CIP record is available from the British Library.

Contents

I   Age at Onset: Mechanisms and Methods

II   Neurodevelopmental Pathways to "Adult" Psychiatric Disorders: Triggers of Disease Onset

III Schizophrenia: Specific Disorders

IV Depression and Anxiety

V Early Prevention of Adult Psychiatric Disorders

Contributors

Judith A. Badner, M.D., Ph.D.
Assistant Professor, Department of Psychiatry, University of Chicago, Chicago, Illinois

William R. Beardslee, M.D.
Department of Psychiatry, Children's Hospital, Harvard Medical School, Boston, Massachusetts

Alan Brown, M.D.
Department of Epidemiology of Brain Disorders, New York State Psychiatric Institute, New York, New York

Gabrielle A. Carlson, M.D.
Professor of Psychiatry and Pediatics and Director, Child and Adolescent Psychiatry, State University of New York at Stony Brook, Stony Brook, New York

Stephanie Ceman, Ph.D.
Research Associate, Howard Hughes Medical Institute and Departments of Biochemistry, Pediatrics and Genetics, Emory University School of Medicine, Atlanta, Georgia

Barton Childs, M.D.
Professor Emeritus, Department of Pediatrics, Johns Hopkins University School of Medicine, Baltimore, Maryland

Sevilla D. Detera-Wadleigh, Ph.D.
Clinical Neurogenetics Branch, National Institute of Mental Health, Bethesda, Maryland

Lisa T. Eyler Zorrilla, Ph.D.
Postdoctoral Fellow, Department of Psychiatry, University of California, San Diego; VA San Diego Healthcare System, San Diego, California

Paul Fearon, M.B., M.R.C.Psych.
Department of Psychological Medicine, Institute of Psychiatry, London, United Kingdom

Elliot S. Gershon, M.D.
Chairman, Department of Psychiatry, University of Chicago, Chicago, Illinois

Richard Harrington, F.R.C.Psych.
Department of Child and Adolescent Psychiatry, Royal Manchester Children's Hospital, Manchester, England

Dilip V. Jeste, M.D.
Professor of Psychiatry and Neurosciences, Department of Psychiatry, University of California, San Diego; Director, Geriatric Psychiatry Interventions Research Center; VA San Diego Healthcare System, San Diego, California

Peter B. Jones, M.B., M.Sc., Ph.D., M.R.C.P., M.R.C.Psych.
Professor, Division of Psychiatry, University of Nottingham, Nottingham, England

Roselind Lieb, Ph.D., Dipl.Psych.
Max Planck Institute of Psychiatry, Munich, Germany

Tom Matte, M.D., M.P.H.
Senior Epidemiologist, Center for Urban Epidemiologic Studies, New York Academy of Medicine, New York, New York; Centers for Disease Control and Prevention, Atlanta, Georgia

Colm McDonald, M.B., M.R.C.Psych.
Department of Psychological Medicine, Institute of Psychiatry, London, United Kingdom

Donna Moreau, M.D.
Associate Clinical Professor of Psychiatry, College of Physicians and Surgeons of Columbia University; Research Scientist, New York State Psychiatric Institute, New York, New York

Robin M. Murray, D.Sc., F.R.C.Psych.
Department of Psychological Medicine, Institute of Psychiatry, London, England

Rob Nicolson, M.D.
Staff Psychiatrist, Child Psychiatry Branch, National Institute of Mental Health, Bethesda, Maryland

David R. Offord, M.D.
Director, Centre for Studies of Children at Risk, Hamilton Health Sciences Corporation; Faculty of Health Sciences, McMaster University, Hamilton, Ontario, Canada

Albertine J. Oldehinkel, Ph.D.
Max Planck Institute of Psychiatry, Munich, Germany

Mark Olfson, M.D.
Associate Professor of Clinical Psychiatry, College of Physicians and Surgeons of Columbia University, New York, New York

Margaret Pekar, M.A.
Research Assistant, Pediatrics and Developmental Neuropsychiatry Branch, National Institute of Mental Health, Bethesda, Maryland

Judith L. Rapoport, M.D.
Chief, Child Psychiatry Branch, National Institute of Mental Health, Bethesda, Maryland

Peter Schuster, Dipl.Psych.
Max Planck Institute of Psychiatry, Munich, Germany

Ezra Susser, M.D., Dr.P.H.
Head, Division of Epidemiology, Mailman School of Public Health at Columbia University, New York, New York; Head, Department of Epidemiology of Brain Disorders, New York State Psychiatric Institute, New York, New York

Susan E. Swedo, M.D.
Chief, Pediatrics and Developmental Neuropsychiatry Branch, National Institute of Mental Health, Bethesda, Maryland

C. Jane Tarrant, B.Med.Sci., B.M., B.S., M.R.C.Psych.
Research Fellow, Division of Psychiatry, University of Nottingham, Nottingham, England

George E. Vaillant, M.D.
Division of Psychiatry, Brigham and Women's Hospital, Boston, Massachusetts

Virginia Warner, M.P.H.
Research Scientist, Division of Clinical and Genetic Epidemiology, New York State Psychiatric Institute, New York, New York

Stephen T. Warren, Ph.D.
William P. Timmie Professor of Human Genetics and Investigator, Howard Hughes Medical Institute and Emory University School of Medicine, Atlanta, Georgia

Myrna M. Weissman, Ph.D.
Professor of Epidemiology in Psychiatry, College of Physicians and Surgeons of Columbia University and New York State Psychiatric Institute, New York, New York

Priya Wickramaratne, Ph.D.
Associate Professor of Biostatistics in Psychiatry, College of Physicians and Surgeons of Columbia University, New York, New York

Hans-Ulrich Wittchen, Ph.D., Dipl.Psych.
Max Planck Institute of Psychiatry, Munich, Germany

Introduction

This volume contains presentations from the 87th meeting of the American Psychopathological Association (APPA), held in March 1998 in New York City. It meant a great deal, as President, to preside over this meeting. During my research training years, the APPA scholarly presentations, together with the informality and lively exchanges, had a major and nourishing influence on me and on numerous other aspiring clinician researchers.

The theme for the 1998 meeting, "Childhood Onset of 'Adult' Psychiatric Disorders," reflected the growing body of data on very early forms of depression, criminality, alcoholism, schizophrenia, and anxiety. Age at onset has classically determined major categories of illness. Today, our interest is also propelled by the last few decades of genetic research in which consideration of age at onset for a variety of disorders has led to identification of unique genes and, in some cases, physiologically different disorders. For example, in diabetes mellitus, the independent familial aggregation of childhood-onset cases was one clue that led to the identification of insulin-dependent diabetes mellitus and non–insulin-dependent diabetes mellitus as the two major forms of the illness.

Our introductory section on genetics begins with a discussion of models for age at onset of illness by Drs. Judith Badner, Sevilla Detera-Wadleigh, and Elliot Gershon (Chapter 1). One major point made by the authors is that when early-onset illness is under separate genetic influence, one expects to see independent familial aggregation of prepubertal-onset cases in sibs of patients, a pattern reminiscent of that seen with insulin-dependent diabetes mellitus. The authors propose specific research strategies for examining age-at-onset effects within linkage studies and demonstrate some of these strategies by presenting their own findings within a large bipolar pedigree.

An initial overview of genetics and age at onset is provided by Dr.

Barton Childs (Chapter 2), a pediatrician and geneticist who has been writing about early age at onset for the past two decades. He reviews the larger picture of the significance of age at onset in terms of individual variability and the evolutionary significance of disease. More to the point, as Dr. Childs notes, age at onset is one aspect of that individuality. Age at onset is noted to be a function of genetic vulnerability, experiential factors, and developmental state. Dr. Childs gives many examples of the greater heritability of early-onset illness and implications for future programs of prevention.

Drs. Stephanie Ceman and Stephen Warren (Chapter 3) give us a lucid illustration of what is the most clear purely biological manner in which early-onset disorder progresses: trinucleotide expansion in the *FMR1* gene that causes the fragile X syndrome. In this remarkable story, parental carriers can themselves have normal mental development while carrying an intermediate expansion of the *FMR1* gene on the X chromosome. Fragile X is the best understood of such conditions, but considerable research will be needed to find out what makes FMRP, the protein which this gene produces, critical for normal mental development.

Drs. Jane Tarrant and Peter Jones (Chapter 4), from Nottingham, England, begin the next section on neurobiological pathways from childhood to adult disorders with a sweeping review of biological markers that are precursors to schizophrenia. They review studies of markers of individual diversity of the central nervous system. From Fish's classic observations of "pandevelopmental retardation" in the development of high-risk infants, to Walker's home movies during the childhood of individuals with adult-onset schizophrenia and developmental data from two British cohort studies, it is clear that subtle but abnormal nervous system development precedes the onset of schizophrenia in many, though not all, cases. Neurological "soft signs" and various dermatoglyphic and other minor physical abnormalities are also indirect evidence of impaired nervous system early in development. These, too, have an association with schizophrenia. The authors then grapple in a most lucid way with the fact that these associations are nonspecific — that is, are associated with a variety of other disorders — and that this limits the models that can be derived from them.

Dr. Susan Swedo and Ms. Margaret Pekar (Chapter 5) present

evidence for a very different pathway—that for childhood-onset obsessive-compulsive disorder (OCD). Historical reports prompted a series of studies of Sydenham's chorea as a medical model for OCD. In Sydenham's chorea, a sequel of rheumatic fever, autoimmune response to Group A β-hemolytic streptococcus infection appears to produce a rather localized effect on the basal ganglia, particularly the caudate and globus pallidus. Since 70% of Sydenham's chorea patients have full or partial OCD, the studies have gone on to look at this group with brain imaging studies, and immunosuppressant treatment has lent considerable excitement to this group's work.

Another pathway to adult disorder is through prenatal and perinatal adverse events, which have been studied extensively and are reviewed here by Drs. Ezra Susser, Alan Brown, and Tom Matte (Chapter 6). The concept of *life course epidemiology* is put forth as a broader, more dynamic view in which multiple classes of developmental impairments may interact over the course of a lifetime to produce certain disease outcomes in adulthood. The example of prenatal exposure to diethylstilbestrol and development of vaginal cancer in female offspring in their teens and twenties represents such a medical model. In a variety of studies of prenatal influenza and rubella infections and exposure to famine conditions, the association with adult-onset schizophrenia has been demonstrated. As with the data reviewed by Drs. Tarrant and Jones's, the issues of delayed onset and of the nonspecificity of precursors remain important factors in modeling developmental pathways to schizophrenia. Ongoing studies with large U.S. birth cohorts whose members are now past the age of maximum risk for psychosis will further refine these models.

It is easy for child psychiatrists to forget that late age at onset of disorder is just as pertinent to the understanding of disease etiology. Drs. Lisa Zorrilla and Dilip Jeste (Chapter 7) begin the section on schizophrenia with a review of their studies of late-onset disorder. Patients with late-onset schizophrenia have better premorbid functioning and less marked neuropsychological and brain abnormalities (as seen with magnetic brain imaging) than patients with earlier onset. One interpretation of these data is that individuals with late-onset schizophrenia have a greater "dose" of a protective factor against the neurodevelopmental abnormalities that are part of schizophrenia.

At the other extreme from Drs. Zorrilla and Jeste's project is the study of very early-onset schizophrenia, defined as onset by age 12 years. Dr. Rob Nicolson and I (Chapter 8) outline the evidence suggesting that childhood-onset schizophrenia is truly the same as schizophrenia seen in adult years. It appears that the clinical and neurobiological measures of the childhood- and adult-onset forms are very similar. It is probable that in childhood-onset cases the disorder is more severe and the outcome is poorer. The most interesting part of this project—the evidence for greater number or unique salience of risk factors—is just starting. Genetic factors are clearly important in childhood-onset illnesses, because the group with these illnesses has increased rates of schizophrenia and, strikingly, schizotypal personality in their first-degree relatives. There are also increased rates of abnormal smooth pursuit eye movements and cytogenetic abnormalities. Most striking is the absence of abnormalities in obstetrical records of these individuals relative to both their well siblings and control subjects from the literature. Thus, all signs point to increased genetic risk, but as ever, the issue of disease-specific versus -nonspecific protective factor(s) as the model for early onset is unresolved.

Dr. Robin Murray, with his colleagues Dr. Colm McDonald and Paul Fearon (Chapter 9), reviews the evidence for the neurodevelopmental hypothesis of schizophrenia, which they conclude is now overwhelming. Moreover, the authors believe that the nature of the abnormalities place the brain insult timing early in fetal life. The developmental hypothesis has its limitations, however. The onset in adolescence or adulthood remains unexplained, although a number of factors, such as gender and early developmental problems and obstetrical risk, are statistically related. One theme that we saw throughout the earlier chapters on risk factors is reiterated: the brain-imaging abnormalities, minor anomalies, and so forth are subtle and relatively nonspecific. Thus, it remains unclear exactly how neurodevelopment contributes to psychosis and how much of the variance can be explained in this fashion.

Dr. Richard Harrington (Chapter 10) reviews the diagnosis of depression in young children. Of particular interest, however, is that, counterintuitively, earlier age at onset seems to be associated with a lower risk of subsequent depression. Equally surprising are some preliminary data that very early onset (i.e., prepubertal) depression is associated with fewer familial and more striking environmental adversities. Similarly, neurobiological studies indicate that depression of very early onset may be discontinuous from depression of later (i.e., adolescent) onset. These remarkable results, if replicated, provide a striking instance in which age at onset is crucial for understanding the causes and treatment of an illness. Prepubertal depression may be a separate disorder.

The findings for anxiety and affective disorders, the topic of an entire section of this volume, are perhaps the most confusing and controversial.

Dr. Myrna Weissman and coauthors (Chapter 11) review their studies of offspring who are at high risk for developing depressive disorder or anxiety by virtue of their parents' depression. The offspring had a higher risk for major depressive disorder and anxiety, and poorer overall functioning. Prepubertal onset occurred more often in the high-risk group. Interestingly, early age at onset for major depressive disorder correlated with early parental age at onset of the disorder (defined in these studies as before age 20 years).

Dr. Hans-Ulrich Wittchen and coauthors (Chapter 12) remind us of how important methodology is to age-at-onset research by comparing longitudinal prospective measures of first symptoms with the onset of the full syndrome. The early onset of anxiety disorders is well documented, although when criteria for the full syndrome are used as the basis for diagnosis, onset occurs somewhat later. The importance of standardizing the type of symptom (vs. the full syndrome) across disorders, which is not done in the Composite International Diagnostic Interview or the Diagnostic Interview Schedule, becomes apparent when the relative onset ages are compared.

Perhaps the most controversial issue at the meeting on which this volume is based involved very early onset of bipolar disorder and its possible relation to attention-deficit/hyperactivity disorder (ADHD). Dr. Gabrielle Carlson (Chapter 13) points out that the criteria for a manic episode are relatively nonspecific and that therefore many clinically referred children meet these criteria. On the other hand, whether meeting the criteria signifies bipolar disorder in childhood is more complex. In her ongoing studies, children with concurrent behavior problems were more likely to have recurrence of mania. Taken together, the data lead her to conclude that it is still premature to identify a particular subtype of childhood behavioral disorder as a precursor to bipolar disorder.

Interest in early onset of "adult" psychopathology is also driven by hopes for prevention. The last three chapters give us very different accounts of efforts to implement preventive programs in childhood. Dr. William Beardslee (Chapter 14) presents unique data from his studies on preventive interventions for childhood depression. The two forms of educational intervention compared in these studies—one didactic and one with more of a family-interactive focus—are based on theoretical models of risk. His models that include encouragement of coping strategies associated with resilience are particularly appealing. Dr. Beardslee reminds us that prevention does not need to wait for further research into developmental psychopathology.

Dr. George Vaillant (Chapter 15) reviews the evidence that alcoholism in itself creates psychiatric disorder. With the possible exception of antisocial personality, it does not seem that other disorders such as anxiety or depression predispose to alcoholism, but exactly the opposite. Surprisingly, there is little evidence that familiality per se leads to earlier onset of alcoholism once family breakdown and number of antisocial relatives are taken into account. As for preventive interventions in childhood, the most clear effect is for social training of moderation in alcohol intake. Dr. Vaillant's compelling descriptions of alcohol-related behaviors across cultures support the powerful role of social ritual and cultural values in restricting alcohol intake.

Finally, Dr. David Offord (Chapter 16) reviews the concepts behind community prevention efforts. His chapter is a model for thoughtful decision making in considering which prevention option is most appropriate for a specific disorder. His target of antisocial behavior is the most difficult and yet the area in which broad social issues are most fully inextricable from preventive strategy. No one should contemplate such an effort without being absolutely conversant with these issues.

Judith L. Rapoport, M.D.

Age at Onset: Mechanisms and Methods

CHAPTER 1

Genetics of Early-Onset Manic-Depressive Illness and Schizophrenia

Judith A. Badner, M.D., Ph.D.
Sevilla D. Detera-Wadleigh, Ph.D.
Elliot S. Gershon, M.D.

Genetic Epidemiology

Prepubertal onset of either bipolar illness or schizophrenia is a rare event. Of the patients with bipolar disorder, the proportion with bipolar disorder of childhood onset is estimated to be less than 0.5% (Biederman and Faraone 1995), while the population prevalence of bipolar disorder is approximately 1%. The population prevalence of prepubertal schizophrenia is estimated to be between 1 and 20 per 10,000 (Gottesman 1991).

It is generally accepted that the childhood-onset form of either illness does not represent a separate familial disease from the adult form — that is, that there is a *continuum* of genetic and environmental factors that encompasses both forms of illness. Still, there have been few family studies that tested whether there is an independent familial aggregation of the childhood- and adult-onset forms of these illnesses. If such independent aggregation were found, it would imply an opposite hypothesis — namely, that the childhood- and adult-onset forms represent two genetically distinct disorders. This proved to be the case with diabetes mellitus, in which the independent familial aggregation of the childhood-onset disorder was a crucial clue that led to the identification of insulin-dependent diabetes mellitus (usually of childhood onset) and non–insulin-dependent diabetes mellitus (usually of onset in maturity) as the two major genetic forms of the illness (Simpson 1962).

In bipolar illness, in contrast to diabetes, relatives of patients with adult-onset bipolar disorder have an excess number of relatives who have childhood-onset bipolar disorder (Todd et al. 1996), and persons with childhood-onset bipolar disorder have numerous adult relatives with the illness (Strober et al. 1988; Todd et al. 1993). The earlier-onset cases are associated with the highest prevalences of affective illness in relatives, and this suggests a genetic continuum, in which the same type of genetic/familial liability is present to a greater degree in the earliest-onset cases (Strober et al. 1988; Todd et al. 1993). However, Todd et al. (1993) observed marginally significant coaggregation of early-onset bipolar relatives and probands with early-onset bipolar disorder, and the possibility remains that in a subset of cases there is a familial childhood-onset disease.

The study of schizophrenia was complicated for some years by the inclusion of infancy-onset autism as a category of schizophrenia. As convincingly argued by Gottesman (1991), the absence of psychosis in the parents of the children in these very early-onset cases argues against these cases being on a continuum with schizophrenia, and cases in which onset occurs before 5 years of age are no longer included in the diagnostic category of schizophrenia (American Psychiatric Association 1994). A careful review of all the reported prevalences of schizophrenia in relatives of persons with childhood-onset psychosis supported the continuum hypothesis of schizophrenia only tentatively, since the family study data were somewhat ambiguous and decidedly meager (Hanson and Gottesman 1992). One major early study (Kallman and Roth 1956) clearly showed independent familial aggregation of prepubertal-onset cases in siblings of patients—a finding reminiscent of the data on insulin-dependent (type I) diabetes mellitus—which we, unlike the authors of that study, would interpret as not supporting a continuum hypothesis for all the causes of schizophrenia. Although not following modern diagnostic criteria, this study had the largest number of siblings observed in childhood of any study on which to base estimates of risk.

If we adopt the continuum hypothesis as a working assumption in our search for genetic factors in early onset, we can think of the variation in age at onset in several ways. First, we can conceive of a purely random variation around a mean age in which there are no genetic or environmental differences between childhood-onset and late-onset illness. But we can also think of a susceptibility that has its own mean age at onset that is modified by specific genetic and environmental factors that can shift the onset to earlier or later ages, including shifts to childhood. Observed age at onset could be considered as a quantitative trait in a straightforward manner (cf. Li and Huang 1997). Among affected individuals in the same family, one could look for genes that are linked to differences in age at onset, for example—an approach illustrated in this chapter with data for bipolar illness. Nonetheless, it is useful to consider a range of genetic strategies that could be employed to investigate age at onset, because the working assumption—that a *continuum* of genetic and environmental factors encompasses these illnesses—may not be true.

Either genetic or environmental factors could be modifying a continuum diathesis toward illness to produce onset of the disorder in childhood. In this chapter, we focus on genetic factors because, at present, specific genetic factors in illness are more detectable with epidemiological and molecular methods than are environmental factors. It is our expectation that the identification of specific genetic mechanisms will facilitate research into environmental mechanisms.

Strategies for Investigating Genetic Mechanisms for Early Onset of Disease

With the discovery of genetic anticipation (i.e., progressively earlier onset of illness in successive generations) associated with expanding trinucleotide repeats, one strategy for finding genetic causes of early onset to any illness, particularly illnesses of the central nervous system (CNS), is to look for trinucleotide repeats. A second strategy is to use linkage knowledge gained from age-unrelated genomic scans of pedigrees with illness and determine if these linkages can be connected to variation in age at onset. Such information could be obtained from, for example, cytogenetic studies, which can be considered a form of genomic scan. A variant on this strategy, described earlier in this chapter, is to use the linkage data from affected relative pairs, disregard the role of the gene in illness, and simply look for linkage to age at onset, which is considered a quantitative variable. Yet another strategy is to study candidate genes for illness on the basis of their association with risk factors for schizophrenia or their relationship to neuropharmacology of illness and determine if any of these genes are related to early onset. In this chapter, we consider each of these strategies in turn.

Anticipation and Expanding Trinucleotide Repeat Sequences

Expansion of DNA trinucleotide repeat sequences can occur as germ cells are formed and in early stages of embryonic development. This expansion has been found to be the disease mutation in several CNS-related diseases, including Huntington's disease and mental retardation due to fragile X syndrome, and has been proposed to exist in psychiatric illnesses (Ross et al. 1993). A clinical feature of these diseases is *anticipation*, which refers to an increase in disease severity and/or earlier age at onset in successive generations; this feature is correlated with progressively greater expansions of the trinucleotide repeats.

It has been argued (Grigoroiu-Serbanescu et al. 1995, 1997; McInnis et al. 1993) that anticipation occurs in bipolar disorder and in schizophrenia (Chotai et al. 1995; Thibaut et al. 1995; Yaw et al. 1996) and that trinucleotide repeat expansion may thus prove to be the basis of the genetic predisposition (Petronis et al. 1996; Ross et al. 1993). Using the repeat expansion detection method of Schalling et al. (1993), in which the size of the largest trinucleotide (triplet) repeats in a genome is nonspecifically reported, some investigators have found increased prevalence of expansions up to 180 triplets in length in persons with bipolar disorder or schizophrenia (Burgess et al. 1997; Lindblad et al. 1995; Morris et al. 1995; O'Donovan et al. 1996); others, however, have not found such an increase (Petronis et al. 1996). Until recently, no method that identifies an actual gene had consistently shown a gene with increased triplet repeat expansion in either disorder (cf. Bowen et al. 1996; Cardno et al. 1996; Gaitonde et al. 1997). The lack of such evidence was a serious shortcoming, since there are expanded genes without any known phenotype, and it has become possible to use the results of a nonspecific test, such as repeat expansion detection, to clone the actual expanded gene (Koob et al. 1997; Lindblad et al. 1997). Recently, Schalling et al. (1998) reported evidence that two specific genes account for much of the observed increase in long trinucleotide repeats in persons with bipolar disorder and in children with schizophrenia or multidimensional impairment. One of the two, *CTG18.1*, occurred with increased frequency in individuals with bipolar disorder and in the children with schizophrenia or multidimensional impairment, with marginal statistical significance. However, the increased frequency of the gene appeared to be associated with a stable polymorphism, rather than a trinucleotide repeat whose expansion was observed in the patients' families.

Genomic Scan Strategies

Susceptibility Genes Discovered Through Linkage Mapping and Their Relation to Early Onset

The field of linkage studies of bipolar disorder and schizophrenia is in flux, with considerable competition between methods on the basis of major locus detection in large pedigrees, often from isolates, and common disease genes with small effects, detected in large numbers of affected-relative pairs with nonparametric analyses. Table 1–1, modified from a recent review by Gershon et al. (1998), summarizes the published and replicated findings of linkage studies of these disorders that met significance criteria. (For each initial study in Table 1–1 there also existed nonreplications, which may have occurred because of the limited power to detect small-effects genes with the sample sizes studied; see Gershon et al. 1998 for details.) All of these findings are from studies that used nonparametric affected-relative-pair methods; however, the reader is reminded that other findings, including impressive single-locus findings, have been presented at meetings and may soon be published.

The significance threshold for replication is less stringent because the probability of a false positive result in a genomewide scan need not

TABLE 1–1.   *Linkage studies of bipolar disorder and schizophrenia with positive findings for linkage or probable linkage and at least one replication*

Initial report	Region	Replication	Corroboration[a]
Bipolar (manic-depressive) illness			
Berrettini et al. 1994; Berrettini et al. 1997[b]	18p	Stine et al. 1995	Nothen et al. 1996; Wildenauer et al. 1996; Nothen et al. 1997
Straub et al. 1994	21q	Gurling et al. 1995; Detera-Wadleigh et al. 1996, 1997; Smyth et al. 1997[c]	
Schizophrenia			
Straub et al. 1995[d]; Wang et al. 1995[e]	6p	Schwab et al. 1995; Moises et al. 1995a; Schizophrenia Linkage Collaborative Group 1996[f]	
Cao et al. 1997	6q	Cao et al. 1997[g]	

Note. Table includes published findings as of February 1998. Studies listed were those with positive findings that met the significance thresholds for definite or suggestive linkage recommended by Lander and Kruglyak (1995) ($P < 2.2 \times 10^{-5}$ or $P < 7.4 \times 10^{-4}$; thresholds are for affected sib-pairs) and for which there was at least one confirmatory report at the significance threshold for replication ($P < 0.01$). In each instance there also existed nonreplications, which may have occurred because of the limited power to detect small-effects genes with the sample sizes studied (see Gershon et al. 1998). All findings in this table are from studies that used nonparametric affected-relative-pair methods.
[a]Studies in which the significance criterion was not met or was met only with some qualification of the phenotype definition.
[b]Same data set as in Berrettini et al. 1994.
[c]Same data set as in Gurling et al. 1995.
[d]For analysis of data in this study, see Kruglyak 1996.
[e]Same data set as in Straub et al. 1995.
[f]Overlapping data in these three studies.
[g]Two data sets studied.

be accounted for. We include as "corroborative" studies those in which the significance criterion was not met or was met only with some qualification of the phenotype definition. For example, Wildenauer et al. (1996) studied schizophrenia and related conditions, including recurrent major depression, in the families of schizophrenia probands. They found suggestive linkage and association evidence in the same area of chromosome 18 as that identified by Berrettini et al. (1994), which implies that the phenotype related to this gene may be a very inclusive one. These findings can be studied for preferential presence or absence in families with early-onset forms of bipolar disorder or schizophrenia, including those of prepubertal onset.

Cytogenetic Abnormality on Chromosome 22 and Possible Association With Disease and Early Onset

The clinical syndrome associated with hemizygous deletions within 22q11 has been characterized by several names, including DiGeorge syndrome and velocardiofacial syndrome, for the cardiac defects, cleft palate, characteristic facial appearance, and learning disabilities. Psychiatric disturbances in persons with this syndrome have long been noted. Examinations of patients known to have this deletion have suggested associations with both schizophrenia and bipolar disorder (Carlson et al. 1997; Karayiorgou et al. 1995; Papolos et al. 1996). Examination of 100 schizophrenia patients from a register revealed 2 with deletions in this region (Lindsay et al. 1995). There is modest evidence of linkage of this region of deletion with schizophrenia (Moises et al. 1995b; Polymeropoulos et al. 1994) and with bipolar disorder (Lachman et al. 1997) and of association of markers at some distance (20–40 cM) from that region with schizophrenia (Moises et al. 1995b; Polymeropoulos et al. 1994). Papolos et al. (1996) suggested that this deletion is specifically associated with bipolar illness of onset in late childhood or early adolescence. If this association with childhood onset is confirmed, and stronger linkage results become available, the region of this deletion would be a candidate for a single susceptibility gene that predisposes both to the major psychiatric illnesses (bipolar disorder and schizophrenia) and to childhood onset.

Determination of Whether Genes for Age at Onset Are Independent of Genes for Illness

One way to determine whether genes for age at onset are independent of genes for illness is with a quantitative trait locus approach. With this approach, the ages at onset in pairs of ill relatives are known, and a genomic scan is analyzed for linkage to age of onset. Susceptibility to illness itself may be disregarded in this analysis.

We analyzed a panel of 20 multiplex, unilineal bipolar pedigrees. Diagnostic and ascertainment methods for these pedigrees have been described elsewhere (Berrettini et al. 1991). (Age at onset was not recorded for two of the pedigrees.) A minimum of four affected individuals per kindred were included, under the broad affection model (ASM II), which included bipolar disorder (both I and II, with major depression), schizoaffective illness, and recurrent unipolar depression with impairment in general functioning. The narrow affection model (ASM I) had the same diagnoses, except that recurrent unipolar depression was not included. In this pedigree series, as well as in two additional pedigrees, we found evidence of linkage to chromosome 18 (Berrettini et al. 1994) and chromosome 21 (Detera-Wadleigh et al. 1996). (Genotypes were kindly made available for this analysis by Drs. Berrettini and Detera-Wadleigh.)

The ASM II model pertained to 144 individuals. Data on age at onset of affective illness were present for 119 of these individuals (89 of whom were affected under ASM I). Definition of age at onset was age at first symptoms of mania or depression. The distributions of the ages at onset for this sample according to affection status model are presented in Figure 1–1.

We analyzed 59 chromosome-11 markers, 22 chromosome-18 markers, 18 chromosome-21 markers, 38 chromosome-5 markers, and 33 chromosome-1 markers. Only those markers for which the nominal P value for linkage to age at onset was less than 0.05 for either affection status model are presented in Table 1–2. The lowest P value observed was 0.00065, at D11S2002. At D21S266, for which there was also some evidence in earlier studies consistent with linkage to disease (Detera-Wadleigh et al. 1996), there were also interesting P values for linkage to age at onset (0.0033 for ASM I and 0.01 for ASM II). In order to

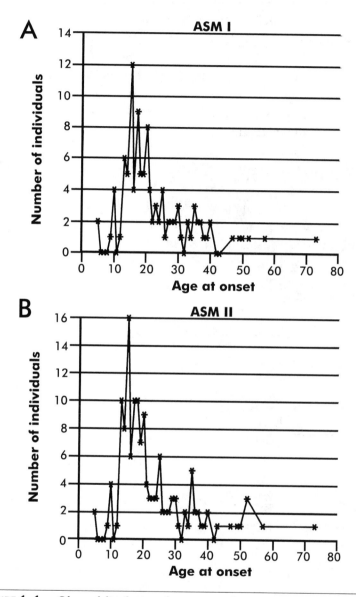

FIGURE 1–1.   *Observed distribution of ages at onset for NIMH Clinical Neurogenetics Branch sample according to affection status model.* (**A**) Narrow affection model (ASM I), which included bipolar disorder (both I and II, with major depression) and schizoaffective illness. (**B**) Broad affection model (ASM II), which included bipolar disorder (both I and II, with major depression), schizoaffective illness, and recurrent unipolar depression with impairment.

Source. Data from Berrettini et al. 1994.

correct for the number of markers tested, a nominal P value of 0.0003 would be required to accept linkage. One of these markers, D11S2002, was shown to fit the accepted criteria for suggestive linkage in a genome-wide scan (Lander and Kruglyak 1995). If replicated, these findings would be an important clue to the mechanism of disease onset.

Age at onset was analyzed as a quantitative trait. Only data for affected sib-pairs were analyzed. The data were analyzed with the Haseman-Elston statistic (Haseman and Elston 1972) as implemented in the SIBPAL program of the SAGE computer package (SAGE 1997). SIBPAL estimates the proportion of alleles shared identical by descent at a single marker by a sib-pair. (*Identical by descent* means that each sibling inherited the same allele from their parent.) The squared sib-pair difference for the quantitative trait is linearly regressed on this estimated proportion to detect a possible linkage to the marker.

TABLE 1–2. *Linkage of markers to age at onset of affective illness as a quantitative trait locus*

Marker	Chromosomal location[a]	No. of affected sib-pairs			
		ASM I	P	ASM II	P
D1S552	22.4	60	0.037	111	0.2
D18S482	13.9	54	0.015	103	0.08
D11S2002	101.9	59	0.021	111	0.00065
D11S1332	107.2	55	0.042	98	0.07
D11S923	110.1	61	0.06	113	0.01
D11S4078	114.4	65	0.027	117	0.06
D11S1327	114.9	63	0.03	116	0.08
D11S4122	114.9	61	0.09	113	0.04
D11S1998	121.3	59	0.023	111	0.038
D21S266[b]	47.3	65	0.0033	114	0.01

Note. ASM I = narrow affection model; ASM II = broad affection model.
[a]Composite location in the Location Database (Collins et al. 1996).
[b]Evidence of linkage in all affected sib-pairs (P < 0.05).

Candidate Genes Based on Physiology or Pharmacology of Illness

Genes related to specific physiological or pharmacological features of illness have been studied for their role in determining susceptibility, but not for their role in determining age at onset. Genetic studies of onset are feasible, as described earlier, and some of the reasonable candidates to consider are reviewed here.

Genes for CNS Dysfunctions Associated With Schizophrenia

Two neurophysiological abnormalities associated with schizophrenia have been linked to specific chromosomal regions, and these could be studied for association with early onset. Freedman et al. (1997) studied inheritance of a neurophysiological abnormality associated with schizophrenia: a defect in the normal decrease of a cortical evoked potential (P50) after repeated auditory stimuli. A genomewide scan of the P50 abnormality was done in members of nine schizophrenia pedigrees without respect to affection status with schizophrenia. When a single-locus model of the trait was used, linkage was found to markers on chromosome 15, very close to the gene for the $\alpha7$ subunit of the nicotinic cholinergic receptor. Similarly, the smooth pursuit eye tracking abnormalities observed in schizophrenia have been linked to a region on the short arm of chromosome 6 (6p21–23) (Arolt et al. 1996).

Separate Analyses of Families With and Without Clinical Risk Factors

Obstetrical complications have long been associated with increased risk of schizophrenia. Verdoux et al. (1997) carried out a meta-analysis on data from a large series of patients with schizophrenia ($N = 874$) and found a correlation between increased obstetrical complications and earlier onset (prior to age 22). No significant correlation between perinatal complications and family history was found. It is still possible, however, that there is an inherited vulnerability to schizophrenia as a result of perinatal complications and that this vulnerability is also associated with early onset. Separate molecular linkage and association studies could detect such a vulnerability. Similar subdivision of families according to season of birth and prenatal infections (cf. Wright et al. 1995) could be used to analyze for genetic factors associated with early onset.

Neuropharmacologically Derived Candidate Genes

Candidate genes related to the processes of monoamine synaptic transmission and signal transduction are appealing because of the enormous utility, for therapeutic drug development, of the dopamine hypothesis of psychosis and the norepinephrine/serotonin/dopamine hypotheses of depression and anxiety. Acetylcholine, γ-aminobutyric acid (GABA), glycine, and aspartate/glutamate transmission systems have also been the basis for candidate gene hypotheses.

In evaluating these candidate gene studies, some methodological points should be raised. Testing a candidate gene hypothesis by linkage rather than association is rational but entails choosing the method with weaker statistical power (Risch and Merikangas 1996). On the other hand, one can have more confidence from a linkage result that the genomic region containing the gene is in fact scanned, and linkage is robust to the presence of multiple ancestral mutations.

Among studies testing a candidate gene hypothesis by association, within-family association studies are less subject to hidden population stratification than comparisons of patients and control subjects (Lander and Schork 1994; Spielman and Ewens 1996). Depending on which molecular strategy is applied to a candidate gene, the results will have greater or lesser biological meaning. In association studies, testing a single polymorphism, such as length of a repeat sequence or a base-pair substitution, does not necessarily serve as a statistical scan of the entire gene (including the introns, intron/exon junctions, exons, and promoter region). For a single polymorphism to serve as a valid test of a mutation elsewhere in the gene, it would have to be demonstrated that there is an abnormality in the gene that leads to disturbed expression of the gene or function of its product.

Lastly, the issue must be raised of the correct statistical significance criterion for association tests of candidate genes when the candidate is based on a hypothesis only (i.e., no prior evidence that the gene product is abnormal). Significance testing of a result by an observed *P* value in a study of one such gene must be corrected by taking into account the very large number of genes that could have been tested (Crowe 1993; Risch and Merikangas 1996) or by testing and replication in several independent series to generate a single result. It is misleading to test association with one gene, such as one of the dopamine receptor genes in schizophrenia, using a nominal *P* value of 0.05 as the significance threshold.

Unique reasons for testing a particular gene can always be advanced, such as the affinity of clozapine for the D_4 dopamine receptor. Nonetheless, the investigator in such a study should remind himself or herself that the number of potential candidates includes all the genes that interact with the cellular signal reception and transduction systems affected by any of the psychotropic drugs useful in the treatment of an illness. This interaction can be direct or indirect (e.g., downstream in a cascade of signal transduction events). Many of these genes have potential as candidate genes.

For less than 0.05 probability that the observation is a false positive to be attained, the threshold for a significant observed *P* value in a single association study should be set at 0.05 divided by the number of genes that might just as reasonably have been considered. This is a standard that has yet to be met in research on manic-depressive illness and schizophrenia, but it might be prudent to adopt such a standard to protect the field from false positives. This standard, if adopted, would be analogous to the significance criteria adopted for linkage to protect against false positives in genome scans.

Dopamine receptor genes.   In a brief review such as this one, we cannot provide a comprehensive discussion of all candidate gene studies in the major psychiatric disorders. The genes for the dopamine receptor molecules on the synapse have been the most appealing candidates in investigating disease susceptibility. Two subfamilies of dopamine receptors have been identified, each having different pharmacology, signal transduction, and genomic organization. Receptors in the D_1-like subfamily (D_1 and D_5) couple to G_s proteins, whereas receptors in the D_2-like subfamily (D_2, D_3, and D_4) couple to G_i proteins (Gingrich and Caron 1993).

Dopamine receptor molecules were the subject of the largest number of candidate gene studies in schizophrenia found by us in a computerized literature search with *MEDLINE* in February 1997. (We also reviewed issues of *American Journal of Medical Genetics [Neuropsychiatric Genetics]* through February 1997.) The molecules involved in postreceptor signal transduction events, such as subunits of heterotrimeric G proteins, also represent plausible candidates for a dopamine-based hypothesis (Ram et al. 1997).

Among the association studies of dopamine receptor genes to date, only a few complete molecular scans of the entire gene have been performed (see, e.g., Gejman et al. 1994). By and large, the association studies are group comparisons, not within-family transmission tests. The entire molecular investigation of many studies consists of one polymorphism. Even for a negative conclusion that none of the genes are associated with disease, the evidence is modest because of the methods used. Also, few sequence variants have been tested for functional differences (as was done by Asghari et al. [1994] and Cravchik et al. [1996]).

In nearly all of the studies, no association or linkage of schizophrenia with the dopamine receptor genes studied was detected. For the dopamine receptor D_2 gene (*DRD2*), we found 12 studies (references omitted for reasons of space). In only one (Arinami et al. 1994) was nominal significance reported. For the dopamine receptor D_4 gene (*DRD4*), there are 11 studies, with one (Catalano et al. 1993) reporting a nominally significant association with delusional disorder but not with schizophrenia. Even when one takes into account the possibility that one of these genes could have a very weak effect, the large number of studies with negative findings, coupled with the fact that the positive findings could not be replicated in subsequent analyses, implies that there is no valid association.

For the dopamine receptor D_3 gene (*DRD3*), the picture is mixed. A possibly valid weak positive finding might be contained within two reports. An initial study (Crocq et al. 1992) did not find an allelic association with a bi-allelic polymorphism of *DRD3* that codes for a serine-to-glycine amino acid substitution. Further examination of the data suggested a genotypic association with genotype 1-1 ($P < 0.008$) and with homozygosity ($P = 0.0001$). We were able to find 16 studies of *DRD3* association with schizophrenia after this initial report. Disregarding studies that retrospectively subdivided their sample or that pooled findings from samples in published reports with findings from new samples, only one study (Shaikh et al. 1996) replicated the initial finding. The French and English sample in this study was similar to that in the study by Crocq et al. (1992). Shaikh et al. found an association of schizophrenia with the 1-1 genotype ($P = 0.003$), as in Crocq et al., and also an association of illness with allele 1, which Crocq et al. did not find in their sample. Despite all the nonreplications, it would appear worthwhile to do further studies, including molecular scanning studies of the entire receptor gene in some families and functional studies of the known variant and of others that may be discovered.

Serotonin transporter gene. Several associations of polymorphisms of the serotonin transporter gene with bipolar disorder have been reported, but there is little consistency among them. Two major polymorphisms have been identified: a variable number of tandem repeats (VNTR) in the second intron of the gene (variants have 9, 10, and 12 repeats) and a 44-bp insertion/deletion in the promoter region. In the United Kingdom, although preliminary results in one series initially suggested an increase of the 12-repeat allele in bipolar disorder (Collier et al. 1996), the same group of investigators (Ogilvie et al. 1996), in a later analysis, found that the allele frequency of the 9-repeat VNTR was associated with unipolar, but not bipolar, affective disorder. In an extension of the same series, Battersby et al. (1996) reported a slight increase in the 9-repeat VNTR allele in Scottish bipolar patients versus control subjects (3.1% vs. 1.2%), as well as in unipolar patients vs. control subjects (4.2% vs. 1.2%). This association was not observed in Germany (Stober et al. 1996) or Japan (Kunugi et al. 1996). The Japanese group later reported that the 12-repeat allele was slightly increased (93% vs. 89%), and the 10-repeat allele slightly decreased, in the patients with bipolar disorder (Kunugi et al. 1997). In another British sample, an increase in allele 12 in bipolar patients was reported (Rees et al. 1997). Molecular sequencing of the messenger RNA of this gene from a few of the bipolar patients failed to reveal any abnormalities relative to the mRNA of this gene from control subjects (Lesch et al. 1995), and a linkage study (Kelsoe et al. 1996a) was interpreted as not supporting the presence of a susceptibility disorder. Although additional molecular scanning may be warranted, it does not appear that the evidence so far would favor an association of the serotonin transporter gene with bipolar disorder. For schizophrenia, the association evidence has been consistently negative (Bellivier et al. 1997; Bonnet-Brilhault et al. 1997).

Dopamine transporter gene. One pedigree study (Kelsoe et al. 1996b) found modest evidence for linkage and association of bipolar disorder with the dopamine transporter gene; however, this association was not detected in another study (Manki et al. 1996). For schizophrenia, there appears to be no association or linkage (Bodeau-Pean et al. 1995; Daniels et al. 1995; Inada et al. 1996; Maier et al. 1996; Persico and Macciardi 1997; Persico et al. 1995).

We conclude that there are no well-established associations of the neuropharmacologically derived candidate genes with bipolar disorder or schizophrenic disorders—neither among the genes reviewed here or among other genes that could not be encompassed in a brief review article. The search for clues to early onset could conceivably still be aided by study of these genes, but the data so far are not encouraging.

Conclusion

We can consider two possible ways to look at childhood-onset bipolar disorder: as specific to the physiology (including gene expression) and/ or environment of childhood or as a manifestation of events (whether genetic, environmental, or random variation) that, given a susceptibility to illness due to other factors, can shift onset to an earlier age by an incremental amount. At present, there are data consistent with genetic or environmental events for bipolar disorder and schizophrenia, but none is definitive. The evidence for linkage to age at onset described in this chapter in the data for bipolar disorder, if corroborated, would imply that childhood onset is an extreme instance along an onset curve that can extend well into middle age. The data on anticipation in schizophrenia and in bipolar disorder would have a similar implication. On the other hand, if the velocardiofacial syndrome association with childhood-onset bipolar disorder is confirmed, a gene specific to childhood onset will have been established.

The molecular and statistical technologies available to study age at onset have advanced faster than the actual collection of data. It would be very desirable to have access to sizable sets of families identified by probands with childhood onset of a specific major psychiatric disorder, such as bipolar disorder or schizophrenia (cf. Todd et al. 1993). As shown by Risch and Zhang (1996), extreme differences in age at onset between affected relative-pairs would provide the greatest power to detect linkage to this variable. Other disorders with cases of childhood and adult onset in the same families could reasonably be studied, such as obsessive-compulsive disorder, panic disorder, and unipolar depression, but there is even less information on specific genetic susceptibility to these disorders than for the diseases we have considered. Finally, data on families with uncharacteristically early onset of illness in multiple members, if such families could be located, would constitute a most valuable resource.

References

American Psychiatric Association: Diagnostic and Statistical Manual of Mental Disorders, 4th Edition. Washington, DC, American Psychiatric Association, 1994

Arinami T, Itokawa M, Enguchi H, et al: Association of dopamine D2 receptor molecular variant with schizophrenia (see comments). Lancet 343:703–704, 1994

Arolt V, Lencer R, Nolte A, et al: Eye tracking dysfunction is a putative phenotypic susceptibility marker of schizophrenia and maps to a locus on chromosome 6 in families with multiple occurrence of the disease. Am J Med Genet 67:564–579, 1996

Asghari V, Schoots O, van Kats S, et al: Dopamine D4 receptor repeat: analysis of different native and mutant forms of the human and rat genes. Mol Pharmacol 46:364–373, 1994

Battersby S, Ogilvie AD, Smith CA, et al: Structure of a variable number tandem repeat of the serotonin transporter gene and association with affective disorder. Psychiatr Genet 6:177–181, 1996

Bellivier F, Laplanche JL, Leboyer M, et al: Serotonin transporter gene and manic depressive illness: an association study. Biol Psychiatry 41:750–752, 1997

Berrettini WH, Goldin LR, Martinez MM, et al: A bipolar pedigree series for genomic mapping for disease genes: diagnostic and analytic considerations. Psychiatr Genet 2:125–160, 1991

Berrettini WH, Ferraro TN, Goldin LR, et al: Chromosome 18 DNA markers and manic-depressive illness: evidence for a susceptibility gene. Proc Natl Acad Sci U S A 91:5918–5921, 1994

Berrettini WH, Ferraro TN, Goldin LR, et al: A linkage study of bipolar illness. Arch Gen Psychiatry 54:27–35, 1997

Biederman J, Faraone SV: Childhood mania revisited. Isr J Med Sci 31:647–651, 1995

Bodeau-Pean S, Laurent C, Campion D, et al: No evidence for linkage or association between the dopamine transporter gene and schizophrenia in a French population. Psychiatry Res 59:1–6, 1995

Bonnet-Brilhault F, Laurent C, Thibaut F, et al: Serotonin transporter gene polymorphism and schizophrenia: an association study. Biol Psychiatry 42:634–636, 1997

Bowen T, Guy C, Speight G, et al: Expansion of 50 CAG/CTG repeats excluded in schizophrenia by application of a highly efficient approach using repeat expansion detection and a PCR screening set. Am J Hum Genet 59:912–917, 1996

Burgess CE, Lindblad E, Sidransky E, et al: CAG expansions and childhood-onset schizophrenia (abstract). Am J Hum Genet 61:A305, 1997

Cao Q, Martinez M, Zhang J, et al: Suggestive evidence for a schizophrenia susceptibility locus on chromosome 6q and a confirmation in an independent series of pedigrees. Genomics 43:1–8, 1997

Cardno AG, Murphy KC, Jones LA, et al: Expanded CAG/CTG repeats in schizophrenia. A study of clinical correlates. Br J Psychiatry 169:766–771, 1996

Carlson C, Papolos D, Pandita RK, et al: Molecular analysis of velo-cardio-facial syndrome patients with psychiatric disorders. Am J Hum Genet 60:851–859, 1997

Catalano M, Nobile M, Novelli E, et al: Distribution of a novel mutation in the first exon of the human dopamine D4 receptor gene in psychotic patients. Biol Psychiatry 34:459–464, 1993

Chotai J, Engstrom C, Ekholm B, et al: Anticipation in Swedish families with schizophrenia. Psychiatr Genet 5:181–186, 1995

Collier DA, Stober G, Li T, et al: A novel functional polymorphism within the promoter of the serotonin transporter gene: possible role in susceptibility to affective disorders (see comments). Mol Psychiatry 1:453–460, 1996

Collins A, Frezal J, Teague J, et al: A metric map of humans: 23,500 loci in 850 bands. Proc Natl Acad Sci U S A 93:14771–14775, 1996

Cravchik A, Sibley DR, Gejman PV: Functional analysis of the human D2 dopamine receptor missense variants. J Biol Chem 42:26013–26017, 1996

Crocq MA, Mant R, Asherson P, et al: Association between schizophrenia and homozygosity at the dopamine D3 receptor gene (see comments). J Med Genet 29:858–860, 1992

Crowe RR: Candidate genes in psychiatry: an epidemiological perspective. Am J Med Genet (Neuropsychiatr Genet) 48:74–77, 1993

Daniels J, Williams J, Asherson P, et al: No association between schizophrenia and polymorphisms within the genes for debrisoquine 4-hydroxylase (CYP2D6) and the dopamine transporter (DAT). Am J Med Genet 60:85–87, 1995

Detera-Wadleigh SD, Badner JA, Goldin LR, et al: Affected-sib-pair analyses reveal support of prior evidence for a susceptibility locus for bipolar disorder on 21q. Am J Hum Genet 58:1279–1285, 1996

Detera-Wadleigh SD, Badner JA, Yoshikawa T, et al: Initial genome scan of the NIMH Genetics Initiative bipolar pedigrees: chromosomes 4, 7, 9, 18, 19, 20, and 21q. Am J Med Genet 74:254–262, 1997

Freedman R, Coon H, Myles-Worsley M, et al: Linkage of a neurophysiological deficit in schizophrenia to a chromosome 15 locus. Proc Natl Acad Sci U S A 94:587–592, 1997

Gaitonde EJ, Sivagnanasundaram S, Morris AG, et al: The number of triplet repeats in five brain-expressed loci with CAG repeats is not associated with schizophrenia. Schizophr Res 25:111–116, 1997

Gejman PV, Ram A, Gelernter J, et al: No structural mutation in the dopamine D2 receptor gene in alcoholism or schizophrenia. Analysis using denaturing gradient gel electrophoresis. JAMA 271:204–208, 1994

Gershon ES, Badner JA, Goldin LR, et al: Closing in on genes for manic-depressive illness and schizophrenia. Neuropsychopharmacology 18:232–242, 1998

Gingrich JA, Caron MG: Recent advances in the molecular biology of dopamine receptors. Annu Rev Neurosci 16:299–321, 1993

Gottesman II: Schizophrenia Genesis: The Origins of Madness, New York, WH Freeman, 1991, p 39

Grigoroiu-Serbanescu M, Nothen M, Propping P, et al: Clinical evidence for genomic imprinting in bipolar I disorder. Acta Psychiatr Scand 92:365–370, 1995

Grigoroiu-Serbanescu M, Wickramaratne PJ, Hodge SE, et al: Genetic antic-ipation and imprinting in bipolar I illness. Br J Psychiatry 170:162–166, 1997

Gurling H, Smyth C, Kalsi G, et al: Linkage findings in bipolar disorder (letter). Nat Genet 10:8–9, 1995

Hanson DR, Gottesman II: Schizophrenia, in The Genetic Basis of Common Diseases. Edited by King RS, Rotter JI, Motulsky AR. New York, Oxford University Press, 1992, pp 816–836

Haseman JK, Elston RC: The investigation of linkage between a quantitative trait and a marker locus. Behav Genet 2:3–19, 1972

Inada T, Sugita T, Dobashi I, et al: Dopamine transporter gene polymorphism and psychiatric symptoms seen in schizophrenic patients at their first ep-isode. Am J Med Genet 67:406–408, 1996

Kallman FJ, Roth BR: Genetic aspects of preadolescent schizophrenia. Am J Psychiatry 112:599–606, 1956

Karayiorgou M, Morris MA, Morrow B, et al: Schizophrenia susceptibility as-sociated with interstitial deletions of chromosome 22q11. Proc Natl Acad Sci U S A 92:7612–7616, 1995

Kelsoe JR, Remick RA, Sadovnick AD, et al: Genetic linkage study of bipolar disorder and the serotonin transporter. Am J Med Genet 67:215–217, 1996a

Kelsoe JR, Sadovnick AD, Kristbjarnarson H, et al: Possible locus for bipolar disorder near the dopamine transporter on chromosome 5. Am J Med Genet 67:533–540, 1996b

Koob MD, Benzow KA, Day JW, et al: Rapid cloning of expanded trinucleotide repeat sequences from genomic and cDNA samples (abstract). Am J Hum Genet 61:A312, 1997

Kruglyak L: Thresholds and sample sizes (letter; comment). Nat Genet 14:132–133, 1996

Kunugi H, Hattori M, Kato T, et al: Serotonin transporter gene polymorphisms: ethnic difference and possible association with bipolar affective disorder. Mol Psychiatry 2:457–462, 1997

Kunugi H, Tatsumi M, Sakai T, et al: Serotonin transporter gene polymorphism and affective disorder (letter; comment). Lancet 347:1340, 1996

Lachman HM, Kelsoe JR, Remick RA, et al: Linkage studies suggest a possible locus for bipolar disorder near the velo-cardio-facial syndrome region on chromosome 22. Am J Med Genet 74:121–128, 1997

Lander E, Kruglyak L: Genetic dissection of complex traits: guidelines for in-terpreting and reporting linkage results (see comments). Nat Genet 11:241–247, 1995

Lander ES, Schork NJ: Genetic dissection of complex traits. Science 265:2037–2048, 1994

Lesch KP, Gross J, Franzek E, et al: Primary structure of the serotonin transporter in unipolar depression and bipolar disorder. Biol Psychiatry 37:215–223, 1995

Li H, Huang J: Incorporation of age of onset into multipoint linkage analysis using pseudolikelihood (abstract). Genet Epidemiol 14:533, 1997

Lindblad K, Nylander PO, De bruyn A, et al: Detection of expanded CAG repeats in bipolar affective disorder using the repeat expansion detection (RED) method. Neurobiol Dis 2:55–62, 1995

Lindblad K, Burgess CE, Yuan Q-P, et al: A strategy for identification of sequence flanking trinucleotide repeat expansion loci (abstract). Am J Hum Genet 61:A313, 1997

Lindsay EA, Morris MA, Gos A, et al: Schizophrenia and chromosomal deletions within 22q11.2 (letter). Am J Hum Genet 56:1502–1503, 1995

Maier W, Minges J, Eckstein N, et al: Genetic relationship between dopamine transporter gene and schizophrenia: linkage and association. Schizophr Res 20:175–180, 1996

Manki H, Kanba S, Muramatsu T, et al: Dopamine D2, D3 and D4 receptor and transporter gene polymorphisms and mood disorders. J Affect Disord 40:7–13, 1996

McInnis MG, McMahon FJ, Chase GA, Simpson SG, et al: Anticipation in bipolar affective disorder (see comments). Am J Hum Genet 53:385–390, 1993

Moises HW, Yang L, Kristbjanarson H, et al: An international two-stage genome-wide search for schizophrenia susceptibility genes. Nat Genet 11:321–324, 1995a

Moises HW, Yang L, Li T, et al: Potential linkage disequilibrium between schizophrenia and locus D22S278 on the long arm of chromosome 22. Am J Med Genet 60:465–467, 1995b

Morris AG, Gaitonde EJ, McKenna PJ, et al: CAG repeat expansions and schizophrenia: association with disease in females and with early age-at-onset. Hum Mol Genet 4:1957–1961, 1995

Nothen M, Cichon S, Craddock N, et al: Linkage studies of bipolar disorder to chromosome 18 markers (abstract). Biol Psychiatry 39:615–615, 1996

Nothen M, Cichon S, Franzek E, et al: Systematic search for susceptibility genes in bipolar affective disorder—evidence for disease loci at 18p and 4p (abstract). Am J Hum Genet 61:A288, 1997

O'Donovan MC, Guy C, Craddock N, et al: Confirmation of association between expanded CAG/CTG repeats and both schizophrenia and bipolar disorder. Psychol Med 26:1145–1153, 1996

Ogilvie AD, Battersby S, Bubb VJ, et al: Polymorphism in serotonin transporter gene associated with susceptibility to major depression (see comments). Lancet 347:731–733, 1996

Papolos DF, Faedda GL, Veit S, et al: Bipolar spectrum disorders in patients diagnosed with velo-cardio-facial syndrome: does a hemizygous deletion of chromosome 22q11 result in bipolar affective disorder? Am J Psychiatry 153:1541–1547, 1996

Persico AM, Macciardi F: Genotypic association between dopamine transporter gene polymorphisms and schizophrenia. Am J Med Genet 74:53–57, 1997

Persico AM, Wang ZW, Black DW, et al: Exclusion of close linkage of the dopamine transporter gene with schizophrenia spectrum disorders. Am J Psychiatry 152:134–136, 1995

Petronis A, Bassett AS, Honer WG, et al: Search for unstable DNA in schizophrenia families with evidence for genetic anticipation. Am J Hum Genet 59:905–911, 1996

Polymeropoulos MD, Coon H, Byerley W, et al: Search for a schizophrenia susceptibility locus on human chromosome 22. Am J Med Genet (Neuropsychiatr Genet) 54:93–99, 1994

Ram A, Guedj F, Cravchik A, et al: No abnormality in the gene for the G protein stimulatory alpha subunit in patients with bipolar disorder. Arch Gen Psychiatry 54:44–48, 1997

Rees M, Norton N, Jones I, et al: Association studies of bipolar disorder at the human serotonin transporter gene (hSERT; 5HTT). Mol Psychiatry 2:398–402, 1997

Risch N, Merikangas K: The future of genetics studies of complex human diseases. Science 273:1516–1517, 1996

Risch N, Zhang H: Mapping quantitative trait loci with extreme discordant sib pairs: sampling considerations. Am J Hum Genet 58:836–843, 1996

Ross CA, McInnis MG, Margolis RL, et al: Genes with triplet repeats: candidate mediators of neuropsychiatric disorders. Trends Neurosci 16:254–260, 1993

SAGE. Statistical Analysis for Genetic Epidemiology, 3.0. Department of Biometry and Biostatistics, Rammelkamp Center for Education and Research, Case Western Reserve University, Cleveland, OH, 1997

Schalling M, Hudson TJ, Buetow KH, et al: Direct detection of novel expanded trinucleotide repeats in the human genome. Nat Genet 4:135–139, 1993

Schalling M, et al: Repeat expansion in neuropsychiatric disorders. Paper presented at the Park City Molecular Psychiatry Conference, Park City, Utah, February 2, 1998

Schizophrenia Linkage Collaborative Group for Chromosomes 3, 6 and 8: Additional support for schizophrenia linkage on chromosomes 6 and 8: a multicenter study. Am J Med Genet (Neuropsychiat Genet) 67:580–594, 1996

Schwab SG, Albus M, Hallmayer J, et al: Evidence for susceptibility gene for schizophrenia on chromosome 6p by multipoint affected-sib-pair linkage analysis. Nat Genet 11:325–327, 1995

Shaikh S, Collier DA, Sham PC, et al: Allelic association between a Ser-9-Gly polymorphism in the dopamine D3 receptor gene and schizophrenia. Hum Genet 97:714–719, 1996

Simpson NE: The genetics of diabetes: a study of 233 families of juvenile diabetics. Ann Hum Genet 26:1–12, 1962

Smyth C, Kalsi G, Curtis D, et al: Two-locus admixture linkage analysis of bipolar and unipolar affective disorder supports the presence of susceptibility loci on chromosomes 11p15 and 21q22. Genomics 39:271–278, 1997

Spielman RS, Ewens WJ: The TDT and other family-based tests for linkage disequilibrium and association (invited editorial). Am J Hum Genet 59:983–989, 1996

Stine OC, Xu J, Koskela R, et al: Evidence for linkage of bipolar disorder to chromosome 18 with a parent of origin effect. Am J Hum Genet 57:1384–1394, 1995

Stober G, Heils A, Lesch KP: Serotonin transporter gene polymorphism and affective disorder (letter; comment). Lancet 347:1340–1341, 1996

Straub RE, Lehner T, Luo Y, et al: A possible vulnerability locus for bipolar affective disorder on chromosome 21q22.3. Nat Genet 8:291–296, 1994

Straub RE, MacLean CJ, O'Neill FA, et al: A potential vulnerability locus for schizophrenia on chromosome 6p24–22: evidence for genetic heterogeneity. Nat Genet 11:287–293, 1995

Strober M, Morrell W, Burroughs J, et al: Family study of bipolar I disorder in adolescence. J Affect Disord 15:255–268, 1988

Thibaut F, Martinez M, Petit M, et al: Further evidence for anticipation in schizophrenia. Psychiatry Res 59:25–33, 1995

Todd RD, Neuman R, Geller BFLW, et al: Genetic studies of affective disorders: should we be starting with childhood onset probands? J Am Acad Child Adolesc Psychiatry 32:1164–1171, 1993

Todd RD, Reich W, Petti TA, et al: Psychiatric diagnoses in the child and adolescent members of extended families identified through adult bipolar affective disorder probands. J Am Acad Child Adolesc Psychiatry 35:664–671, 1996

Verdoux H, Geddes JR, Takei N, et al: Obstetric complications and age at onset in schizophrenia: an international collaborative meta-analysis of individual patient data. Am J Psychiatry 154:1220–1227, 1997

Wang S, Sun CE, Walczak CA, et al: Evidence for a susceptibility locus for schizophrenia on chromosome 6pter–p22. Nat Genet 10:41–46, 1995

Wildenauer DB, Hallmayer J, Albus M, et al: Searching for susceptibility genes in schizophrenia by genetic linkage analysis. Cold Spring Harb Symp Quant Biol 61:845–850, 1996

Wright P, Takei N, Rifkin L, et al: Maternal influenza, obstetric complications, and schizophrenia (see comments). Am J Psychiatry 152:1714–1720, 1995

Yaw J, Myles-Worsley M, Hoff M, et al: Anticipation in multiplex schizophrenia pedigrees. Psychiatr Genet 6:7–11, 1996

CHAPTER 2

Genetics, Evolution, and Age at Onset of Disease

Barton Childs, M.D.

Why should a pediatrician–geneticist be invited to contribute to this record of a meeting of psychiatrists? Perhaps it is because the concerns of pediatrics are *always* expressed in the context of development, and development is clearly the matrix of psychopathology. For its part, genetics is expressed in individuality, itself shaped by experiences mediated by development. So genes and development are conjoint, and it is to genes, development, and experiences that we owe the individuality that distinguishes us as us and no other and that characterizes our diseases as it does our noses, stature, and competencies. I will return to the question of the contribution of pediatrics–genetics later in this chapter.

Individuality

The shaping of individuality is manifest in behavioral properties, some of which bring some of us to the psychiatrist because of behavior that

---

This chapter is adapted from the author's Zubin award lecture, presented at the 87th meeting of the American Psychopathological Association, March 1998, in New York City.

transcends some standard. Such a behavior is characterized by its history, signs, and symptoms and their impact on the patient's well-being and ability to carry on in life. Diagnostic tests explore the origins of signs and symptoms in biochemical or physiological properties, and the disorder is given a name. Then, today, a search is made for the presumably nonstandard genes whose products lie at the root of the named disorder. Such molecules are expected to reveal an association with some homeostatic device and, perhaps, to become a target for pharmacological ventures that will lead to new treatments. But there is a level of understanding that lies between these reductive exercises and the behavioral property they are supposed to explain. That is, there are rules of biology that both determine and constrain disease. I think of that middle zone as *individuality*, a word expressive of outcome of the interactions of the products of genotypes with conditions of the environment that take place in a developmental matrix.

Development is a historical process: what we are today is conditioned by what we were yesterday, and tomorrow's events will go forward in the context of biological memories of today. This continuity is preserved by the constancy of the genes that specify the protein elements of the homeostatic devices that promote growth and maintain the steady state. It is the variable qualities of these protein gene products, and their integration into the systems of cells and organs, that form a matrix within which the products interact with elements of the environment to express the individuality of both health and disease. Among these expressions is the *age at onset* of disease, and it is to conjure with this and other such expressions of individuality that is the aim of this chapter.

Sources of Individuality

Some Revealing Questions

If you were to say to a physician, "You have 10 seconds in which to cite the most important questions in medicine," the most likely response is, "What disease does the patient have and how do I treat it?" with the "it" referring to the disease, not the patient. In saying these things without thought, the physician reflects a deeply embedded concept of medicine:

the body is a machine that breaks and needs a doctor to fix it. To this end, medicine has appropriated from biology whatever is relevant to its conventional missions. But in so doing, the wherewithal to answer other questions is omitted—questions no less germane to those conventional missions, but inclusive, as the standard questions are not, of the individuality of the patient. These questions are

a. What is disease and why does it exist?
b. Why does this particular person have this particular disease?
c. Why has the disease appeared at this moment in the patient's life?

These questions transcend the first two in stressing the individuality of the patient and calling into question the sufficiency of the machine mentality. It is not that "What is the disease?" and "How do I treat it?" are not germane—they are, and critically. It is simply that they stop short of questions whose answers extend their scope to form the basis for a synthesis, catalyzed by genetics, of the thinking of medicine and biology.

Answers

What Is Disease, and Why Do We Have It?

The answer to the questions "What is disease, and why do we have it?" might be, a successful species maintains a store of variation that is generated at meiosis, is constrained by natural selection, and is revealed in a gene pool that reflects its evolutionary origin. This variation is expressed in the specification, by the genes, of alternative protein gene products, each of which assumes a place in homeostasis determined by its specificity, and its variation is reflected in its relative efficiency in its function, whether in development, in maintenance, or in coping with stress. When it fails in any of these missions, it becomes a point of vulnerability—a risk factor—that, given the appropriate conditions, may become a proximate cause of disease.

So disease is defined as a consequence of incongruence between a vulnerable homeostasis and specific experiences of the environment. That is, it is a by-product of the means a species has of creating new variation. Let us not forget that that store of variation is no less the wherewithal for normal individuality than for abnormal, and the range of options for both mutation and for kinds and degrees of experiences of the environment is so great that it makes all variability, including that of disease and normality, continuous. But this continuity is no news to the psychiatrist, whose phenotypes often differ only quantitatively from behavior that, however odd, is still perceived as "normal."

Why This Person, This Disease?

The answers to the questions "Why this particular person?" and "Why this disease?" flow directly from the answers to the questions discussed above. If there is variability in the gene pool, it is distributed into individuals according to demography, ethnic groups, mating systems, and Mendelian laws, so that some people are, by chance, endowed with this allele, some with that, and if one of these represents vulnerability, incongruence may lead to disease. And because the action or inaction of different genes in different cells is the essence of differentiation, the vulnerability allele may express its incompetence in some cells and not in others, thereby influencing the choice of signs and symptoms and thus the name of the disease. So events at meiosis in one generation influence lives in later generations, but that influence is always contingent on the unique development of those lives.

Why Now?

The third question is "Why now?" "Why is one disease expressed early in life, another late?" and "Why should there be variation in onset within diseases too?" To the machine mentality, age at onset is a useful diagnostic flag. It is acknowledged in the classification of diseases and in the organization of hospitals, medical schools, and specialties. But to the geneticist, age at onset is an expression of individuality at work in the dynamics of the life history. We perceive human growth and development as embracing the first 20 years or so and aging as beginning, however subtly, in the third decade. Growth, development, and aging are words with historical content representing together a single life trajectory that characterizes the individual. The engines of life are the protein gene products that are integrated into the homeostasis of cells and whole organisms—a homeostasis that development brings into being—while aging entails its slow undoing. Development and aging simply represent stages in that evolving matrix in which the moment-to-moment interactions between homeostatic devices and experiences of the environment take place. If this matrix evolves with time, how can there fail to be differences in ages at onset? If the substrate for the action of the agents of disease changes, so must the ages optimal for those actions vary (Childs and Scriver 1986).

Age at Onset and a Selective Gradient

Three elements account for age at onset: 1) the qualities and extent of the genetic vulnerabilities, 2) the kind, intensity, and duration of experiences, and 3) the moment-to-moment state of the developmental matrix. Let us consider first the empirical evidence. Distributions of mortality rates according to age are U shaped. Everyone knows that the causes of disease and death on the two sides of the bottom of the U are different, and these differences can be seen in Table 2–1. Our question is, Why should there be these differences in the qualities of the diseases that afflict the young, the old, and those in between. We already have a partial answer: the generation of variation at meiosis. Life at meiosis is uncoupled from that after fertilization; the gametes possess the whole range of mutational exuberance, which at fertilization is exposed to natural selection. Variation begins at one extreme, with lethal losses of whole chromosomes, and ends at the other, with harmless base-pair substitutions, and is enhanced by recombination in which new associations of vulnerabilities are assembled. Obviously, the most damaging mutants must fall to the earliest selection, so that a great deal of human disease and mortality occurs not late in life, but at the beginning, and it occurs out of sight and mostly out of the medical purview. But if we keep in mind the variety in the gene pool and the principle of continuity, we will think of the individuality of the survivors and the certainty of other mutants more compatible with later life.

A Gradient of Selective Effect

These observations suggest a gradient of selective effect—most rigorous early on and dwindling through life—an idea most easily understood in

TABLE 2–1.   *Differences in the characteristics of diseases of prepubertal and postpubertal onset*

Characteristic	Prepubertal	Postpubertal
Mode of inheritance	Monogenic	Multifactorial
Age at onset	Early	Late
Frequency	Rare	Frequent
Latency	Short	Long
Affected relatives	Numerous	Few
Diagnostic specificity	High	Low
Number of diseases	Very many	Fewer
Burden	Great	Less
Sex differences	Occasional	Frequent
Influence of migration	No	Yes
Secular change	No	Yes
Effects of socioeconomic status	Some	More
Success in treatment	Some	More

the context of a cohort of conceptuses. To the degree that the selective gradient is genetic, its effect is most intense early in the career of the cohort. Nearly all of the mutants that interfere with intrauterine development are capable of doing so in all environments, but that indifference diminishes over the life span with increasing exposure to experiences.

This reciprocity in the relative contributions of genes and experiences is demonstrated in Figure 2–1, a diagram that mimics, and in part explains, actual mortalities. That is, it demonstrates that the heritability of disease declines with the age of the cohort. Heritability is a property of the extent of genetic contribution to the variability expressed in a population. It is characteristic of populations, not individuals, and is clearly evident in the contrasts between the qualities of diseases in the young and the old, particularly in the greater variation in postpubertal disease of the effects of migration, socioeconomic status, and secular change as well as in sex differences and success of ameliorative treatments. But the change in heritability is not monotonic; mortality changes with developmental phase (Figure 2–2). On the left are the

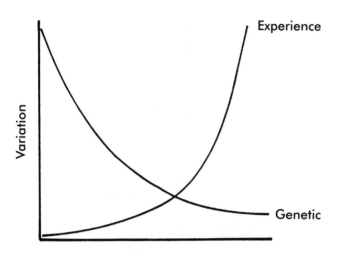

FIGURE 2–1.   *Contribution to disease of experience and genes according to age at onset.*

intrauterine losses, which are greatest during embryogenesis and which decline toward birth. These early intrauterine losses are genetic, the later have to do with the maternal environment. After birth, there is a spate of genetic deaths, which decline toward puberty; more than 80% of all inborn errors have had onset by 10 years. Again, the early-onset deaths are genetic, whereas those of later childhood are more likely to be from accidents and homicide. After puberty, premature mortality is more likely to be genetic than is that of old age.

The gradient of selective effect is observed within diseases too; the early-onset cases are more likely to be familial than the later. Cancers of the breast and of the prostate, as well as deficiency of the LDL (low-density lipoprotein) receptor in premature heart attack, are familiar examples (Carter et al. 1992; Couch and Weber 1998; Goldstein et al.

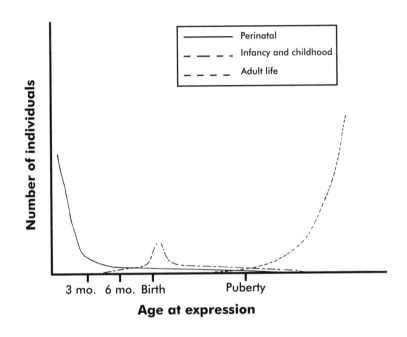

FIGURE 2–2.   *Morbidity and mortality in three developmental phases according to age at onset.*

1994). Nor are psychiatric diseases immune. Weissman and colleagues (1984) demonstrated an inverse relationship of familial aggregation with age at onset.

Figure 2–2 reveals something else about the selective gradient: its own variation. Symptoms of anomalous development, most evident early in life, may appear later or not at all. For example, the absence of one kidney may be fatal to a patient with nephritis or diabetes but may be evident only at the autopsy of, say, a centenarian of robust health who died after being hit by a bicycle messenger in New York City. The figure also makes plain that monogenic disorders, characteristic of early life, may have onset in late life, while multigenic disorders, characteristic of late life, may have early onset.

A Rationale for Prevention

Age at onset, then, is one more exemplar of the continuity of health and disease. Onset marks that moment when incongruence, long manifested only as vulnerability, is raised to expressions that bring the individual to the doctor. It is that moment when homeostatic devices intended to preserve the steady state have, perhaps after long resistance, succumbed to pressures they cannot continue to contain. And, as we have seen, the steady state is dependent on the gene-specified qualities of the protein unit steps of homeostasis and the receptiveness or resistance of the developmental matrix to the experiences of the moment. Any one of these three factors can override the others to bring vulnerability to the level of disease. But it is the variation in each that conspires with that of the others to determine outcomes, whether disease—severe, mild, or subclinical—or none at all.

So it is that emphasis on the genes and their products displaces medical concentration from an exclusive attention to onset of expression to the elements of incongruence, whether genetic or of experience, or of the developmental matrix. That is, we are beginning to pay more attention to those subclinical expressions that represent disease in its formative stages, a time that puts us in the best position to prevent the overt break in the machine. Today we are learning of both genes and their molecular products that tell us where in homeostasis the incongruence lies, with implications for prevention. So, armed with the fruits of the Human Genome Project, is it not likely that the primary aim of medicine will shift slowly toward prevention? Is it not likely that the primary aim of medicine will be to drive the heritability of disease toward 1.0?

An Analysis of Disease in the Context of Prevention

The synthesis of medical and genetic thinking, prompted perhaps by answers to the comprehensive questions asked earlier in this chapter, has given us a rationale for prevention. How does such an analysis work?

The outcome of the Human Genome Project will be lists of variant genes with the variant proteins they specify, and some of the latter will impart some degree of vulnerability to the device of which they are a part. These genetically specified protein variants represent points of union of the clinician, whose analysis goes from signs and symptoms downward, and the molecular geneticist, whose analysis goes upward from the gene to its product. They also represent the point where chemical structure is transmuted into function, where individuality is given molecular substance, and where reductionist information begins its path into such emergent expressions of individuality as specific behaviors.

Such lists of variant genes and their products have an immediate and obvious role in the solution of monogenic disorders. But the bulk of illness does not segregate. One way to investigate multifactorial illness, as I've already mentioned, is a genome search for linkage and then identification of genes, their products, and relevant homeostatic devices. In this way, one or more genes may be identified. These methods have been successful in diabetes, hypertension, and atherosclerosis and heart attack and are also being applied in psychiatric disorders. But how can they be used in clarifying these disorders? In particular, how do we accommodate heterogeneity and individuality? No one expects all cases of any disease of complex origin to have all of the genes that have been identified in populations of cases. Such genes will differ in frequency and in relation to the selective gradient, so we should expect some to be more prominent in their effects, and others to add to vulnerability— or to resistance. We must also expect diverse distributions of relevant genes from case to case. Some genes may turn up frequently in some populations, and we can group cases around these, keeping in mind always that they represent one subtype, one grouping in the heterogeneity of cause.

Now, having found a list of genes and having shown how they are distributed among cases and their families, and having set in motion the effort to identify the gene product and its homeostatic home, what's next? We analyze the disorder according to the distribution in cases, of the genes, experiences of the environment, and the developmental matrix. Some such analysis is going on in relation to atherosclerosis and heart attack (Hood 1992; Keating and Sanguinetti 1996). The genes involved in these conditions are many, with variant products that contribute to such apparently unrelated homeostatic elements as the endothelial lining of the arteries, cholesterol transport, growth factors and immune responses to arterial damage, and the clotting mechanism (itself influenced by other systems), and this list is by no means complete. The products differ in relation to the selective gradient. The LDL receptor mutant that is strongly selective is rivaled by at least one APOE allele. Variants of platelet factor and fibrinogen, as well as a mutant of homocysteine synthase, enhance the likelihood of thrombosis. These are some of the variant unit steps of homeostasis that constitute vulnerability to heart attack—that is, incongruence with factors of the developmental matrix. For example, heart attacks are most likely to occur in the morning in consonance with the diurnal rhythm of platelet factors (Miller et al. 1989). It would be interesting to contrast properties in the three columns in Table 2–2 in people whose heart attack occurred in the morning with those in people whose thrombosis occurred during the opposite phase of the platelet factor diurnal rhythm. Similarly, epidemiologists have begun to suspect that the propensity for heart attack dates from intrauterine life, and epidemiological evidence has been adduced to test the idea (Barker 1992). So, again, we should contrast cases who have the fetal factors with those who lack them in the context of the genes and other factors.

TABLE 2–2.   *Elements contributing to the individuality of phenotypes*

Genes	Developmental matrix	Environment (experiences)
Major gene modifiers	Age	Geography
	Sex	Time
	Parental effects	Climate
	Ethnic group	Education
	Cognition	Occupation
	Behavioral attitudes	Diet
		Habits
		Socioeconomic status
		Disease

The point is that in each case there is a unique array of factors that in their aggregate account for age at onset and other clinical expression, and it is the balance of vulnerabilities with those of resistance that determines outcomes. Such a balance is revealed in women whose estrogen protects them from heart attacks until after the menopause (Menger 1985). But women who have a premenopausal coronary thrombosis, when compared with men of the same age, carry a far heavier load of risks in all three categories than the men, and the outcome for these women is bleaker too. The mission is not to find risk factors that purport to represent vulnerability for everyone, but to find subtypes whose risks relate most strongly to them. In the end it will be seen that everyone's risk is unique, but economy requires that we group affected individuals into subtypes according to risk for prevention and treatment.

This is where we stand at the moment. It is a time of great promise—which prompts me to return to the question of why the pediatrician-geneticist was asked to participate. I already mentioned, as one reason, the emphasis on development shared by pediatrics and psychiatry and explained by genetics. Another reason is that genetics entered medicine by way of pediatric problems—namely, inborn errors and anomalies of development. But this point of entry was nothing but an accident of the prominence in the selective gradient of monogenic disease, which is highly familial, of heavy burden, and with onset early in life.

Psychiatrists are dealing competently with a range of genetic issues, and this suggests that a psychiatric geneticist, or indeed a urological, ophthalmological, or geriatric geneticist or any double-barreled designation you prefer, might have done as well. The point is that genes are indifferent to a classification of specialties that is no more than a human concoction representing human convenience. We are on the threshold of a genetic medicine in which disease is perceived not as pediatric or psychiatric, but as exemplary of the individuality of the patient. Once that concept becomes the core of our thinking, then we have the wherewithal for a synthesis of medical and genetic thought that can provide a *framework of coherence* within which to describe and to understand the qualities of all diseases, no matter how they are classified in textbooks or in medical organization.

Genetics has effected such syntheses before, notably with evolutionary biology to produce neo-Darwinism and with embryology to form developmental biology. So, in the synthesis of medicine and genetics, we can think first of how genes specify products that constitute homeostatic devices whose variations, interacting with those of experience and development, are differentiated by age at onset, burden as exemplified in threat to life, curtailment of fertility and permanent disability. Once these fundamentals are embedded in the medical lore, then it is possible to be a pediatrician or a psychiatrist without having lost sight of what makes us all physicians. And given the origins of individuality in variations of genes, development, and experiences, how can we ignore this aspect of our patients' lives?

Reductive medicine exerts a centrifugal dispersion to specialism and patient anonymity. The synthetic view exerts a centripetal counterforce to reveal that individuality partakes of variation in qualities common to all diseases. The reductive eye is on the disease, the synthetic eye is on the patient. This is easy to say, but not to convey; the machine mentality is deeply embedded in us all. But efforts to integrate genetic and developmental themes into psychiatry are shaking up the machine mentality. So, we may ask how the examples of development and individuality under discussion here can be used in constructing a conceptual framework that teaches how the machine and its disorders are best described in principles of increasing generality traceable in the end to biology's most comprehensive ideas.

References

Barker DJP: Fetal and Infant Origins of Adult Disease. London, BMJ Press, 1992

Carter BS, Beaty TH, Steinberg GD, et al: Mendelian inheritance of familial prostate cancer. Proc Natl Acad Sci U S A 89:3367–3371, 1992

Childs B, Scriver CR: Age at onset and causes of disease. Persp Biol Med 29:437–459, 1986

Couch FJ, Weber BL: Breast cancer, in The Genetic Basis of Human Cancer. Edited by Vogelstein B, Kinzler KW. New York, McGraw-Hill, 1998, pp 537–564

Goldstein JL, Hobbs HH, Brown MS: Familial hypercholesterolemia, in The Metabolic and Molecular Bases of Inherited Disease, 7th Edition. Edited by Scriver CR, Beaudet AL, Sly WS, et al. New York, McGraw-Hill, 1994, pp 1981–2030

Hood L: Biology and medicine in the 21st century, in The Code of Codes. Edited by Keveles DJ, Hood L. Cambridge, MA, Harvard University Press, 1992, pp 136–163

Keating MT, Sanguinetti MC: Molecular genetic insights into cardiovascular disease. Science 272:681–685, 1996

Menger N: Coronary disease in women. Annu Rev Med 36:285–294, 1985

Miller JE, Tofler GH, Stone PH: Circadian variation and triggers of onset of acute cardiovascular disease. Circulation 79:733–743, 1989

Weissman MM, Wickramaratne P, Merikangas KR, et al: Onset of major depression in early adulthood: increased familial loading and specificity. Arch Gen Psychiatry 41:1136–1143, 1984

CHAPTER 3

Trinucleotide Expansion in the *FMR1* Gene and Fragile X Syndrome

Stephanie Ceman, Ph.D.

Stephen T. Warren, Ph.D.

Fragile X syndrome is the most common form of inherited mental retardation. The prevalence of fragile X syndrome is estimated to be approximately 1 per 4,000 males (Morton et al. 1997; Turner et al. 1996). This syndrome is unique because the affected X chromosome has a visible constriction under specific culture conditions at the location of a gene. Positional cloning led to the identification of this gene, *FMR1*, which has a unique CGG repeat tract in the 5′ untranslated region (UTR) that varies in size among individuals. When the number of repeats is larger than 200, the region is hypermethylated and the gene is no longer expressed. The protein encoded by *FMR1*, FMRP, binds messenger RNA (mRNA) and assembles with ribosomes. FMRP is found primarily in the cytoplasm but can also be found in the nucleus. Staining of neurons has shown that FMRP localizes to the dendrites, and this suggests that it may control expression of certain mRNAs on receipt of a specific, as yet undefined signal.

History of X-Linked Mental Retardation

In an 1897 address to the Association of Medical Officers of American Institutions for Idiotic and Feeble-Minded Persons, G. E. Johnson cited 1890 census figures showing that there were 24% more males than females among retarded individuals (Johnson 1897, as reviewed in Lehrke 1974). At the end of his talk, Johnson went on to speculate that "idiocy is due in the majority of cases to some hereditary taint . . ." A genetic mechanism to explain this preponderance of mental retardation in males would be provided more than 50 years later by Martin and Bell (1943), with their presentation of the first extensive family pedigree indicating that some forms of mental retardation segregate in an X-linked manner.

An actual physical defect in the X chromosome was described 26 years later in 1969 when H. A. Lubs noted an unusual secondary constriction at the end of the X chromosome in all affected males and in two unaffected females in a family with X-linked mental retardation. He called this cytogenetically distinct chromosome "marker X chromosome" and proposed that a gene, whose absence resulted in mental retardation, was located at or near the constriction (Lubs 1969) (Figure 3–1). This marker X chromosome was described again in 1971 by Escalante and co-workers in their characterization of a family with three mentally retarded brothers and later by others (Giraud et al. 1976; Harvey et al. 1977).

The ability to consistently detect the constriction on the X chromosome required specific culture conditions in which the availability of pyrimidine nucleotide triphosphate (specifically, thymidine) was limited. To enhance expression of the fragile site, inhibitors of thymidine monophosphate synthesis, such as 5-fluorodeoxyuridine or methotrexate, were used (Glover 1981; Sutherland et al. 1983). Once researchers were able to consistently induce the fragile X site, they were able to demonstrate that about 40% of families with two or more retarded brothers had the "marker X" or fragile X chromosome (for review, see Brown et al. 1986).

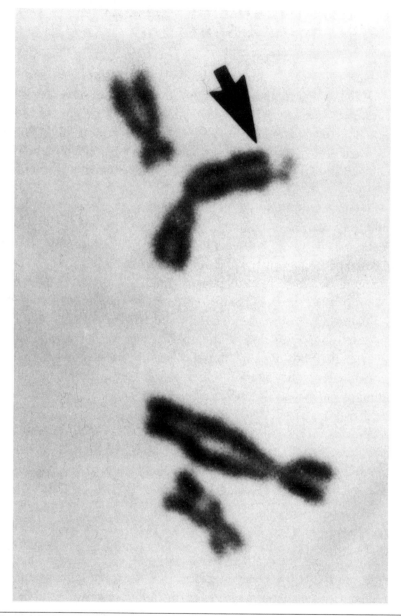

FIGURE 3–1. *Partial karyotype of Giemsa-stained human chromosomes showing the fragile site (arrow).*
Source. Reprinted with permission from Warren ST, Nelson DL: "Advances in Molecular Analysis of Fragile X Syndrome." *JAMA* 271:536–542, 1994. Copyright 1994, American Medical Association.

Clinical Features of Patients With Fragile X Syndrome

The most significant features of the fragile X syndrome are developmental delays and mental retardation. Affected males show a range of mental retardation from profound to borderline, with an average IQ in the moderately retarded range (20–60) (Pennington et al. 1991). Males with fragile X syndrome may also have behavior problems, showing avoidance, similar to that in autism, as well as hyperactivity and attention deficits.

Fragile X syndrome is difficult to diagnose in newborns, with the subtle facial features becoming more apparent with age (Figure 3–2). Affected males generally have a long, narrow face with a moderately increased head circumference (>50th percentile). They may also have a prominent forehead and jaw and large, mildly dysmorphic ears (Butler et al. 1991a, 1991b, 1992). Some of the phenotype is reminiscent of a mild connective tissue disorder, with affected individuals exhibiting hyperextensible joints, high-arched palate, and mitral valve prolapse (Loehr et al. 1986). Probably the most significant physical feature of affected males is the enlarged testicular volume (macroorchidism) in postpubescent males. Almost 90% of such males have testicular volumes in excess of 25 mL (Butler et al. 1992).

Females with fragile X syndrome are usually much more mildly affected than males. Physical signs may be absent or mild, and the mental retardation is less severe, with most female patients having IQs falling in the mild-to-borderline range.

Genetics of Fragile X Inheritance

In the late 1970s, the specific region of the X chromosome where the fragile site is located was mapped near the interface of Xq27 and 28 (for review, see Brookwell et al. 1982) and then specifically at Xq27.3 (Krawczun et al. 1985). Identification of the gene's location, however, did not provide an explanation for the complex inheritance of this disorder. Fragile X differs from all known X-linked, inherited diseases

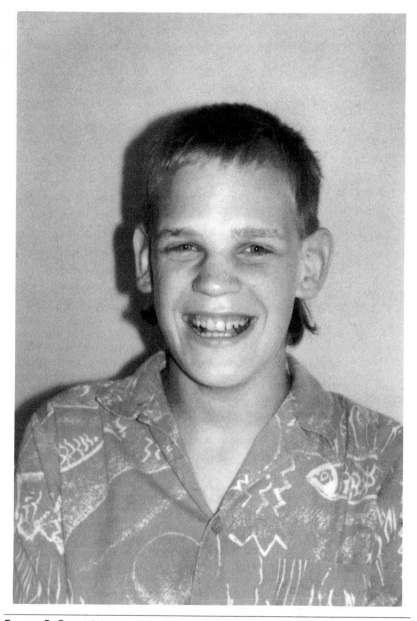

FIGURE 3–2.   *Adolescent male with fragile X syndrome and associated mental retardation.*
Source. Reprinted with permission from Warren ST, Nelson DL: "Advances in Molecular Analysis of Fragile X Syndrome." *JAMA* 271:536–542, 1994. Copyright 1994, American Medical Association.

in two ways: 1) there is a relatively high frequency of nonpenetrant carrier males, and 2) the mothers and daughters of transmitting males, although similar in phenotype, express the gene differently in their offspring. The unaffected daughters of transmitting males are much more likely to have affected offspring than are the mothers of transmitting males (Sherman et al. 1984, 1985). This phenomenon is called the *Sherman paradox*. A satisfactory explanation for this complex pattern of inheritance would not be provided until the gene was cloned and characterized.

Cloning the Fragile X Gene

The line of investigation that would ultimately lead to isolation of the fragile X gene began with somatic cell hybrids (Warren and Davidson 1984). On the X chromosome, the fragile X site is flanked by two genes, those for hypoxanthine-guanine phosphoribosyltransferase (HGPRT) and glucose-6-phosphate dehydrogenase (G6PD), both of which can be assayed. When human cells expressing both of these enzymes were fused with hamster cells deficient for both, a hybrid containing the markers could be selected for. Such a cell has at least the portion of the human X chromosome containing HGPRT, the intervening fragile X site, and G6PD (Warren et al. 1987). Warren and co-workers isolated somatic cell hybrids that contained translocations between the fragile X site and rodent chromosomes, indicating that the fragile site had a tendency to promote breakage. Such a chromosome facilitated mapping and cloning of the fragile X site through the use of probes for species-specific DNA repeats.

  Human YAC clones were identified that spanned the fragile X site–induced translocation break points. A gene, *FMR1*, was identified within a four-cosmid contig of YAC DNA and was shown to be expressed in the human brain as a 4.8-kilobase mRNA (Verkerk et al. 1991). A complementary DNA (cDNA) clone was isolated containing a CGG repeat at the 5′ end. It was speculated that the fragile X variation and break-point clustering might involve this repeat, which is 220 base pairs distal to a CpG island that is methylated in patients with fragile X syndrome.

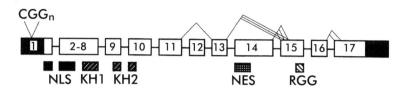

FIGURE 3–3.   *The* FMR1 *gene and encoded protein.* Exons 1–17 are shown as boxes connected by lines representing introns with alternative splicing shown at the 3′ end. The first exon contains the CGG repeat in the 5′ untranslated region that undergoes expansion in individuals with fragile X syndrome. The nuclear localization signal (NLS), K-protein homology (KH) domains, nuclear export signal (NES), and RGG box of the *FMR1*-encoded protein, FMRP, are shown.

Fine Structure of *FMR1* and Resolution of the Sherman Paradox

The *FMR1* gene consists of 17 exons (Eichler et al. 1993) (Figure 3–3). The first exon contains the CGG repeat, which is upstream of the translation initiation site (Ashley et al. 1993a). The size of the repeat is normally highly polymorphic, ranging from 6 to 54 repeats, with a mode of 30 (Jacobs et al. 1993; Snow et al. 1993). When the repeat is expanded, as in patients with fragile X syndrome, it ranges in size from 230 to more than 1,000 repeats. As a result, the gene, the repeat, and the CpG island become abnormally methylated (Hornstra et al. 1993; Oberle et al. 1986), and this results in transcriptional silencing of *FMR1* (Pieretti et al. 1991; Sutcliffe et al. 1992). Therefore, an *FMR1* gene with up to 54 repeats expresses normal levels of protein, whereas a gene with more than 230 repeats is transcriptionally silent.

Inheritance of a fragile X chromosome is much more complicated, however, than whether one inherits a gene that falls into either of the aforementioned categories. A more complex inheritance was indicated earlier by the Sherman paradox, which described an increased risk of mental retardation depending on where an individual was located within the pedigree. An explanation for this increasing risk was provided by characterization of a third category of *FMR1* based on repeat size, called the *premutation allele,* which has between 54 and 200 repeats.

Individuals carrying premutation alleles are unaffected; however, these genes are meiotically unstable (Kremer et al. 1991; Oberle et al. 1986; Yu et al. 1991). An example of this meiotic instability is shown in Figure 3–4. The grandmother of an affected male has a normal allele with 25 repeats and a premutation allele with 94 repeats. Passage of the premutation allele through her daughter leads to expression of a full mutation in the affected grandson. Another example of the instability of the premutation allele is shown in the first generation, where it varies in size among siblings, who have repeat numbers of 94, 86, 90, and 85, while the normal allele is inherited stably at 25 repeats (Warren and Nelson 1994). This instability shows a distinct parent-of-origin effect whereby expansion to full mutation occurs only in maternal transmission (Fu et al. 1991; Snow et al. 1993).

Exactly how a premutation allele expands to a full mutation is unknown, although CGG repeats can form unusual DNA structures in vitro (Gacy et al. 1995). Interruption of the repeat tract with a different triplet may enhance genomic stability. Certain haplotypes, which contain more nearly pure CGG repeat tracts, are overrepresented on fragile X chromosomes, suggesting that alleles with long, perfect repeat tracts are predisposed to expansion (Hirst et al. 1994; Kunst and Warren 1994; Snow et al. 1994).

The specific point during embryonic development when repeat expansion occurs is unknown, although it has been proposed that repeat expansion occurs during a fixed window of time between days 5 and 20 of early human development (Devys et al. 1993; Reyniers et al. 1993; Wohrle et al. 1993). Somatic mosaicism is often observed in fragile X males who contain both premutation and multiple full mutation alleles (Fu et al. 1991). Although these expanded CGG repeats are mitotically stable in somatic tissues (Wohrle et al. 1993), only premutation alleles are found in the sperm of males with the full mutation. To explain this observation, it was initially proposed that repeat expansion might occur after segregation of the germ tissue; however, careful analysis of the gonadal tissue from fetuses with the full mutation showed that full-mutation alleles were present in the germ cells. This result suggested that the premutation sperm in males with the full mutation have a selective advantage caused by contraction of the repeat length (Malter et al. 1997). The presence of FMRP is not an absolute requirement for viable

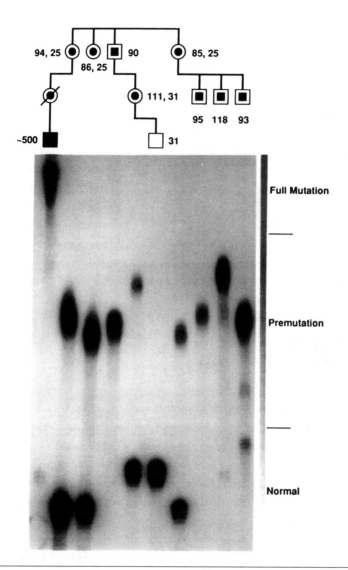

FIGURE 3–4. *Polymerase chain reaction analysis of DNA from members of a fragile X family probed with the CGG oligonucleotide.* The partially filled circles (female) and squares (male) indicate nonpenetrant carriers, closed square indicates penetrant male, open square indicates normal male, and partially filled circle with slash indicates deceased family member.

Source. Reprinted with permission from Warren ST, Nelson DL: "Advances in Molecular Analysis of Fragile X Syndrome." *JAMA* 271:536–542, 1994. Copyright 1994, American Medical Association.

sperm production, however, because *FMR1* knockout mice have normal fertility. These mice may be able to produce sperm lacking FMRP because there are no competing spermatogonia expressing FMRP (Consortium D-BFX 1994).

With regard to the 3′ end of the gene, cDNA cloning revealed the existence of different *FMR1* isoforms based on alternative splicing (Ashley et al. 1993a). It has been observed that the splice donors and acceptors in the 5′ portion of the gene demonstrate greater adherence to consensus sequences than those in the 3′ end of the gene, with this difference providing a possible explanation for the presence of the alternative splice forms (Eichler et al. 1993). One splice variant results in the loss of exon 12, which eliminates a major hydrophobic segment. Another splice form eliminates exon 14 and introduces a frameshift that results in a novel carboxy terminus. Determination of whether certain isoforms exhibit distinct cellular or subcellular locations awaits the development of isoform-specific antibodies.

Other Trinucleotide Repeat Disorders

Currently, there are 12 diseases known to be caused by trinucleotide repeat expansions (Table 3–1). Triplet repeats can be found in regions of the gene encoding either 5′ or 3′ untranslated regions (fragile X or myotonic dystrophy, respectively), in spliced-out intronic sequences (Friedreich's ataxia), and in coding exonic sequences (the dominant ataxias) (for review, see Wilmot and Warren 1998). In general, the noncoding repeats are able to undergo massive expansions from a normal number of repeats (6–40) to an abnormal range of many hundreds or thousands of repeats. Such expansions lead to either transcriptional suppression (fragile X syndrome) or abnormal RNA processing (myotonic dystrophy). In contrast, expansions in coding regions undergo more modest increases, likely constrained by the ability to form a functional protein containing the repeat. All of the CAG expansions appear to reflect a gain or alteration of function leading to neurodegeneration (Warren 1996). Repeat sizes other than triplets have been shown to exhibit expansion that leads to pathology. One example is an

TABLE 3–1. *Summary of diseases caused by trinucleotide repeat expansions*

Disorder	Inheritance	Gene/Locus	Chromosomal localization	Protein product	Expansion size		Repeat location	Mutation type	Parental sex bias
					Normal	Mutant			
Fragile X syndrome	X-linked dominant	FMR1 (FRAXA)	Xq27.3	FMRP	$(CGG)_{6-52}$	$(CGG)_{60-200}$ (premutation) $(CGG)_{230-1000}$ (full)	5'-UTR	LOF Fragile site	Maternal
Fragile XE mental retardation	X-linked ? dominant	FMR2 (FRAXE)	Xq28	FMR2 protein	$(GCC)_{7-35}$	$(GCC)_{130-150}$ (premutation) $(GCC)_{230-750}$ (full)	5'-UTR	LOF Fragile site	ND
Friedreich's ataxia	Autosomal recessive	X25	9q13–21.1	Frataxin	$(GAA)_{6-34}$	$(GAA)_{80}$ (premutation) $(GAA)_{112-1700}$ (full)	Intron 1	LOF (partial)	Maternal
Myotonic dystrophy	Autosomal dominant	DMPK	19q13	Myotonic dystrophy protein kinase	$(CTG)_{5-37}$	$(CTG)_{50-3000}$	3'-UTR	? Dominant negative	Maternal

TABLE 3–1. *Summary of diseases caused by trinucleotide repeat expansions* (continued)

Disorder	Inheritance	Gene/Locus	Chromosomal localization	Protein product	Expansion size		Repeat location	Mutation type	Parental sex bias
					Normal	Mutant			
Spinobulbar muscular atrophy (Kennedy disease)	X-linked recessive	AR	Xq13–21	Androgen receptor	$(CAG)_{11-33}$	$(CAG)_{38-66}$	Coding	GOF LOF(partial)	ND
Huntington's disease	Autosomal dominant	IT15	4p16.3	Huntingtin	$(CAG)_{6-39}$	$(CAG)_{36-121}$	Coding	GOF	Paternal
Dentatorubral-pallidoluysian atrophy/Haw River syndrome	Autosomal dominant	DRPLA (B37)	12p13.31	Atrophin-1 (drplap)	$(CAG)_{6-35}$	$(CAG)_{51-88}$	Coding	GOF	Paternal
Spinocerebellar ataxia									
Type 1	Autosomal dominant	SCA1	6p23	Ataxin-1	$(CAG)_{6-39}$	$(CAG)_{41-81}$	Coding	GOF	Paternal
Type 2	Autosomal dominant	SCA2	12q24.1	Ataxin-2	$(CAG)_{14-31}$	$(CAG)_{35-64}$	Coding	GOF	Paternal
Type 3/Machado-Joseph disease	Autosomal dominant	SCA3 (MJD1)	14q32.1	Ataxin-3	$(CAG)_{12-41}$	$(CAG)_{40-84}$	Coding	GOF	Paternal

TABLE 3–1. *Summary of diseases caused by trinucleotide repeat expansions* (continued)

Disorder	Inheritance	Gene/Locus	Chromosomal localization	Protein product	Expansion size		Repeat location	Mutation type	Parental sex bias
					Normal	Mutant			
Spinocerebellar ataxia (continued)									
Type 6/ episodic ataxia type 2	Autosomal dominant	CACNA1A	19p13	a_{1A}-voltage-dependent calcium-channel subunit	$(CAG)_{7-18}$	$(CAG)_{20-23}$ (EA2) $(CAG)_{21-27}$ (SCA6)	Coding	ND	ND
Type 7	Autosomal dominant	SCA7	3p12–13	Ataxin-7	$(CAG)_{7-17}$	$(CAG)_{38-130}$	Coding	GOF	Paternal

Note. GOF = gain of function; LOF = loss of function; ND = not determined; UTR = untranslated region.
Source. Reprinted from Wilmot GR, Warren ST: "A New Mutational Basis for Disease," in *Genetic Instabilities and Hereditary Neurological Diseases.* Edited by Wells RD, Warren ST. San Diego, CA, Academic Press, 1998. Used with permission.

unstable dodecamer repeat upstream of cystatin B whose expansion leads to progressive myoclonus epilepsy (Lalioti et al. 1997).

It is likely that more diseases caused by repeat expansions will be identified, since new experimental techniques have been developed for their identification, including library screening; repeat expansion detection, or RED; direct identification of repeat expansion and cloning technique, or DIRECT; and reactivity with a monoclonal antibody that recognizes expanded polyglutamine domains (for review, see Wilmot and Warren 1998).

FMR1-Encoded Protein (FMRP)

RNA Binding Domains

Figure 3–3 (see earlier in chapter) shows the functional domains that have been identified in *FMR1* on the basis of homology searches with small regions of the *FMR1*-encoded protein, FMRP. Nucleic acid binding assays of in vitro translated FMRP indicate that FMRP is an RNA binding protein that binds to its own transcript with high affinity (K_d = 5.7 nM) and, to a lesser extent, to a pool of RNAs from human fetal brain. We estimate that approximately 4% of the messages are bound by FMRP. In addition, weak binding of FMRP to both single-stranded and double-stranded DNA was observed (Ashley et al. 1993b).

The region of FMRP responsible for RNA binding has not been precisely identified; however, an isoleucine-to-asparagine mutation in the second heterogeneous ribonucleoprotein (hnRNP) K-protein homology (KH) domain was observed in a severely affected patient with fragile X syndrome (De Boulle et al. 1993). This mutation eliminates binding to poly(U) RNA under high-salt conditions (Siomi et al. 1994; Verheij et al. 1995). Three-dimensional solution structure of the KH domain folding suggests that this region may be very important for RNA binding. The carboxy terminus of FMRP containing the RGG box has also been shown to be important, because truncation results in a protein that is unable to bind mRNA (Price et al. 1996; Siomi et al. 1993).

FMRP is associated with translating ribosomes in an RNA-dependent manner (Eberhart et al. 1996; Khandjian et al. 1995; Tamanini et al. 1996). EDTA treatment, which dissociates ribosomal subunits, releases FMRP from ribosomes into a large (>669 kilodalton) particle containing both poly(A)+ mRNA and protein (Eberhart et al. 1996; Feng et al. 1997a). Such particles are referred to as messenger ribonucleoprotein (mRNP) particles. These complexes are formed in the cytoplasm after the hnRNP proteins, which accompany the mRNA from the nucleus to the cytoplasm, are exchanged for mRNP proteins (for review, see Dreyfuss et al. 1993). However, some cytoplasmic RNA binding proteins are identical to those found in the nucleus (Hamilton et al. 1993). Thus, some proteins seem to remain associated with mRNAs regardless of the subcellular localization of the complex. mRNPs may constitute a unique set of polypeptides as well as several common polypeptides like the poly(A)-binding protein and some eukaryotic initiation factors (for review, see Bag and Wu 1996). The proteins associated with the mRNA may control many aspects of mRNA expression, such as translation initiation, intracellular transport, localization, and conservation and degradation of the mRNA (for review, see Spirin 1996).

Nuclear Localization and Export Sequences

FMRP has been localized primarily to the cytoplasm by intracellular staining (Devys et al. 1993; Feng et al. 1995; Verheij et al. 1993). However, immunogold studies have shown nucleocytoplasmic shuttling of FMRP and have identified its location in transit in the nuclear pores (Feng et al. 1997b). To characterize subcellular localization motifs encoded in the protein sequence, different groups have derived truncated forms of FMRP (Devys et al. 1993; Eberhart et al. 1996; Sittler et al. 1996). In addition, the isoform of *FMR1* (Iso4), in which exon 14 is spliced out and a novel carboxy terminus is created, localizes to the nucleus (Eberhart et al. 1996; Sittler et al. 1996), suggesting that exon 14 contains a nuclear export sequence (NES).

Eberhart and co-workers (1996) defined this NES further by showing that the first 17 amino acids of exon 14 (425–441) can direct nuclear export of a fusion protein. Because the carboxy terminal truncation forms of FMRP are retained in the nucleus, it was inferred that the amino terminal portion of the protein must contain a nuclear localization sequence (NLS). Eberhart and co-workers demonstrated that FMRP contains an NLS by showing nuclear translocation of a fusion protein comprising the amino terminal portion of FMRP and a cytoplasmic protein (Eberhart et al. 1996). This result confirmed the data of Devys and co-workers (1993), which suggested that the first 284 amino acids of FMRP contain a NLS. Because FMRP is primarily localized to the cytoplasm, the NLS signal must be overridden by the NES, possibly because the NES is much stronger. Exactly how this regulation occurs is unknown, although identification of FMRP-associating proteins may give insight into the nature of this control.

Homologs of *FMR1*

With the yeast two-hybrid system, two proteins, FXR1P and FXR2P, were identified that interact with FMRP (Siomi et al. 1995; Zhang et al. 1995). Both proteins are very similar in overall structure to FMRP (about 60% amino acid identity) and have two KH domains and a putative NLS. In addition, FXR1P and FXR2P also bind RNA and associate with ribosomes (Siomi et al. 1996). FXR1P, FXR2P, and FMRP have been shown to associate with one another when expressed simultaneously (Zhang et al. 1995); however, the significance of this observation is unclear because the tissue distribution of *FXR1* expression is distinct from that of *FMR1* (Coy et al. 1995). At this time, it is unknown whether the absence of either FXR1P or FXR2P would result in mental impairment. Unlike *FMR1*, *FXR1* and *FXR2* are both encoded on autosomes (Siomi et al. 1995; Zhang et al. 1995).

Models for FMRP Protein Function

FMRP is a protein that is able to bind RNA, associate with ribosomes, and move in and out of the nucleus. In addition, it is present in dendritic branch points, at the origin of spine necks, and in spine heads—all known locations of neuronal polysomes (Feng et al. 1997b). Because the absence of this protein results in mental retardation, its interaction with mRNAs and proteins must be critical to the development of higher mental function. One model for FMRP function would be that it trafficks to the nucleus, where it associates with specific mRNAs, assembling into an mRNP. In the cytoplasm, as a part of a large protein/mRNA complex, FMRP associates with ribosomes, where translation of the mRNAs may be modulated depending on the signal received by the neuron. FMRP may function as a "masking protein"—that is, a protein within the mRNP that prevents translation of mRNAs until a specific signal is received.

Alternatively, the presence of FMRP in the mRNP may direct the intracellular transport and localization of certain mRNAs to polysomes in the dendrites. Finally, FMRP may affect the conservation or degradation of the mRNAs with which it forms an mRNP, thus controlling the longevity of the mRNA.

The characterization of both the mRNAs and proteins that FMRP associates with will provide more insight into how this protein, which is critical for normal mental development, functions.

References

Ashley CT, Sutcliffe JS, Kunst CB, et al: Human and murine FMR-1: alternative splicing and translational initiation downstream of the CGG repeat. Nat Genet 4:244–251, 1993a

Ashley CT, Wilkinson KD, Reines D, et al: FMR1 protein: conserved RNP family domains and selective RNA binding. Science 262:563–566, 1993b

Bag J, Wu J: Translational control of poly(A)-binding protein expression. Eur J Biochem 237:143–152, 1996

Brookwell R, Daniel A, Turner G, et al: The fragile X(q27) form of X-linked mental retardation: FUdR as an inducing agent for fra(X)(q27) expression in lymphocytes, fibroblasts, and amniocytes. Am Med Genet 13:139–148, 1982

Brown WT, Jenkins EC, Krawczun MS, et al: The fragile X syndrome. Ann N Y Acad Sci 477:129–150, 1986

Butler MG, Allen A, Haynes JL, et al: Anthropometric comparison of mentally retarded males with and without the fragile X syndrome. Am J Med Genet 38:260–268, 1991a

Butler MG, Mangrum T, Gupta R, et al: A 15-item checklist for screening mentally retarded males for the fragile X syndrome. Clin Genet 39:347–354, 1991b

Butler MG, Brunschwig A, Miller LK, et al: Standards for elected anthropometric measurements in males with the fragile X syndrome. Pediatrics 89:1059–1062, 1992

Consortium D-BFX: FMR1 knockout mice: a model to study fragile X mental retardation. Cell 78:23–33, 1994

Coy JF, Sedlacek Z, Bachner D, et al: Highly conserved 3'UTR and expression pattern of FXR1 points to a divergent gene regulation of FXR1 and FMR1. Hum Mol Genet 4:2209–2218, 1995

De Boulle K, Verkerk AJMH, Reyniers E, et al: A point mutation in the FMR-1 gene associated with fragile X mental retardation. Nat Genet 3:31–35, 1993

Devys D, Lutz Y, Rouyer N, et al: The FMR-1 protein is cytoplasmic, most abundant in neurons, and appears normal in carriers of the fragile X premutation. Nat Genet 4:335–340, 1993

Dreyfuss G, Matunis MJ, Pinol-Roma S, et al: hnRNP proteins and the biogenesis of mRNA. Annu Rev Biochem 62:289-321, 1993

Eberhart DE, Malter HE, Feng Y, et al: The fragile X mental retardation protein · is a ribonucleoprotein containing both nuclear localization and nuclear export signals. Hum Mol Genet 5:1083–1091, 1996

Eichler EE, Richards S, Gibbs RA, et al: Fine structure of the human FMR1 gene. Hum Mol Genet 2:1147–1153, 1993

Escalante JA, Grunspun H, Frosa-Pessoa O: Severe sex-linked mental retardation. J Genet Hum 19:137–140, 1971

Feng Y, Zhang F, Lokey LK, et al: Translational suppression by trinucleotide repeat expansion at FMR1. Science 268:731–734, 1995

Feng Y, Absher D, Eberhart DE, et al: FMRP associates with polyribosomes as an mRNP, and the I304N mutation of severe fragile X syndrome abolishes this association. Mol Cell 1:109–118, 1997a

Feng Y, Gutekunst C-A, Eberhart DE, et al: Fragile X mental retardation protein: nucleocytoplasmic shuttling and association with somatodendritic ribosomes. J Neurosci 17:1539–1547, 1997b

Fu Y-H, Kuhl DP, Pizzuti A, et al: Variation of the CGG repeat at the fragile X site results in genetic instability: resolution of the Sherman paradox. Cell 67:1047–1058, 1991

Gacy AM, Goellner G, Juranic N, et al: Trinucleotide repeats that expand in human disease form hairpin structures in vitro. Cell 81:533–540, 1995

Giraud F, Ayme S, Mattei F, et al: Constitutional chromosomal breakage. Hum Genet 34:125–136, 1976

Glover TW: FUdR induction of the X chromosome fragile site: evidence for the mechanism of folic acid thymidine deprivation. Am J Hum Genet 33:234–242, 1981

Hamilton BJ, Nagy E, Malters JS, et al: Association of heterogeneous nuclear ribonucleoprotein A1 and C proteins with reiterated AUUUA sequences. J Biol Chem 268:8881–8887, 1993

Harvey J, Judge C, Wiener S: Familial X-linked mental retardation with an X chromosome abnormality. J Med Genet 14:46–50, 1977

Hirst MC, Grewal PK, Davies KE: Precursor arrays for triplet repeat expansion at the fragile X locus. Hum Mol Genet 3:1553–1560, 1994

Hornstra IK, Nelson DL, Warren ST, et al: High resolution methylation analysis of the FMR1 gene trinucleotide repeat region in fragile X syndrome. Hum Mol Genet 2:1659–1665, 1993

Jacobs PA, Bullman H, Macpherson J, et al: Population studies of the fragile X: a molecular approach. J Med Genet 30:454–459, 1993

Johnson GE: Contribution to the psychology and pedagogy of feebleminded children. Journal of Psycho-Asthenics 2:26–32, 1897

Khandjian EW, Fortin A, Thibodeau A, et al: A heterogenous set of FMR1 proteins is widely distributed in mouse tissues and modulated in cell culture. Hum Mol Genet 4:783–789, 1995

Krawczun MS, Jenkins EC, Brown WT: Analysis of the fragile-X chromosome: localization and detection of the fragile site in high resolution preparations. Hum Genet 69:209–211, 1985

Kremer EJ, Pritchard M, Lynch M, et al: Mapping of DNA instability at the fragile X to a trinucleotide repeat sequence p(CCG)n. Science 252:1711–1714, 1991

Kunst CB, Warren ST: Cryptic and polar variation of the fragile X repeat could result in predisposing normal alleles. Cell 77:853–861, 1994

Kunst CB, Zerylnick C, Karickhoff L, et al: FMR1 in global populations. Am J Hum Genet 58:513–522, 1996

Lalioti MD, Scott HS, Buresi C, et al: Dodecamer repeat expansion in cystatin B gene in progressive myoclonus epilepsy. Nature 386:847–851, 1997

Lehrke RG: X-linked mental retardation and verbal disability. Birth Defects Original Article Series 10c:1–100, 1974

Loehr JP, Synhorst DP, Wolfe RR, et al: Aortic root dilatation and mitral valve prolapse in the fragile-X syndrome. Am J Med Genet 23:89–194, 1986

Lubs JA Jr: A marker X chromosome. Am J Hum Genet 21:231–244, 1969

Malter HE, Iber JC, Willemsen R, et al: Characterization of the full fragile X syndrome mutation in female gametes. Nat Genet 15:165–169, 1997

Martin JP, Bell J: A pedigree of mental defect showing sex linkage. J Neurol Neurosurg Psychiatry 6:154–157, 1943

Morton JE, Bundey S, Webb TP, et al: Fragile X syndrome is less common than previously estimated. J Med Genet 34:1–5, 1997

Oberle I, Heilig R, Moisan JP, et al: Fragile-X mental retardation syndrome with two flanking polymorphic DNA markers. Proc Natl Acad Sci U S A 83:1016–1020, 1986

Pennington BF, O'Connor RA, Sudhalter V: Toward a Neuropsychology of Fragile X Syndrome. Baltimore, MD, Johns Hopkins University Press, 1991

Pieretti M, Zhang F, Fu YH, et al: Absence of expression of the FMR-1 gene in fragile X syndrome. Cell 66:817–822, 1991

Price DK, Zhang F, Ashley CT, et al: The chicken FMR1 gene is highly conserved with a CCT 5′ untranslated repeat and encodes an RNA-binding protein. Genomics 31:3–12, 1996

Reyniers E, Vits L, De Boulle K, et al: The full mutation in the FMR-1 gene of male fragile X patients is absent in their sperm. Nat Genet 4:143–146, 1993

Sherman SL, Morton NE, Jacobs PA, et al: The marker (X) syndrome: a cytogenetic and genetic analysis. Ann Hum Genet 48:21–37, 1984

Sherman SL, Jacobs PA, Morton NE, et al: Further segregation analysis of the fragile X syndrome with special reference to transmitting males. Hum Genet 69:289–299, 1985

Siomi H, Matunis MJ, Michael WM, et al: The pre-mRNA binding K protein contains a novel evolutionarily conserved motif. Nucl Acid Res 21:1193–1198, 1993

Siomi H, Choi M, Siomi MC, et al: Essential role for KH domains in RNA binding: impaired RNA binding by a mutation in the KH domain of FMR1 that causes fragile X syndrome. Cell 77:33–39, 1994

Siomi M, Siomi H, Sauer WH, et al: FXR1, an autosomal homolog of the fragile X mental retardation gene. EMBO J 14:2401–2408, 1995

Siomi MC, Zhang Y, Siomi H, et al: Specific sequences in the fragile X syndrome protein FMR1 and the FXR proteins mediate their binding to 60S ribosomal subunits and the interactions among them. Mol Cell Biol 16:3825–3832, 1996

Sittler A, Devys D, Weber C, et al: Alternative splicing of exon 14 determines nuclear or cytoplasmic localisation of fmr1 protein isoforms. Hum Mol Genet 5:95–102, 1996

Snow K, Doud LK, Hagerman R, et al: Analysis of a CGG sequence at the FMR-1 locus in fragile X families and in the general population. Am J Hum Genet 53:1217–1228, 1993

Snow K, Tester DJ, Kruckeberg KE, et al: Sequence analysis of the fragile X trinucleotide repeat: implications for the origin of the fragile X mutation. Hum Mol Genet 3:1543–1551, 1994

Spirin AS: Masked and Translatable Messenger Ribonucleoproteins in Higher Eukaryotes. Cold Spring Harbor, NY, Cold Spring Harbor Laboratory Press, 1996

Sutcliffe JS, Nelson DL, Zhang, et al: DNA methylation represses FMR-1 transcription in fragile X syndrome. Hum Mol Genet 1:397–400, 1992

Sutherland GR, Jacky PB, Baker E, et al: Heritable fragile sites on human chromosome, X: new folate-sensitive fragile sites: 6p23, 9p21, 9q32, 11q23. Am J Hum Genet 35:432–437, 1983

Tamanini F, Meijer N, Verheij C, et al: FMRP is associated to the ribosomes via RNA. Hum Mol Genet 5:809–813, 1996

Turner G, Webb T, Wake S, et al: Prevalence of fragile X syndrome. Am J Med Genet 64:196–197, 1996

Verheij C, Bakker CE, de Graaff E, et al: Characterization and localization of the FMR-1 gene product associated with fragile X syndrome. Nature 363:722–724, 1993

Verheij C, de Graaff E, Bakker CE, et al: Characterization of FMR1 proteins isolated from different tissues. Hum Mol Genet 4:895–901, 1995

Verkerk AJMH, Pieretti M, Sutcliffe JS, et al: Identification of a gene (FMR-1) containing a CGG repeat coincident with a breakpoint cluster region exhibiting length variation in fragile X syndrome. Cell 65:905–914, 1991

Warren ST: The expanding world of trinucleotide repeats. Science 271:1374–1375, 1996

Warren ST, Davidson RL: Expression of fragile X chromosome in human-rodent somatic cell hybrids. Somat Cell Mol Genet 10:409–413, 1984

Warren ST, Nelson DL: Advances in molecular analysis of fragile X syndrome. JAMA 271:536–542, 1994

Warren ST, Zhang F, Licameli GR, et al: The fragile X site in somatic cell hybrids: an approach for molecular cloning of fragile sites. Science 237:420–423, 1987

Wilmot GR, Warren ST: A new mutational basis for disease, in Genetic Instabilities and Hereditary Neurological Diseases. Edited by Wells RD, Warren ST. San Diego, CA, Academic Press, 1998, pp 3–12

Wohrle D, Hennig I, Vogel W, et al: Mitotic stability of fragile X mutations in differentiated cells indicates early post-conceptional trinucleotide repeat expansion. Nat Genet 4:140–142, 1993

Yu S, Pritchard M, Kremer E, et al: Fragile X genotype characterized by an unstable region of DNA. Science 252:1179–1181, 1991

Zhang Y, O'Connor JP, Siomi MC, et al: The fragile X mental retardation syndrome protein interacts with novel homologs FXR1 and FXR2. EMBO J 14:5358–5366, 1995

Neurodevelopmental Pathways to "Adult" Psychiatric Disorders: Triggers of Disease Onset

Biological Markers as Precursors to Schizophrenia: Specificity, Predictive Ability, and Etiological Significance

C. Jane Tarrant, B.Med.Sci., B.M., B.S., M.R.C.Psych.

Peter B. Jones, M.B., M.Sc., Ph.D., M.R.C.P., M.R.C.Psych.

The development of the central nervous system (CNS) is a complex process that involves the production of a functional network of neurons. As discussed by Murray and colleagues in Chapter 9 of this volume, the syndrome of schizophrenia may result from abnormal connectivity, so uncovering the reasons for this abnormal connectivity may give us insight into the causes of schizophrenia.

Unfortunately, such a model hardly narrows our search for these causes. Individual diversity of the CNS lies in the modification of the multiplicity of events that occur at different stages and in different areas during the developmental process (Nowakowski 1987). Development of nervous tissue begins in the middle of the third week postconception

Work on this review was supported by the Medical Research Council of Great Britain and the Stanley Foundation.

but is by no means confined to gestation. Most neurons are produced within the first 9 months of life, but growth and organization continue long after. Myelination is an important part of the maturational process, continuing through adolescence into early adulthood; cortical-hippocampal relays, for instance, are myelinated in late adolescence (Benes 1989). Synaptogenesis, the basis of connectivity, is an ongoing process throughout life and occurs in two phases. *Target selection* is an early phase in which neuroblasts and neurons form indiscriminate synaptic contacts. *Address selection* occurs when competition from different axons for the same postsynaptic cell leads to the degeneration of some synapses and the reinforcing of others (Huttenlocher 1979).

The most naive evidence for a developmental perspective on the syndrome of schizophrenia comes from the age incidence distribution characteristic of this syndrome. Bearing in mind the methodological concerns of cross-sectional incidence studies (Pogue-Geile 1997), large epidemiological studies have clearly shown that the risk of developing schizophrenia varies with age and is subject to gender bias (Hafner et al. 1989, 1993; Hambrecht et al. 1992; Jablensky et al. 1992). For men, the increase in risk begins in the late teens, reaches a peak in the early twenties, and diminishes through the thirties. For women, there is an approximately 5-year differential in the age at onset, with the greatest risk occurring in the late twenties. After age 45, women are at greater risk of developing the schizophrenia syndrome than are men (Castle et al. 1993; Hafner et al. 1993). The sex ratio, which has a male bias in early-onset cases, appears to reverse later in life. Overall, however, the sex ratio when the whole age range is considered appears to be equal (Castle et al. 1993; Hambrecht et al. 1992).

Weinberger (1987) and Murray and Lewis (1987) proposed that a static brain lesion occurs early in life in people with schizophrenia, perhaps in utero, in an area of the brain that becomes functionally mature only in adolescence. This congenital defect largely remains silent until, through an interaction with the normal processes of development leading to the mature brain, a psychotic illness becomes manifest. Meehl (1989) suggested a different theory to account for the delay in symptoms from the initial early insult. He hypothesized that an accumulation of adverse events during the intervening years would lead to the onset of psychosis, with a threshold of adversity needing to be crossed before the symptoms of a congenital vulnerability would become apparent in early adulthood.

Others believe that there may be processes that occur later but that still involve alterations in the ongoing development of the CNS. These theories do not have to explain a delay in the onset of the illness. Feinberg (1982–1983, 1997) considered that aberrations may arise from the maturational changes in the brain that take place in the second decade, for instance, the synaptic pruning of neural elements. If this process were abnormal, there would be a disruption of integration and modulation of neuronal circuits within the brain. It is also known that different genes can be expressed at different times in development (Plomin 1986), so that the brain abnormalities in schizophrenia may be due to either the expression of abnormal genes or a change in expression in the genes encoding for brain development in young adulthood (Jones and Murray 1991; Pogue-Geile 1991).

Against this complex biological background, we have set out in this chapter to consider the nature of precursors of the syndrome and to review the evidence regarding the specificity of a selection of precursors. We also discuss the implications of precursors for nosology regarding lack of specificity; first, in terms of a multiplicity of outcomes for any one precursor, and, second, in terms of any one outcome (in this case schizophrenia) having a variety of nonspecific precursors.

Precursors and Risk Factors

The term *precursor* is a general one. It can be applied to any characteristic that occurs prior to an event or clinical outcome. Figure 4–1 is a schematic representation of life prior to the onset of a psychotic syndrome. The term precursor could be, and is, applied to any feature that might otherwise be referred to as a "risk factor."

It is useful in the development of causal and mechanistic models to subdivide these precursors or risk factors. Some may be genuine *risk modifiers*, intimately associated with causation. (The risk modifiers are represented by the upward-pointing arrows in Figure 4–1.) If they were removed, risk of the outcome would decrease. Other precursors are better formulated as *risk indicators*, perhaps being manifestations of

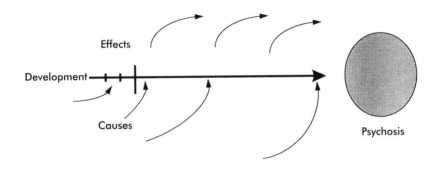

FIGURE 4–1.   *Timing and manifestations of early risk in the development of schizophrenia.*

other risk-modifying precursors. (The risk indicators are represented by the rightward-pointing arrows above the development line in Figure 4–1.) However, they are not intimately related to causation, and reduction in their frequency will not result in reduction of disease frequency. They may or may not be considered a longitudinal aspect of the disease phenotype; their relative frequency and the strength of their association with the psychotic syndrome might determine whether they are.

The inclusion of a time element to the representation in Figure 4–1 allows a third class of precursor to be identified: *the abnormal developmental mechanism* that precedes and leads to the adverse outcome (represented by the horizontal line). This mechanism is impinged on by the risk modifiers that, analogous to predisposing and precipitating causes, may act proximally or distally. Subsequent abnormalities in development may produce both the precursors manifest as risk indicators (perhaps abnormal behavior). They may also lead to psychosis, but perhaps only if further insults occur.

The abnormal mechanism as a "precursor" may not itself be manifested in terms of current measures or knowledge, but it can be modeled statistically or in other ways. A further feature of this model of precursors is that there may be some blurring of the distinction between distal causes and developmental effects. These latter manifestations may themselves impinge on the developmental process. (Schematically, in Figure 4–1, the arrows leading away from the line may curve around and become risk modifiers themselves, acting from below.) In practical terms, one might consider a situation in which a distal risk modifier leads to an aberration of development manifested as abnormal behavior. This behavior may itself alter the environment in which a child functions, with the alteration leading to altered experience and further abnormality in the ongoing developmental process. The extent to which this happens, including whether it happens at all, may be subject to other factors, including chance. Consideration of these factors increases the complexity of a developmental model and is one way in which lack of specificity in precursors can be accommodated. The model is a dynamic one, facilitating what we have referred to elsewhere as a "self-perpetuating cascade of abnormal function" and development prior to onset of schizophrenia (P. B. Jones et al. 1994).

Developmental Markers—
Longitudinal Studies

Research into developmental markers in schizophrenia and other psychoses has been conducted with different types of longitudinal samples, including genetic, opportunistic, or otherwise high-risk groups, and general population samples. Over the last two decades numerous reports have provided evidence suggesting that the neurobiological state of children who go on to develop schizophrenia as adults differs from that of children who do not. Indeed, empirical data echo the observations of Kraepelin and Bleuler. Some of the first such data came from the cohort of child guidance clinic attendees studied by O'Neal and Robins (1958). These authors found that difficulty in walking was an early sign that differentiated children who went on to develop schizophrenia from those who did not. Also, 7% of the boys who had attended the child guidance clinic for a variety of psychopathology, including antisocial behavior, were found at follow-up as an adult to have developed schizophrenia, whereas none of the control sample had (Robins 1966).

Genetic High-Risk Studies

Fish (1975, 1977; Fish et al. 1992), in reviewing "high risk" studies (i.e., studies of individuals at high risk of developing schizophrenia), reported on the New York Infant Study. This study followed the progress of 12 infants at high risk of developing schizophrenia by merit of being born to parents with the illness. The infants were compared with 12 control subjects. Initial results led to the hypothesis by Fish that in the high-risk infants there was a major disorganization in the normal process of development in many areas of CNS function. This disorganization, which occurred in a subgroup of the high-risk population in infancy, included abnormalities in physical growth, in gross motor, visual-motor, and cognitive development, in proprioceptive and vestibular responses, and in muscle tone. Fish coined the term *pandevelopmental retardation* to describe the delay in achieving milestones and the poor integration of CNS functioning.

These findings from the New York Infant Study were reinforced by data from the Israeli School-Age Study (Marcus 1970, 1974; Rosenthal 1971, 1974) and the Jerusalem Infant Developmental Study (Marcus et al. 1981). Fish et al. (1992) reported a partial replication of the findings from the Jerusalem study. The authors found that on follow-up at 10 years, pandevelopmental retardation was significantly related to a parental diagnosis of schizophrenia and to ongoing cognitive and neurointegrative deficits—a finding that suggests continuity of deficit through maturation. However, researchers have not yet been able to establish a link between early childhood abnormalities and adult schizophrenia because the study group has not yet lived through the risk period for onset of the illness. In contrast, the subjects in the New York Infant Study have been followed up to ages 20–22. All seven subjects who were diagnosed as having either schizophrenia or schizotypal personality disorder had pandevelopmental retardation in infancy.

Fish et al. (1992) concluded that pandevelopmental retardation can act as a marker of inherited neurointegrative defects and may provide a strategy for looking at at-risk individuals prior to onset of adult psychopathology. This approach would be a good example of the precursor as a mechanism, as set out in the earlier discussion of Figure 4–1.

Studies With Opportunistic Samples

Walker et al. (1994) undertook blind ratings of neuromotor behavior in home videos of families in which one child later developed schizophrenia. Compared with siblings who remained healthy, toddlers and children who developed schizophrenia were rated as showing poorer motor skills as children and a higher rate of neuromotor abnormalities. These abnormalities were seen predominantly on the left side of the body. The differences in the groups were only significant for the first 2 years of life, and this suggests that the differences are transitory and that affected individuals "catch up."

General Population Birth Cohort Studies

Genetic and opportunistic studies provide evidence of childhood developmental deviance before the onset of schizophrenia. Although the studies reported are prospective in design, they are being carried out with singular samples or small high-risk groups and thus beg the question as to whether their results are relevant to all persons with schizophrenia.

Studies of samples of the general population identified at birth (i.e., birth cohorts), which follow subjects systematically through life, provide unbiased and prospective data. Several have collected relevant data on child development, have followed subjects into or through the period of risk of developing schizophrenia, and have been large enough to yield sufficient cases for analysis.

P. B. Jones and colleagues (Jones and Done 1997; Jones et al. 1994) reported on the Medical Research Council National Survey of Health and Development. The cohort in this survey was derived from a stratified, random sample of births occurring in Britain during a week in March 1946 (Wadsworth 1991). In this survey 5,362 children were followed at regular intervals, including 11 contacts up to the age of 16 years. Since that time there have been 9 contacts, with the most recent at age 43. The data were collected in numerous domains by a variety of workers, including health visitors (senior nurses trained to visit at home), doctors, teachers, and parents, as well as by the subjects themselves. A shortened version of the Present State Examination was completed at age 36, and a derivative of this instrument, the Psychiatric Symptom Frequency, was completed at age 43 years. Cases of schizophrenia were identified on the basis of information from the cohort questionnaires, the Present State Examination at age 36, and the Mental Health Enquiry, a central, independent register of psychiatric hospital admissions. Of 4,746 subjects alive and living in the United Kingdom at age 16, 30 subsequently met the DSM-III-R criteria for schizophrenia. The remaining 4,716 subjects were considered to have been at risk and were used as control subjects.

The children who later developed schizophrenia were shown to have a significant delay in achieving developmental milestones over the first 2 years of life. At age 2 years they were less likely to have attained all the milestones of sitting, standing, walking, and talking. Walking and talking showed the greatest differences, with the case subjects experiencing an average delay of 1.2 months for each. Between ages 2 and 15 years, speech problems were significantly more frequent in the case subjects.

The case subjects had consistently poorer results on cognitive tests, conducted at ages 8, 11, and 15 years, compared with the control subjects. Particular areas in which deficits were observed were verbal, nonverbal, and mathematical skills. The differences between groups appeared to widen in adolescence, although the significance of this divergence was statistically uncertain. The children who later developed schizophrenia preferred to play on their own at ages 4 and 6 years and showed a statistically significant linear trend for being more socially anxious as teenagers. There was no indication that disadvantaged home circumstances or low social class was associated with the later development of schizophrenia.

The specificity of these precursors to schizophrenia and affective disorder has been examined. Van Os et al. (1997b), using the same birth cohort of 5,362 people, established two groups: 1) those with childhood affective disturbance at ages 13 and/or 15 (identified by teacher questionnaires), and 2) those with adult affective disorder at ages 36 and/or 43 (identified from Present State Examination and Psychiatric Symptom Frequency data). Illness persistence for those with childhood affective disturbance was defined as presence of the disturbance at both ages 13 and 15 years. Illness persistence in those with adult affective disorder was defined as evidence of chronic or recurrent affective symptoms between the ages of 36 and 42.

Van Os et al. (1997b) found that 195 subjects met the criteria for childhood affective disturbance. Of these, only 34, or 17.4%, were later classified as being depressed in adulthood. The authors also found that

270 subjects met the criteria for adult affective disturbance, and nearly 30% of these achieved "affective disorder caseness" at both ages 36 and 43, indicating possible persistence of illness. Female gender and lower scores on childhood cognitive tests predicted later depression in the total group of subjects. Subjects who developed childhood affective disturbance exhibited significantly different characteristics in attainment of later motor milestones and more twitches and grimaces at age 15 years compared with control subjects. Those with adult affective disturbance who did not have childhood affective disturbance did not show these developmental delays and abnormal movements. Thus, although there were similarities between developmental effects in affective disorder and schizophrenia, the magnitude of these effects was persistently lower in affective disorder and appeared to be more specific for those who showed an earlier onset of affective disturbance.

Findings from the study of another British birth cohort have been reported by Done and colleagues (Done et al. 1994; Jones and Done 1997). The National Child Development Study followed up on subjects born during a week in March 1958. Data were collected at birth and at ages 7, 11, 16, and 23 years. At ages 7, 15,398 subjects were traced. Cases were identified by means of the Mental Health Enquiry, and Present State Examination diagnoses were made from ratings of medical notes. By 1994, 29 of the subjects received a diagnosis of "narrow schizophrenia," 29 were considered to have undergone an affective psychosis, and 71 were judged to have had a neurotic illness. A control group comprised a randomly selected sample (10%) of cohort members who had never received psychiatric treatment.

Ratings of motor function and neurological soft signs were made at ages 7 and 11 years. At age 7, the subjects who went on to develop narrowly defined ("narrow") schizophrenia and affective psychoses showed significantly more abnormal coordination and clumsiness than did the control subjects. At age 11, differences in hand preference/relative hand skill, coordination, and CNS impairment were apparent in the schizophrenia group compared with the control group. However, some abnormalities in coordination, CNS impairment, and tics and twitches were also associated with later development of affective psychosis.

Poorer educational achievement was found in the group who went on to develop schizophrenia. The deficits in performance encompassed a wide range of tasks, and there was no change in the relative difference between the case subjects and control subjects from ages 7 to 16. Only minor cognitive deficits were measured in the subjects with affective psychosis prior to development of their illness. There were, however, more marked abnormalities in the group who went on to develop neurotic illness and evidence of a decline in function in the females with age. Social disadvantage did account for some of the difference within this group.

In a large cohort of men conscripted into the Swedish army and given cognitive assessments at age 18 years, David et al. (1997) demonstrated lower performance in these tests as a risk factor. This was specific to schizophrenia and was not found for other psychoses. As in the British 1946 cohort (Jones et al. 1994), this IQ effect was not confined to a subgroup within schizophrenia. Rather, there was evidence of a population shift in those who went on to develop the disorder, compared with the total cohort.

Birth Cohort Studies of Precursors to Schizophrenia as Risk Modifiers

Associations between schizophrenia and antecedents of possible etiological significance have been investigated in birth cohort studies. E. Susser and colleagues (Susser and Lin 1992; Susser et al. 1996) tested the hypothesis that exposure of a fetus to malnutrition early in gestation is associated with the later development of schizophrenia (see Chapter 6, this volume). The population in their study was drawn from people born in the Netherlands between 1944 and 1946, a period that included the Dutch Hunger Winter of 1944/45. Three birth cohorts were compared: 1) subjects who were exposed to low food rations during the first trimester, 2) subjects who were conceived at the height of the famine and who, like the subjects in the first birth cohort, were exposed to low food rations during the first trimester, and 3) subjects who were not exposed to nutritional deficiencies. Cases of schizophrenia were obtained from the Dutch National Psychiatric Registry, and both "narrow" and "broad" definitions of schizophrenia according to ICD-9 were used for separate analyses. The risk of "narrow" schizophrenia in the second cohort was significantly higher than in the unexposed group (relative risk = 2.0, with no gender differences). The authors commented on the high specificity of their findings. Later development of schizophrenia was associated with low food rations during the first trimester and conception at the height of the famine.

Although there is much evidence of schizophrenia's link with prenatal exposure to infection, less is known about the link with exposure to infection after birth. Rantakallio et al. (1997) used the 1966 birth cohort in northern Finland to investigate the association between CNS infection in childhood (up to the age of 14 years) and the later development of schizophrenia or other psychoses. The general population sample yielded 11,017 subjects alive and living in Finland at age 15 years. Cases of CNS infection were identified by hospital admissions and from the Finnish Hospital Discharge Register; 145 of the sample had had CNS infections in childhood, with 102 of the infections viral. Cases of psychoses in subjects up to the age of 27 years were identified also from the Finnish Hospital Discharge Register and were classified according to DSM-III-R criteria; 76 of the subjects had schizophrenia and 53 had other psychoses. Four subjects who had been exposed to CNS infection (viral in all four cases) developed schizophrenia. This association between childhood viral CNS infection and later schizophrenia was significant, with an adjusted odds ratio of 4.8. In the two cases of other psychoses in which the subject had childhood CNS infection, the subject had had a bacterial CNS infection. The association between other psychoses and bacterial CNS infections was also statistically significant, with an adjusted odds ratio of 6.8.

The same northern Finnish cohort, as reported by P. B. Jones et al. (1998), was used to investigate the associations between pregnancy, delivery, and perinatal complications and the later development of schizophrenia. Low birth weight and a combination of low birth weight and short gestational age were more common in the 76 people with schizophrenia. The development of schizophrenia was seven times more likely in subjects with perinatal brain damage than in those who experienced no perinatal brain damage. A general class of obstetric complications was not linked to schizophrenia, nor were numerous individual adverse events. The associations between pregnancy and delivery complications and schizophrenia in the offspring appeared to be specific

TABLE 4–1.   *Developmental markers in schizophrenia: birth cohort studies*

There is strong and consistent evidence of delays in attaining developmental milestones, cognitive deficits, and abnormalities in social functioning that are apparent through childhood, adolescence, and early adulthood.

Both genetic high-risk and birth cohort studies show remarkable confluence of results, with this consistency suggesting that results of the former are relevant to the majority of cases of schizophrenia.

The identified biological markers represent a pattern of developmental shift that, on a population level, can predict later onset of psychopathology.

Impaired neurodevelopment is not specific to schizophrenia. Some features are found in affective disorder, particularly in cases of childhood onset.

Dietary deficiency, CNS infection, and obstetric complications are associated with later development of schizophrenia in birth cohort studies.

to the complications leading to perinatal brain damage that had already been linked to other adverse neurological outcomes such as cerebral palsy and mental retardation (Rantakallio and Von Wendt 1986). Further work will define the specificity of prenatal and perinatal complications to schizophrenia as a psychiatric outcome. It should be noted that perinatal brain damage may itself be a manifestation of earlier events and that its status as a risk indicator or modifier is unclear.

Conclusions

Although direct comparisons between birth cohorts are problematic (P. B. Jones and Done 1997), considerable evidence suggests that subjects who later develop schizophrenia have a variety of quantitative and qualitative features that differentiate them from control subjects (Table 4–1). Delay in reaching developmental milestones is present, and ongoing deficits in cognitive and social functioning are apparent throughout childhood, adolescence, and early adulthood. These changing biological markers represent a pattern of developmental shift that is associated, on a population basis, with later onset of psychopathology. These findings are not completely specific to schizophrenia, although effects are most dramatic in the group of subjects with this disorder. Because of this lack of specificity and the overlap with a normal variation in developmental attainment and CNS integration, a viable prediction of future illness cannot, as yet, be made on an individual basis.

Neurological Soft Signs

The meaning of neurological deviance in schizophrenia is a matter of debate (Chua and McKenna 1995), and a number of questions remain. What is the deviance, and is it an inherent part of the disease process with a spectrum of severity? Does it have etiological significance by acting as a marker of earlier neurological insult? Is it a corollary of the earlier, widespread developmental delay illustrated in the developmental studies? What is clear is that neurological soft signs remain consistent and intriguing clinical observations. In this section, we consider the significance and implications of neurological soft signs for schizophrenia.

Classification of Neurological Abnormalities

Neurological abnormalities have been classified into two categories. "Hard" signs are indicative of damage to specific regions in the nervous system, whereas "soft" signs are considered to be indications of more generalized and nonspecific pathology. Both can be elicited in the basic clinical examination. The neurological soft signs that occur in schizophrenia show some meaningful groupings with consistently occurring abnormalities in the areas of integrative sensory function, motor coordination, and motor sequencing (Heinrichs and Buchanan 1988). We consider these signs to be precursors to the disorder and, in all likelihood, indicators of risk.

Specificity to Schizophrenia

Numerous studies have demonstrated that soft signs are associated with schizophrenia. Quitkin et al. (1976) found evidence to support the hypothesis that individuals with "process schizophrenia" (defined as schizophrenia with poor premorbid functioning, poor response to neuroleptics, and poor prognosis) and "unstable character disorders" (defined as presence of antisocial and impulsive character traits with unpredictable mood swings) have an increased number of neurological and behavioral soft signs. Subsequently, Woods et al. (1986) examined four groups of subjects: those with diagnoses of schizophrenia, manic depression, or drug or alcohol abuse, and a group of psychiatrically healthy volunteers. The subjects with schizophrenia had significantly more neurological abnormalities than the other groups. Subjects with either manic depression or drug abuse, however, also had significantly more abnormalities than the control subjects. Mohr et al. (1996) compared 143 people with schizophrenia with 78 alcoholic subjects and 57 control subjects. Subjects with schizophrenia had more impairment in terms of neurological soft signs than control subjects, but the only significant difference between the alcoholic subjects and those with schizophrenia lay in the tests for motor coordination. Ismail et al. (1998) found at least one neurological abnormality in 100% of 60 patients with schizophrenia but in only 45% of the 75 control subjects. When the criterion was changed to a cutoff score, abnormality being indicated with seven or more neurological signs, 67% of the patients were affected compared with none of the control subjects.

It can be concluded from these studies that neurological soft signs occur more frequently in persons with schizophrenia than in the general population. However, neurological dysfunction also occurs in manic depression, personality disorder, and alcohol dependence, although not to the same extent and with different symptom profiles.

Prevalence in Schizophrenia

The prevalence of neurological soft signs in patients with schizophrenia was estimated to be between 50% and 65%, compared with 5% in control groups (Heinrichs and Buchanan 1988). However, it has been difficult to compare studies assessing neurological soft signs in psychiatric patients because of the different scales that have been adapted and used (Buchanan and Heinrichs 1989; Quitkin et al. 1976; Rossi et al. 1990; Schroder et al. 1992). A structured and reliable procedure for rating neurological soft signs is needed. Other methodological concerns include low sample sizes, reliability, temporal stability of signs, medication effects, and the presence of other confounding variables such as age. In view of the differing scales and methods of scoring with arbitrary cutoffs to decide absence or presence of pathology, Ismail et al. (1998) felt, and illustrated with their work, that prevalence figures can be a function of the defining criteria used.

Associations With Clinical Symptoms of Schizophrenia

Many variables have been investigated in the search for associations between neurological soft signs and schizophrenia. Some authors found evidence for different subtypes of disease being particularly associated with such signs. Schroder et al. (1992) found that neurological soft signs were related to certain symptom clusters (as measured by the Brief Psychiatric Rating Scale), such as thought disorder. Liddle and Morris (1991) proposed that there are three independent syndromes within schizophrenia: psychomotor poverty, disorganization, and reality distortion. These syndromes were validated with confirmed changes in cerebral blood flow among the groups that signified localized brain changes in function. The authors went on to report different relationships among the groups with neurological soft signs (Liddle et al. 1993). Psychomotor poverty was strongly associated with dyspraxia and then agnosia. Disorganization was less strongly associated with neurological soft signs and had the strongest correlation with agnosia. Reality distortion had no associations with neurological soft signs (Liddle et al. 1993). Malla et al. (1997) attempted but failed to replicate these results in a study of 100 patients with schizophrenia. In the few relationships found between syndromes and neurological soft signs, these seemed to be more important for the women; men had no associations that were independent of illness duration.

Temporal Stability of Neurological Soft Signs and Medication Effects

Mohr et al. (1996) reported that neurological soft signs in schizophrenia were significantly increased in the group with a chronic illness—results that replicated the findings of Torrey (1980). In a longitudinal study of schizophrenia from acute states to either chronic or remitting states, Schroder et al. (1992) found that during the clinical course both groups showed a significant decrease in the number of neurological soft signs but that this decrease was most pronounced for the group with remitting course. There was a highly significant difference in the magnitude of decrease in these two groups of patients; however, there remained a significant increase in neurological soft signs in both groups compared with control subjects at follow-up.

Kolakowska et al. (1985), however, concluded that neurological soft signs and outcome were not related in their sample, and others have proposed that the association between chronicity and increased neurological soft signs could be explained by other factors, such as duration or extent of medication treatment. Some studies have found weak effects of medication on neurological soft signs (King et al. 1991), but the general consensus of findings is of no relationship between neurological soft signs and medication (Heinrichs and Buchanan 1988). Gupta et al. (1995) looked at neurological soft signs in a group of patients who were drug naive and a group of those who were not. A higher rate of soft signs was found in the group who had been treated with medication, although all patients had a higher frequency of neurological soft signs compared with control subjects. However, the authors were unable to determine the role of the medication in this effect from the role of other features of the treated group, particularly age. They concluded that although neurological soft signs are present independent of medication, the prevalence of such signs may potentially be increased by neuroleptic medication.

Thus, there appears to be little evidence on which to draw in determining whether neurological soft signs have temporal stability. Kolakowska et al. (1985) retrospectively linked the presence of neurological soft signs in schizophrenia to a history of developmental abnormalities, suggesting that the abnormalities were present in childhood. Marcus et al. (1985) found that neurological soft signs in a group of offspring of people with schizophrenia who themselves were at high risk of developing schizophrenia did have stability through childhood and adolescence. However, few studies have looked at the progression of neurological soft signs across ages. Walker et al. (1994) indicated that the neuromotor abnormalities found in infancy in subjects who later developed schizophrenia were only significant up to the age of 2 years.

Associations With Cognitive Function

Kolakowska et al. (1985) demonstrated that cognitive impairment was associated with neurodysfunction in their sample. King et al. (1991)

reported on a small group of patients with schizophrenia and noted a similar finding. Mohr et al. (1996) also found significant correlations between neurological soft signs and neuropsychological measurements sensitive to prefrontal function.

Associations With Potential Etiological Factors and Other Biological Markers

Different etiological hypotheses have led other researchers to look at associations between neurological soft signs and potential etiological factors thought to be important in schizophrenia. Lane et al. (1996) found that male patients with schizophrenia whose mothers had experienced obstetric complications had higher scores on examinations for neurological soft signs and that female patients with a family history of schizophrenia also had higher neurological soft sign scores.

Some studies have examined associations between neurological soft signs and schizophrenia in high-risk populations. Kinney et al. (1986) found that the prevalence of neurological soft signs in relatives of individuals with schizophrenia was higher than that in psychiatrically healthy comparison subjects. Rossi et al. (1990) compared 58 patients with schizophrenia with 31 well first-degree relatives and 38 healthy control subjects. The patient group had the greatest number of neurological soft signs, but the first-degree relatives had significantly more neurological abnormalities than the control subjects. Ismail et al. (1998) reiterated this pattern of findings, showing that siblings also had high levels of neurological abnormality across many domains. Rossi et al. (1990) found an association between abnormal smooth pursuit eye movement and neurological soft signs. Smooth pursuit eye movement has been found to be abnormal in relatives of individuals with schizophrenia (Holzman 1987) and has been put forward as a marker of vulnerability to schizophrenia.

Conclusions

It is clear from the available evidence that neurological soft signs are associated with schizophrenia. However, as has been shown, they are not specifically associated with schizophrenia and occur in other patient groups, albeit not to the same extent. Neurological soft signs appear to be an indicator of cerebral dysfunction. There is some evidence that they are associated with developmental abnormalities in childhood, but no prospective data currently exist to indicate temporal stability of this neurodysfunction after the onset of psychosis.

Although neurological soft signs are heterogeneous, evidence has pointed toward a pattern of neurological deficits in motor coordination, sensory dysfunction, and complex sequencing of motor events. It may be that the schizophrenia syndrome includes a motor component. Associations with groups of clinical symptoms and abnormalities in neurocognitive tests have led some to speculate on the significance of the neurological soft signs according to localized function, such as in prefrontal and parietal areas. However, imaging studies have indicated that neurological soft signs are potentially important indicators of dysfunction in other areas, such as the basal ganglia (Mohr et al. 1996; Schroder et al. 1992).

Consistent findings in high-risk groups of relatives being affected indicate that the neurodysfunction is probably family related. Furthermore, links with neurological soft signs and smooth pursuit eye movements in patients and families suggest that they both may be potentially useful as trait markers for schizophrenia. Their presence in drug-naive patients suggests that they are intrinsic to the disease and not due to medication, but it appears that neurological soft signs are not of value in predicting outcome or course of illness.

The significance of neurological soft signs in an etiological context is yet to be clarified. These signs may reflect an interaction between environmental and genetic factors, with families having these in common. Genetic effects may be differentially expressed according to sex, and further work on epigenetic causes is required. Conclusions based on research findings on the association of neurological soft signs and schizophrenia are presented in Table 4–2.

Dermatoglyphic Patterns

Dermatoglyphics refers to the configurations of skin ridges on the palms and soles; each individual has unique patterns. Dermal ridges appear during the second trimester of fetal development. Ectodermal cells

TABLE 4–2.   *Neurological soft signs and schizophrenia*

Neurological soft signs are more common in people with schizophrenia, although they are not specific to this disorder.

Temporal stability of the neurological soft signs is uncertain, although links with developmental abnormalities in childhood have been made.

A pattern of neurological abnormality, with deficits in motor coordination, sensory integration, and motor sequencing, occurs in schizophrenia.

Neurological soft signs appear to be a biological marker of cerebral dysfunction in schizophrenia and may act as a trait marker.

Neurological soft signs do not predict course and outcome.

The significance of neurological soft signs in the etiology of schizophrenia is not currently known.

destined for the palmar surfaces of the hands migrate to their final positions between weeks 14 and 22 of gestation. Ridge count is thought to be affected by fetal size in relation to gestational age. Once formed, the patterns of ridges are permanent and will not be disrupted by postnatal events. Any alterations in adult hand morphology, therefore, act as fairly exact evidence of the time of disruption during intrauterine development.

The migration of dermal cells, although under genetic control, is sensitive to environmental insults, such as ischemia, infection, or toxicity (Schaumann and Alter 1976). The concept of individual right-left asymmetry, or "fluctuating asymmetry," in these characteristics has been used as a marker of developmental disturbance (Van Valen 1962). The second trimester is also the critical time for the massive migration of cortical neurons from the periventricular germinal matrix to the cerebral cortex (Rakic 1988), and this explains the relevance of dermatoglyphics to schizophrenia and other disorders with developmental origins.

Markow and Wandler (1986) initially found that there was an increased fluctuating asymmetry of hand morphology in subjects with schizophrenia compared with subjects with affective disorder and psychiatrically healthy control subjects. They also indicated that this difference was more pronounced in those with an earlier onset of schizophrenia. Mellor (1992), revisiting data from his pioneering study (Mellor

1968a, 1968b) and adopting the concept of fluctuating asymmetry, confirmed that there was a greater degree of asymmetry in the subjects with schizophrenia than in the control group on four independent measures.

Cannon et al. (1994) compared the finger and palm prints of 46 people with schizophrenia with those of an age- and sex-matched control group. Of the ill subjects, 15.2% had abnormal dermatoglyphic patterns characterized by a high density of secondary creases in the prints. None of the subjects in the control group were affected.

Several twin studies have examined the differences in dermatoglyphic patterns between concordant and discordant pairs. Markow and Gottesman (1989) compared fluctuating asymmetry of dermatoglyphic markers in 22 concordant and 19 discordant twin pairs with a psychotic disorder and a group of 9 twin pairs in which the co-twin had a mental illness but not schizophrenia. There were 16 pairs of monozygotic twins in the concordant group, 3 in the discordant group, and 2 in the other group. The authors found that the asymmetry was greatest in the concordant twin group, in which both twins had schizophrenia, and least in the discordant twin group. Bracha et al. (1991) looked at intra-pair discrepancies in monozygotic twins discordant for schizophrenia. The affected co-twin had significantly more minor hand anomalies, and there were significant differences in fingertip ridge count between the co-twins (Bracha et al. 1992).

In another twin study, Van Os et al. (1997a) found that ectodermal hand patterns such as abnormal creases or ridge dissociation were significantly more common in subjects with a psychosis compared with psychiatrically healthy control subjects. These results were in agreement with the finding of Markow and Gottesman (1989) that monozygotic twins concordant for psychosis had higher rates of dermatoglyphic abnormalities than discordant pairs; however, Bracha et al. (1991) did not find any differences between the affected and well co-twins of discordant pairs.

Despite initial uncertainty as to whether the dermatoglyphic patterns in individuals with schizophrenia were different from those in psychiatrically healthy individuals, a change in the way of measuring and analyzing these biological markers has shown that a greater asymmetry exists in individuals with schizophrenia compared with individuals with other mental illnesses and control subjects. Twin studies have found differences between monozygotic and dizygotic pairs who are concordant compared with those who are not. It was initially assumed that dermatoglyphic patterns were linked with the genetic liability to inherit schizophrenia. Livshits and Kobyliansky (1987) found that dermatoglyphic asymmetry was greater with increasing genetic homozygosity in a population. This inbred instability has been thought to signify a lower capacity by the individual to buffer adverse environmental effects that could alter the determined course of development (Van Valen 1962; C. H. Waddington 1957). The greater asymmetry in the monozygotic concordant twin pairs found by Markow and Gottesman (1989) would therefore be concordant with a greater homozygosity, a greater liability to developmental instability, and an impaired ability to buffer potential adverse environmental influences.

However, combinations of external adverse conditions, heat, cold, and protein deprivation have been shown to increase fluctuating asymmetry in laboratory animals (Siegel and Smookler 1973), and research has shown that dermatoglyphic patterns can be affected by second-trimester prenatal insults such as viral infections (Schaumann and Alter 1976). Consistent with these reports is the finding of dermatoglyphic differences between genetically similar monozygotic twins discordant for schizophrenia (Bracha et al. 1992). This discrepancy in dermal ridges between the affected and psychiatrically healthy twins could therefore be explained by differences in events encountered by them in the intrauterine environment during the second trimester while the dermal ridges were forming. Van Os et al. (1997a) have argued that concordant pairs share a common environmental exposure in utero that explains the higher rate of abnormalities in these twins.

Dermatoglyphic abnormalities can be seen as markers of aberrations or adverse events that occurred during the defined intrauterine period when dermal ridges were formed. Their association with schizophrenia may indicate that these adverse events are important factors in the discrepancies of the developmental process of the CNS and in the etiology of the disease. Conclusions based on research findings regarding the association of dermatoglyphic abnormalities and schizophrenia are presented in Table 4–3.

TABLE 4–3.   *Dermatoglyphic abnormalities in schizophrenia*

Altered dermatoglyphic patterns and greater dermatoglyphic asymmetry occur more frequently in people with schizophrenia.

Altered dermatoglyphic patterns and greater dermatoglyphic asymmetry appear to have some specificity for schizophrenia.

Intrapair differences between monozygotic discordant twins suggest that a discrepancy in intrauterine environment during the second trimester may be important in producing both the dermatoglyphic abnormalities and schizophrenia.

Minor Physical Anomalies

According to K. L. Jones (1997), minor physical anomalies are "unusual morphological features that are of no serious medical or cosmetic consequence to the patient" (p. 727) and are most common in the face, ears, hands, and feet. The significance of minor physical anomalies is debated. The significance ascribed to these anomalies varies widely, ranging from their being a sign of normality, and a usual feature within families, to their being indicative of major congenital disorder (Marden et al. 1964). Their presence acts as a biological marker of developmental disturbance within a fetus that can be located in time relative to the normal development of the embryo. We consider them to be indicators of risk.

Craniofacial development is an interaction of genetic instruction and biochemical and physical cell environments. The cell proliferation, differentiation, migration, and organization in a cascade of events lead to a rapidly changing facial profile of the fetus. The morphogenesis of the brain and of the overlying face are "inextricably intertwined" (DeMeyer 1975; see also Diewert et al. 1993); both develop from common embryonic ectoderm during the first or early second trimester. Hence, dysmorphological facial features may act as markers of brain pathology and indicate an etiological process, with disruptive events occurring within the first or early second trimester.

An increased number of minor physical anomalies has been found in individuals with schizophrenia in many studies. Gualtieri et al. (1982) examined 64 adults with schizophrenia and 38 with alcohol dependency and compared them with 95 control subjects. Dysmorphology was rated with the Waldrop scale (Waldrop and Halverson 1971; Waldrop et al. 1968). After adjustment for confounding variables, subjects with chronic schizophrenia had significantly higher weighted scores than either the control group or the subjects with alcohol dependence.

Guy et al. (1983) investigated the relationship between minor physical anomalies in 40 adult males with schizophrenia and age at onset, premorbid functioning, course of illness, and neurological impairment. The sample consisted only of Caucasian males to eliminate racial and gender differences. The authors found that the group had significantly more than the expected number of anomalies in a general population — the average number being 6.9 on the Waldrop scale — and that patients with poorer premorbid functioning had higher anomaly scores. There was no significant relationship between neuropsychological and neurological measures and the number of anomalies.

Green et al. (1987), using data drawn from a group of 50 individuals with schizophrenia, categorized cases of schizophrenia according to age at onset. They found that subjects who developed the illness before the age of 18 had significantly more minor physical anomalies as assessed by a modified Waldrop scale. Enlarging the sample to 67, Green et al. (1989) showed that there was also a pattern of dysmorphology, with mouth abnormalities being the most consistent finding.

Deutsch and Farkas (1990) grouped minor physical anomalies into chronological order in development (i.e., first trimester or later in gestation). Using their own scale, the authors found that the anomalies that they considered to be formed later in gestation were overrepresented in the schizophrenia group. They also found that these anomalies were found consistently in the proband's first-degree relatives.

O'Callaghan et al. (1991) recruited 41 outpatients with a living biological mother to investigate minor physical anomalies and links with a family history of schizophrenia, obstetric complications, and frontal lobe neuropsychological abnormalities. Higher scores on the Waldrop scale overall were associated with a positive family history of schizophrenia, a history of obstetric complications, and male sex. Patients with a family history but whose mothers did not have obstetric complications tended to have more body regions affected by dysmorphological features and were more likely to have abnormalities of the mouth and palate.

Patients who did not have a family history of schizophrenia but whose mothers had obstetric complications had an intermediate number of body regions affected. The association between minor physical anomalies and obstetric complications depended on a history of bleeding early in pregnancy.

McNeil et al. (1992) looked at a sample of 84 children born to women with a history of nonorganic psychoses and compared them with a control sample of 100 children born to women with no history of psychosis and matched for prenatal care, maternal parity, age, social class, and marital status. Information on major and minor congenital malformations was obtained from baby clinic records from the first 3–4 years of life. There was no difference in the prevalence of congenital malformations between the two groups. McNeil et al. (1993) also investigated head circumferences at birth in a sample of individuals with schizophrenia and a control group. "Preschizophrenic" neonates had significantly smaller head circumferences that were disproportionate to their body length. A small head circumference in the subjects with schizophrenia was related to an absence of a family history of psychoses. C. A. H. Jones et al. (1993) piloted their own structured clinical examination with 60 schizophrenic subjects, finding that 75% of the anomalies present occurred around the head and neck.

Lohr and Flynn (1993) assessed the prevalence of minor physical anomalies in 118 patients with schizophrenia, 33 patients with mood disorders, and 31 control subjects. The higher rates of anomalies in the schizophrenia group were not associated with age at onset, severity of psychopathology, or socioeconomic status. Patients with tardive dyskinesia had significantly more anomalies than did those without this condition. Anomaly scores in the group with mood disorders did not differ significantly from the scores of either the control group or the group with schizophrenia.

Cantor-Graae et al. (1994) independently evaluated pregnancy complications and minor physical anomalies in 40 twin pairs from the National Institute of Mental Health investigation of psychosis in monozygotic twins. They found that there was only a trend in the discordant group toward a greater number of anomalies in the ill twin than in the healthy co-twin. Within the whole group there was an association with complications occurring in early pregnancy and minor physical anomalies; this association was particularly strong for the group of discordant twin pairs.

Green et al. (1994a) investigated minor physical anomalies in 46 Caucasians with chronic schizophrenia. They measured the anomalies with the Waldrop scale and used dermatoglyphic measures of fluctuating asymmetry and total ridge count. Patients were more likely to have high scores on the measures of both minor physical anomalies and asymmetry. Green et al. (1994b) also indicated that the prevalence of minor physical anomalies in the siblings of schizophrenic patients was comparable to that of psychiatrically healthy control subjects, as was the rate of minor physical anomalies in patients with bipolar disorder.

Alexander et al. (1994) investigated 41 subjects with schizophrenia, 8 subjects with bipolar disorder, 19 subjects with mental disability, and 14 psychiatrically healthy subjects. All subjects in this study were Caucasian. Ratings were made by those blind to the diagnosis with an adapted Waldrop scale. The anomaly scores differed significantly, with subjects with mental disability having the highest scores. There was a trend for those with schizophrenia to have higher scores than the psychiatrically normal group. Among the subjects with schizophrenia, the Waldrop scale score was significantly negatively correlated with age, a finding that was not replicated in the other groups. There was a trend toward an association between prenatal and perinatal complications and higher scores, as well as a correlation between higher scores and larger third-ventricle width. The authors found no relationships between family history of schizophrenia and minor physical anomalies, age at onset, duration of illness, and poorer premorbid functioning in the schizophrenia group.

Buckley et al. (1994), using magnetic resonance spectroscopy of the left temporal and frontal lobes, evaluated 28 patients with schizophrenia and 20 control subjects to look for neurodevelopmental and cognitive correlates. They found no association between their results on spectroscopy and indices such as obstetric complications, family history of psychoses, and minor physical anomalies. They did, however, note that minor physical anomalies of the head were more prominent in the schizophrenia patients, with the overall presence of qualitative structural abnormalities found on the magnetic resonance imaging (MRI) scans.

O'Callaghan et al. (1995) repeated their previous study (see

O'Callaghan et al. 1991), this time looking for relationships between minor physical anomalies and cerebral structure on MRI scans. The study sample comprised 47 patients with schizophrenia and 24 control subjects. Minor physical anomalies were unrelated to total lateral ventricular volume but were prominent in patients who had qualitative anomalies in some aspect of the ventricular system. Minor physical anomalies tended to be less prominent in those with a family history of schizophrenia, a finding at odds with O'Callaghan et al.'s previous study, and more evident in patients with obstetric complications occurring in the perinatal period—findings that were consistent with the results of earlier research. In the same sample, J. L. Waddington et al. (1995) assessed the patients with tardive dyskinesia and found no difference in the number of minor physical anomalies in those patients with or without tardive dyskinesia.

McGrath et al. (1995), using a modified Waldrop scale, assessed 157 patients in the Camberwell Collaborative Psychosis Study. The group was split into 79 with schizophrenia, 31 with schizoaffective disorder, 24 with mania, 13 with major depression, 8 with unspecified psychosis, and 2 with organic psychosis. There was no overall increase in minor physical anomalies among diagnostic groups. However, minor physical anomalies were more prevalent in patients with schizophrenia compared with control subjects, with the increase being accounted for by a subgroup of patients with a very high number of minor physical anomalies. There were no associations between minor physical anomalies and age at onset, negative symptoms, poorer premorbid functioning, tardive dyskinesia, pregnancy abnormalities or obstetric complications, or volume of lateral ventricles and area of third ventricle as measured on computed tomography scans.

Sigmundsson et al. (1996) investigated the relationship between minor physical anomalies and family history of schizophrenia. Groups of patients with schizophrenia with or without a family history of the disorder and their relatives were compared with psychiatrically healthy controls. Although the authors found no significant differences in minor physical anomalies between the groups, as assessed by mean scores on the Waldrop scale, they pointed out that the schizophrenic patients with a negative family history as a group had significantly higher scores in terms of minor physical anomalies.

Lohr et al. (1997) recruited and compared different groups of patients—those with early-onset and late-onset schizophrenia, Alzheimer's disease, and mood disorder—with a control group. The authors found more anomalies in the group of patients with early- and late-onset schizophrenia and mood disorders than in the control subjects. The patients with Alzheimer's disease, however, did not have more anomalies than the control subjects.

Deutsch et al. (1997), using a new quantitative scale for evaluation of minor physical anomalies, reported excessive dysmorphology in persons with schizophrenia and in their first-degree relatives. Lane et al. (1997), using a detailed anthropometric scale, evaluated 174 patients with schizophrenia and 84 matched control subjects to describe more thoroughly the nature of the dysmorphology. Twelve variables made significant independent contributions to the increased rate of dysmorphology in the case patients and clearly distinguished the patients from the control subjects. The authors found a significant upward shift in the distribution of minor physical anomalies in the case patients compared with the control subjects. They also found an overall narrowing and elongation of the middle and lower facial region, with widening of the skull base and abnormalities of the mouth, ears, and eyes. A comparison was made with the efficacy of the Waldrop scale, which, although showing an increase in abnormalities, failed to give relevant information about the actual topography of the dysmorphology.

So, what conclusions about the association of minor physical anomalies with schizophrenia can be drawn from these studies? The evidence published so far indicates that, overall, there is an increase in minor physical anomalies found in individuals with schizophrenia. However, we know that there is some doubt that minor physical anomalies are specific to schizophrenia. Initially, the actual topography of the dysmorphology was little explored, although some investigators remarked on the prevalence of abnormalities of the mouth and palate. Subsequent research (Lane et al. 1997) has started to clarify this issue with the development of more specific scales of measurement. Individuals with schizophrenia have been shown to have an overall narrowing and elongation of the lower face, along with abnormalities of the eyes, ears, and mouth. Links between minor physical anomalies and other biological markers of developmental disturbance, such as dermatoglyphic patterns, and schizophrenia have been made, with both occurring at increased frequencies in individuals with schizophrenia.

The evidence regarding minor physical anomalies and other characteristics—clinical and etiological—remains contradictory. We do not know whether genetic or epigenetic variables are associated with minor physical anomalies. An earlier age at onset of schizophrenia was found to be significantly associated with a greater number of minor physical anomalies. Subsequent studies in larger groups have not found such a relationship. It appears that the initial links made between minor physical anomalies and poorer premorbid functioning and tardive dyskinesia also may not be confirmed in studies with larger samples. No associations have been found between minor physical anomalies and severity of psychopathology, presence of negative symptoms, and gender.

The importance of a family history of schizophrenia remains unresolved. One set of researchers initially discovered an association, only later to disprove it. Other studies have mostly concurred with the finding of an absence of an association, and indications of a negative correlation with a family history, the exact opposite hypothesis, have yet to be replicated. One study did not find an increase in the number of minor physical anomalies in the relatives of those with schizophrenia, whereas another found evidence of greater dysmorphology in first-degree relatives. However, individuals born with a supposed higher genetic risk of developing psychoses have not shown any differences in the number of minor physical anomalies when compared with control subjects.

Complications in pregnancy, particularly bleeding in early pregnancy, have been associated with minor physical anomalies in individuals with schizophrenia. This has been replicated by the same researchers and has been found by others in a group of discordant twin pairs. However, no such relationship was found in the Camberwell Collaborative Psychosis Study.

Work on neuropsychological abnormalities and links with minor physical anomalies has so far yielded negative findings. Only a limited number of studies have examined associations between brain morphological measures from computed tomography or MRI scans and minor physical anomalies. The types of measurements investigated have involved only ventricle volumes, not other important neuropathological abnormalities known to exist in persons with schizophrenia. Despite the limited availability of data, there is some evidence to support some correlations and to warrant further and more detailed study in specific brain areas. Conclusions based on research findings on the association of minor physical anomalies and schizophrenia are summarized in Table 4–4.

TABLE **4–4.**   *Minor physical anomalies and schizophrenia*

Minor physical anomalies occur with a greater frequency in persons with schizophrenia compared with psychiatrically healthy control subjects.

The greater frequency of minor physical anomalies is not specific to schizophrenia among psychotic disorders.

New scales for measuring minor physical anomalies are allowing the topography of the craniofacial dysmorphology to be described.

Minor physical anomalies and abnormalities in dermatographic measurements, both biological markers of developmental disturbance, occur together more often in persons with schizophrenia.

Evidence from studies of the relation of other variables to minor physical anomalies (e.g., age at onset, family history) appears to be contradictory.

Further research is needed before conclusions about minor physical anomalies and neuropathology can be drawn.

Conclusion

The studies reviewed in this chapter have produced positive evidence for the conclusion that there are different types of measurable biological precursors, each of which is found with an increased frequency in patients with schizophrenia. None of these precursors is completely specific to schizophrenia. Most have also been found in different groups of persons with mental illness, particularly patients with affective or bipolar disorders, to a greater extent than in control subjects, but not to the degree they are found in patients with schizophrenia. Similarly, schizophrenia has a number of nonspecific precursors.

It would appear that a general pattern of a distributional shift in the markers at a population level is relevant, and such a pattern would argue against a specific biological subgroup within the heterogeneous condition of schizophrenia. It is not possible to use these markers to predict future illness onset on an individual basis because complete specificity is lacking and the markers overlap with normal populations. Also, there is no evidence to suggest that these markers can be used clinically to help in predicting disease course and prognosis. However, each of the biological markers discussed has different implications that can tell us more about the etiology and pathogenesis of schizophrenia.

Certainly, the presence of precursors such as minor physical anomalies in schizophrenia and affective disorder suggests that some other aspects of any causal constellation must be in place early in development (Cohen et al. 1993). The intimacy between the formation of craniofacial and cerebral features is further evidence that minor physical anomalies and the psychological disorders may have a common etiology. The lack of specificity of abnormalities in neuroimaging studies is evidence in favor of this biological formulation (Dolan et al. 1985; Elkis et al. 1995; Jeste et al. 1988; O'Callaghan et al. 1995; Videbech 1997).

Thus, we do not have strong evidence of specificity in terms of the outcome of any one precursor or of the precursors of any one outcome, even though the evidence for any precursor is strongest for schizophrenia. How can the model presented in the opening to this chapter accommodate this lack of specificity, and what are the implications in terms of nosology?

First, lack of specificity is, in some sense, intellectually unsatisfactory. Medicine depends heavily on classification, especially in nosology, and its most satisfactory (or satisfying) classification is, traditionally, an etiological one (Susser 1973). However, in other spheres of medicine, lack of specificity of cause and outcome is not considered problematic. For instance, cigarette smoking causes lung cancer. It also causes other cancers by similar mechanisms, and other diseases, such as heart attack, by different mechanisms. We are comfortable with the fact that the risk-modifying precursor is crudely defined; cigarette smoke is a complex mixture of many substances. So, too, are the precursors measured in developmental epidemiology and in clinical research. A milestone can be delayed for many reasons. Childhood behavioral abnormality is manifested and classified in only a limited number of ways—children are traditionally either seen and not heard or naughty.

The underlying mechanisms of these effects in one disorder may be quite different in a neurobiological sense than in another context.

Our crude measures may belie underlying complexity and strict specificity. This is not meant as an apologia for lack of specificity, but merely as a caveat when one is considering evidence from existing research. In terms of nosology, our existing categories of disorder are still as useful as they have always been (a deliberately bland statement). However, we must acknowledge the possibilities that they may be redefined to add a longitudinal view of developmental manifestations and that they may collapse or coalesce when we learn more about common etiologies.

Turning the microscope around so as to encompass the broader, public health perspective, we should not forget that lack of specificity of a cause or risk modifier in terms of a range of outcomes is a blessing; prevent one and you prevent them all. Once developmental epidemiology of the psychoses is sophisticated enough to suggest prediction, prevention, and early interventions, then lack of specificity, and even weak effects in terms of schizophrenia, may be no bad thing if depression and behavior disorders are reduced along the way (see Chapter 16, this volume, for discussion of such efforts).

References

Alexander RC, Mukherjee S, Richter J, et al: Minor physical anomalies in schizophrenia. J Nerv Ment Dis 182:639–644, 1994

Benes FM: Myelination of cortical-hippocampal relays during late adolescence. Schizophr Bull 15:585–593, 1989

Bracha SH, Torrey EF, Bigelow LB, et al: Subtle signs of prenatal maldevelopment of the hand ectoderm in schizophrenia: a preliminary monozygotic twin study. Biol Psychiatry 30:719–725, 1991

Bracha SH, Torrey EF, Gottesman II, et al: Second-trimester markers of fetal size in schizophrenia: a study of monozygotic twins. Am J Psychiatry 149:1355–1361, 1992

Buchanan RW, Heinrichs DW: The Neurological Evaluation Scale (NES): a structured instrument for the assessment of neurological signs in psychiatry. Psychiatry Res 27:335–350, 1989

Buckley PF, Moore C, Long H, et al: H-Magnetic resonance spectroscopy of the left temporal and frontal lobes in schizophrenia: clinical, neurodevelopmental, and clinical correlates. Biol Psychiatry 36:792–800, 1994

Cannon M, Byrne M, Cotter D, et al: Further evidence for anomalies in the hand-prints of patients with schizophrenia—a study of secondary creases. Schizophr Res 13:179–184, 1994

Cantor-Graae E, Mcneil TF, Torrey EF, et al: Link between pregnancy complications and minor physical anomalies in monozygotic twins discordant for schizophrenia. Am J Psychiatry 151:1188–1193, 1994

Castle DJ, Wessely S, Murray RM: Sex and schizophrenia: effects of diagnostic stringency, and associations with premorbid variables. Br J Psychiatry 162:658–664, 1993

Chua SE, McKenna PJ: Schizophrenia—a brain disease? A critical review of structural and functional cerebral abnormality in the disorder. Br J Psychiatry 166:563–582, 1995

Cohen SR, Chen L, Trotman CA, et al: Soft-palate myogenesis: a developmental field paradigm. Cleft Palate Craniofac J 30:441–446, 1993

David AS, Malmberg A, Brandt L, et al: IQ and risk for schizophrenia: a population-based cohort study. Psychol Med 27:1311–1323, 1997

DeMeyer M: Median facial malformations and their implications for brain malformations. Birth Defects XI:155–181, 1975

Deutsch CK, Farkas LG: Dysmorphology in schizophrenia (abstract). Behav Genet 20:717, 1990

Deutsch CK, Price SF, Wussler J, et al: Craniofacial dysmorphology in schizophrenia. Schizophr Res 24:53–54, 1997

Diewert VM, Lozanoff S, Choy V: Computer reconstructions of human embryonic craniofacial morphology showing changes in relations between the face and brain during primary palate formation. J Craniofac Genet Dev Biol 13:184–192, 1993

Dolan RJ, Calloway SP, Mann AH: Cerebral ventricular size in depressed subjects. Psychol Med 15:873–878, 1985

Done DJ, Crow TJ, Johnson EC, et al: Childhood antecedents of schizophrenia and affective illness: social adjustment at ages 7 and 11. BMJ 309:699–703, 1994

Elkis H, Friedman L, Wise A, et al: Meta-analyses of studies of ventricular enlargement and cortical sulcal prominence in mood disorders: comparisons with controls or patients with schizophrenia. Arch Gen Psychiatry 52:735–746, 1995

Feinberg I: Schizophrenia: caused by a fault in programmed synaptic elimination during adolescence? J Psychiatr Res 17:319–334, 1982–1983

Feinberg I: Schizophrenia as an emergent disorder of late brain maturation, in Neurodevelopment and Adult Psychopathology. Edited by Keshavan

MS, Murray RM. New York, Cambridge University Press, 1997, pp 237–252

Fish B: Biologic antecedents of psychosis in children. Res Publ Assoc Res Nerv Ment Dis 54:48–83, 1975

Fish B: Neurobiologic antecedents of schizophrenia in children. Arch Gen Psychiatry 34:1297–1313, 1977

Fish B, Marcus J, Hans SL, et al: Infants at risk for schizophrenia: sequelae of a genetic neurointegrative defect. Arch Gen Psychiatry 49:221–235, 1992

Green MF, Satz P, Soper HV, et al: Relationship between physical anomalies and age at onset of schizophrenia. Am J Psychiatry 144:666–667, 1987

Green MF, Satz P, Gaier DJ, et al: Minor physical anomalies in schizophrenia. Schizophr Bull 15:91–99, 1989

Green MF, Bracha HS, Christenson CD: Preliminary evidence for an association between minor physical anomalies and second trimester neurodevelopment in schizophrenia. Psychiatry Res 53:119–127, 1994a

Green MF, Satz P, Christenson CD: Minor physical anomalies in schizophrenia patients, bipolar patients and their siblings. Schizophr Bull 20:433–440, 1994b

Gualtieri CT, Adams A, Shen CD, et al: Minor physical anomalies in alcoholic and schizophrenic adults and hyperactive and autistic children. Am J Psychiatry 139:640–642, 1982

Gupta S, Andreasen NC, Arndt S, et al: Neurological soft signs in neuroleptic-naïve and neuroleptic-treated schizophrenic patients and in normal comparison subjects. Am J Psychiatry 152:191–196, 1995

Guy JD, Majorski LV, Wallace CJ, et al: The incidence of minor physical anomalies in adult male schizophrenics. Schizophr Bull 9:571–582, 1983

Hafner H, Riecher A, Maurer K, et al: How does gender influence age at first hospitalisation for schizophrenia? A transnational case register study. Psychol Med 19:903–918, 1989

Hafner H, Maurer K, Loffler W, et al: The influence of age and sex on the onset and early course of schizophrenia. Br J Psychiatry 162:80–86, 1993

Hambrecht M, Maurer K, Hafner H: Evidence for a gender bias in epidemiological studies of schizophrenia. Schizophr Res 8:223–231, 1992

Heinrichs DW, Buchanan RW: Significance and meaning of neurological soft signs in schizophrenia. Am J Psychiatry 145:11–18, 1988

Holzman PS: Recent studies of psychophysiology in schizophrenia. Schizophr Bull 13:49–75, 1987

Huttenlocher PR: Synaptic density in human frontal cortex—developmental changes and effects of aging. Brain Res 163:195–205, 1979

Ismail B, Cantor-Graae E, McNeil TF: Neurological abnormalities in schizophrenic patients and their siblings. Am J Psychiatry 155:84–89, 1998

Jablensky A, Sartorius N, Ernberg G, et al: Schizophrenia: Manifestations, Incidence and Course in Different Cultures. A World Health Organisation Ten-Country Study (Psychol Med Monogr Suppl 20). Cambridge, UK, Cambridge University Press, 1992

Jeste DV, Lohr JB, Goodwin FK: Neuroanatomical studies of major affective disorders. A review and suggestions for further research. Br J Psychiatry 153:444–459, 1988

Jones CAH, Bassett AS, McGillivray BD, et al: Physical anomalies in schizophrenia (abstract). Schizophr Res 9:118, 1993

Jones KL: Smith's Recognizable Patterns of Human Malformation, 5th Edition. Philadelphia, PA, WB Saunders, 1997, pp 727–746

Jones PB, Done DJ: From birth to onset: a developmental perspective of schizophrenia in two national birth cohorts, in Neurodevelopment and Adult Psychopathology. Edited by Keshavan MS, Murray RM. New York, Cambridge University Press, 1997, pp 119–136

Jones PB, Murray RM: The genetics of schizophrenia is the genetics of neurodevelopment. Br J Psychiatry 158:615–623, 1991

Jones PB, Rodgers B, Murray RM, et al: Childhood developmental risk factors for adult schizophrenia in the British 1946 birth cohort. Lancet 334:1398–1402, 1994

Jones PB, Rantakallio P, Hartikainen AL, et al: Schizophrenia as a long-term outcome of pregnancy, delivery and perinatal complications: a 28-year follow-up of the 1966 North Finland general population birth cohort. Am J Psychiatry 155:355–364, 1998

King DJ, Wilson A, Cooper SJ, et al: The clinical correlates of neurological soft signs in chronic schizophrenia. Br J Psychiatry 158:770–775, 1991

Kinney DK, Woods BT, Yurgelun-Todd D: Neurologic abnormalities in schizophrenic patients and their families, II: neurologic and psychiatric findings in relatives. Arch Gen Psychiatry 43:665–668, 1986

Kolakowska T, Williams AO, Jambor K, et al: Schizophrenia with good and poor outcome, III: neurological soft signs, cognitive impairment and their clinical significance. Br J Psychiatry 146:348–357, 1985

Lane A, Colgan K, Moynohan F, et al: Schizophrenia and neurological soft signs: gender differences in clinical correlates and antecedent factors. Psychiatry Res 64:105–114, 1996

Lane A, Kinsella A, Murphy P, et al: The anthropometric assessment of dysmorphic features in schizophrenia as an index of its developmental origins. Psychol Med 27:1155–1164, 1997

Liddle PF, Morris D: Schizophrenic syndromes and frontal lobe performance. Br J Psychiatry 158:340–345, 1991

Liddle PF, Haque S, Morris DL, et al: Dyspraxia and agnosia in schizophrenia. Behav Neurol 6:49–54, 1993

Livshits G, Kobyliansky E: Dermatoglyphic traits as possible markers of developmental processes in humans. Am J Med Genet 26:111–122, 1987

Lohr JB, Flynn K: Minor physical anomalies in schizophrenia and mood disorders. Schizophr Bull 19:551–556, 1993

Lohr JB, Caligiuri MP, Alder M: Minor physical anomalies in older patients with neuropsychiatric disorders (abstract). Biol Psychiatry 41 (suppl 7):339, 1997

Malla AK, Norman RMG, Aguilar O, et al: Relationship between neurological soft signs and syndromes of schizophrenia. Acta Psychiatr Scand 96:274–280, 1997

Marcus J: Neurological findings in offspring of schizophrenics. Paper presented at the Seventh Congress of the International Association for Child Psychiatry and Allied Professions, Jerusalem, August 4, 1970

Marcus J: Cerebral functioning in offspring of schizophrenics: a possible genetic factor. International Journal of Mental Health 3:57–73, 1974

Marcus J, Auerbach J, Wilkinson L, et al: Infants at risk for schizophrenia: the Jerusalem Infant Development Study. Arch Gen Psychiatry 38:703–713, 1981

Marcus J, Hans SL, Lewow E, et al: Neurological findings in high-risk children: childhood assessment and 5-year follow-up. Schizophr Bull 11:85-100, 1985

Marden PM, Smith DW, McDonald MJ: Congenital anomalies in the newborn infant, including minor variations. J Pediatr 64:357, 1964

Markow TA, Gottesman II: Fluctuating dermatoglyphic asymmetry in psychotic twins. Psychiatry Res 29:37–43, 1989

Markow TA, Wandler K: Fluctuating dermatoglyphic asymmetry and the genetics of liability to schizophrenia. Psychiatry Res 19:323–328, 1986

McGrath JJ, Van Os J, Hoyos C, et al: Minor physical anomalies: associations with clinical and putative aetiological variables. Schizophr Res 18:9–20, 1995

McNeil TF, Blennow G, Lundberg L: Congenital malformations and structural developmental anomalies in groups at high risk for psychosis. Am J Psychiatry 149:57–61, 1992

McNeil TF, Cantor-Graae E, Nordstrom LG, et al: Head circumference in preschizophrenic and control neonates. Br J Psychiatry 162:517–523, 1993

Meehl PE: Schizotaxia revisited. Arch Gen Psychiatry 46:935–944, 1989

Mellor CS: Dermatoglyphics in schizophrenia. Part 1: qualitative aspects. Br J Psychiatry 114:1387–1392, 1968a

Mellor CS: Dermatoglyphics in schizophrenia, Part II: quantitative study. Br J Psychiatry 114:1393–1397, 1968b

Mellor CS: Dermatoglyphic evidence of fluctuating asymmetry in schizophrenia. Br J Psychiatry 160:467–472, 1992

Mohr F, Hubmann W, Cohen R, et al: Neurological soft signs in schizophrenia: assessment and correlates. Eur Arch Psychiatry Clin Neurosci 246:240–248, 1996

Murray RM, Lewis SW: Is schizophrenia a neurodevelopmental disorder? BMJ 295:681–682, 1987

Nowakowski RS: Basic concepts of CNS development. Child Dev 58:568–595, 1987

O'Callaghan E, Larkin C, Kinsella A, et al: Familial, obstetric and other clinical correlates of minor physical anomalies in schizophrenia. Am J Psychiatry 148:479–483, 1991

O'Callaghan E, Buckley P, Madigan C, et al: The relationship of minor physical anomalies and other putative indices of developmental disturbance in schizophrenia to abnormalities of cerebral structure on magnetic resonance imaging. Biol Psychiatry 38:516–524, 1995

O'Neal P, Robins LN: Childhood patterns predictive of adult schizophrenia: a 30-year follow-up study. Am J Psychiatry 115:385–391, 1958

Plomin R: Development, Genetics and Psychology. Hillsdale, NJ, Lawrence Erlbaum, 1986

Pogue-Geile MF: The development of liability to schizophrenia: early and late developmental models, in Schizophrenia: A Life-Course Developmental Perspective. Edited by Walker EF. New York, Academic Press, 1991, pp 277–298

Pogue-Geile MF: Developmental aspects of schizophrenia, in Neurodevelopment and Adult Psychopathology. Edited by Keshavan MS, Murray RM. New York, Cambridge University Press, 1997, pp 137–177

Quitkin F, Fifkin A, Klein DF: Neurologic soft signs in schizophrenia and character disorders. Arch Gen Psychiatry 33:845–853, 1976

Rakic P: Specification of cerebral cortical areas. Science 241:170–176, 1988

Rantakallio P, Von Wendt L: A prospective comparative study of the etiology of cerebral palsy and epilepsy in a one-year birth cohort from Northern Finland. Acta Paediatr Scand 75:586–592, 1986

Rantakallio P, Jones P, Moring J, et al: Association between central nervous system infections during childhood and adult onset schizophrenia and other psychoses: a 28-year follow-up. Int J Epidemiol 26:837–843, 1997

Robins LN: Deviant Children Grown Up. Baltimore, MD, Williams & Wilkins, 1966

Rosenthal D: A program of research on heredity in schizophrenia. Behav Sci 116:191–201, 1971

Rosenthal D: Prospects for research on schizophrenia, IV: genetic and environmental factors. Hereditary nature of schizophrenia. Neurosci Res Program Bull 10(4):397–403, 1974

Rossi A, De Cataldo S, Di Michelle V, et al: Neurological soft signs in schizophrenia. Br J Psychiatry 157:735–739, 1990

Schaumann B, Alter M: Dermatoglyphics in Medical Disorders. New York, Springer-Verlag, 1976

Schroder J, Niethammer R, Geider F, et al: Neurological soft signs in schizophrenia. Schizophr Res 6:25–30, 1992

Siegel MI, Smookler HH: Fluctuating dental asymmetry and audiogenic stress. Growth 37:35–39, 1973

Sigmundsson T, Griffiths T, Birkitt P: Minor physical anomalies in schizophrenic patients and their rrelatives (abstract). Schizophr Res 18:170, IX.F 4, 1996

Susser E, Lin SP: Schizophrenia after prenatal exposure to the Dutch Hunger Winter of 1944–1945. Arch Gen Psychiatry 49:983–988, 1992

Susser E, Neugebauer R, Hoek HW, et al: Schizophrenia after prenatal famine, further evidence. Arch Gen Psychiatry 53:25–31, 1996

Susser MW: Causal Thinking in the Health Services: Concepts and Strategies in Epidemiology. New York, Oxford University Press, 1973

Torrey EF: Neurological abnormalities in schizophrenic patients. Biol Psychiatry 15:381–388, 1980

Van Os J, Fananas L, Cannon M, et al: Dermatoglyphic abnormalities in psychosis: a twin study. Biol Psychiatry 41:624–626, 1997a

Van Os J, Jones PB, Lewis G, et al: Developmental precursors of affective illness in a general population birth cohort. Arch Gen Psychiatry 54:625–631, 1997b

Van Valen L: A study of fluctuating asymmetry. Evolution 16:125–142, 1962

Videbech V: MRI findings in patients with affective disorder: a meta-analysis. Acta Psychiatr Scand 96:157–168, 1997

Waddington CH: The Strategy of the Genes. New York, Macmillan, 1957

Waddington JL, O'Callaghan E, Buckley P, et al: Tardive dyskinesia in schizophrenia. Br J Psychiatry 167:41–44, 1995

Wadsworth MEJ: The Imprint of Time: Childhood History and Adult Life. Oxford, UK, Clarendon Press, 1991

Waldrop MF, Halverson CF: Minor physical anomalies and hyperactive behavior in young children, in Exceptional Infant. Studies in Abnormalities. Edited by Helmmuth J. New York, Brunner/Mazel, 1971

Waldrop MF, Pedersen FA, Bell RQ: Minor physical anomalies and behavior in pre-school children. Child Dev 39:391–400, 1968

Walker EF, Savoie T, Davis D: Neuromotor precursors of schizophrenia. Schizophr Bull 20:441–451, 1994

Weinberger DR: Implications of normal brain development for the pathogenesis of schizophrenia. Arch Gen Psychiatry 44:660–669, 1987

Woods BT, Kinney DK, Yurgelun-Todd D: Neurologic abnormalities in schizophrenic patients and their families. Arch Gen Psychiatry 43:657–663, 1986

CHAPTER 5

PANDAS: A New "Species" of Childhood-Onset Obsessive-Compulsive Disorder?

Susan E. Swedo, M.D.

Margaret Pekar, M.A.

The first cases of streptococcus-triggered obsessive-compulsive symptoms were described by Sir William Osler more than 100 years ago, when he wrote of a "certain perseverativeness of behaviour" in children with Sydenham's chorea (Osler 1894). At the time, Osler did not realize that the neuropsychiatric symptoms of Sydenham's chorea (also known as Saint Vitus' dance) were related to the carditis and arthritis of rheumatic fever, nor did he recognize that the behavioral changes and neurological symptoms were preceded by episodes of streptococcal pharyngitis. However, his prescient observations did suggest an etiological relationship between psychiatric symptoms (obsessive-compulsive symptoms and emotional lability) and neurological abnormalities (chorea and other adventitious movements), and these observations, as well as those made decades later by Chapman et al. (1958), Grimshaw (1964), and Freeman et al. (1965), provided a foundation for the conceptualization of Sydenham's chorea as a medical model of obsessive-compulsive disorder (OCD).

This perspective eventually led to the identification of a subgroup of

OCD patients in which streptococcal infections trigger exacerbations of obsessions, compulsions, and other neuropsychiatric symptoms (including tics). The subgroup was given the acronym PANDAS to indicate the postulated pathophysiology: Pediatric Autoimmune Neuropsychiatric Disorders Associated with Streptococcal infections. In this chapter, we review the sequence of events leading from Osler's observations to the identification of the PANDAS phenotype and examine research results that suggest that streptococcal infections might contribute to the pathophysiology of OCD and tic disorders. We conclude the chapter with a discussion of the generalizability of these findings and consider the utility of medical models for other forms of OCD.

Clues From Childhood-Onset OCD

During the early and mid-1980s, a large cohort of children with OCD was studied at the National Institute of Mental Health (NIMH) (Swedo et al. 1989b). Subjects ($N = 70$) were enrolled in a 12-week treatment trial examining the effectiveness of clomipramine (Flament et al. 1985; Leonard et al. 1989) and then were followed for an extended period. The results of those investigations demonstrated that the clinical presentation of OCD in children was remarkably similar to that seen in adults and, specifically, that the content of the obsessions and compulsions was essentially the same in the two groups (Swedo et al. 1989b). However, it became clear that individual symptoms changed over time and that the symptoms could wax and wane in severity independently from each other (e.g., one acute exacerbation might be manifested by washing, another by checking) (Rettew et al. 1992). Thus, specific symptom content was unlikely to serve as a clue to etiological subtypes, although the clinical course did offer other insights into the pathophysiology of the disorder. An abrupt onset and specific symptom trigger were reported by a subgroup of children with OCD ($n = 22$, 31%). Historical information suggested that "variability in intensity was common during and across time periods" and that a subgroup of children had "a fluctuating course . . . [in which] the transition from less to greater severity can be either gradual or sudden" (Swedo et al. 1989b, p. 338). Prospective, longitudinal study confirmed these observations and revealed that in some cases the children's obsessions and compulsions would be relatively well controlled for an extended period and then would dramatically increase in severity (Leonard et al. 1993). These exacerbations were frequently associated with upper respiratory tract infections, and it is tempting now to postulate that some of those symptom exacerbations were environmentally triggered.

The NIMH studies provided a second line of evidence suggesting an association between neurological abnormalities and obsessive-compulsive symptoms. At baseline, one-third of the children with OCD had a choreiform syndrome (consisting of pronator drift and/or piano-playing finger movements) (Denckla 1989). At long-term follow-up, the choreiform syndrome was absent (Swedo et al., unpublished data, 1992), raising the question of whether there might be a common etiology for the neurological and psychiatric symptoms. If so, the neurological symptoms would appear to be an acute response to the environmental stressor, while the psychiatric symptoms would represent a more chronic condition maintained by inherent biological deficits. Conversely, the symptom course might suggest that the "dose" required for symptom expression differed (i.e., that the choreiform movements required a larger etiological dose than did the obsessive-compulsive symptoms). If the latter were true, then children with environmentally triggered chorea (i.e., Sydenham's chorea) might have accompanying obsessive-compulsive symptoms appearing shortly before the movement disorder began and lingering after the chorea disappeared. Of course, it is also possible that there was no causal relation between the presence of the choreiform movements and the onset of the obsessive-compulsive symptoms and that the two neuropsychiatric symptom complexes were independent and unrelated. If so, then there would be no increase in obsessive-compulsive symptoms among children with Sydenham's chorea.

Sydenham's Chorea: A Medical Model for OCD?

First described in the late 1600s as Saint Vitus' dance, Sydenham's chorea is now known to be a variant of rheumatic fever. Rheumatic fever is caused by antibodies directed against Group A β-hemolytic streptococcal bacteria (GABHS) that cross-react with host tissue (Froud et al. 1989). This is thought to trigger an autoimmune reaction, which is most frequently directed against cells in the heart and joints and results in carditis and arthritis, respectively, but also can localize to the central nervous system (CNS) and manifest as Sydenham's chorea (in 20%–30% of cases of rheumatic fever) (Nausieda et al. 1980; Zabriskie 1985). In fact, Husby et al. (1976) showed that children with Sydenham's chorea (and less frequently those with rheumatic fever without Sydenham's chorea) had elevated titers of "antineuronal antibodies" recognizing human caudate and subthalamic tissue. The antineuronal antibodies were adsorbed by GABHS cellular components, consistent with the hypothesis that the antibodies had been produced initially in reaction to the foreign streptococcal proteins and then had mistakenly cross-reacted with CNS tissue. Pathological and neuroimaging studies confirmed involvement of the basal ganglia in Sydenham's chorea (Goldman et al. 1993; Kienzle et al. 1991; Thiebaut 1968). Most recently, volumetric analyses of magnetic resonance imaging (MRI) scans revealed selective enlargements of the caudate, putamen, and globus pallidus in a group of 24 children with Sydenham's chorea (Giedd et al. 1995). Taken together, these findings provide strong evidence that Sydenham's chorea is caused by streptococcus-triggered basal ganglia pathology. The regions involved overlap those presumed to be dysfunctional in OCD (Baxter 1992; Insel 1992; Modell et al. 1989; Rapoport and Wise 1989) and provide an anatomic basis for postulates of shared pathophysiology.

Association of Sydenham's Chorea With OCD

Even in the earliest reports (Osler 1894), psychiatric symptoms were considered to be an important part of the diagnosis of Sydenham's chorea. Emotional lability is present in over 90% of patients with Sydenham's chorea and is characterized by unprecipitated bouts of crying or hysterical laughter and increased irritability. Although early clinical reports focused on the "psychotic" nature of the symptoms (Diefendorf 1912), three small case series published in the late 1950s to early 1960s suggested that obsessive-compulsive symptoms were associated with Sydenham's chorea both at the time of acute illness and in subsequent years (Chapman et al. 1958; Grimshaw 1964; Freeman et al.

1965). These anecdotal reports were intriguing, but the signficance of their findings was limited by their study design.

A retrospective study comparing obsessive-compulsive symptoms in children with Sydenham's chorea and those with rheumatic fever without Sydenham's chorea (an appropriate contrast group to control for medical illness and nonspecific autoimmune factors) demonstrated that obsessive-compulsive symptoms were common among children with Sydenham's chorea (Swedo et al. 1989a). Scores on the 20-item Leyton Obsessional Inventory were significantly higher for the 23 children with Sydenham's chorea than for the 14 children with rheumatic fever without Sydenham's chorea. Three children with Sydenham's chorea met the diagnostic criteria for OCD during their choreic disorder, while none of those with rheumatic fever had significant OCD symptoms. Of particular note, it appeared that the obsessive-compulsive symptoms had their onset shortly *before* the chorea began, with this timing suggesting that 1) the obsessive-compulsive symptoms were not a compensatory response to dealing with a serious medical illness (because the children were not yet ill when they began to experience obsessions and compulsive rituals), and 2) the "dose" (titer and/or duration of exposure) required for obsessive-compulsive symptoms might be less than that required for the movement disorder. The retrospective nature of the study limited the conclusions that could be drawn from these findings, and so a prospective, systematic investigation of Sydenham's chorea was undertaken.

The results of that investigation confirmed and extended the historical reports (Swedo 1994; Swedo et al. 1993). Psychopathology was common among the 21 children evaluated and was temporally related to the onset of the Sydenham's chorea. Obsessive-compulsive symptoms were most obvious, but children also complained of new onset of symptoms consistent with separation anxiety and a picture of motoric hyperactivity, distractibility, and impulsivity similar to that seen in attention-deficit/hyperactivity disorder (ADHD). One of the patients with Sydenham's chorea, an 8-year-old girl whose presentation was typical of that of the other patients with this disorder, had an abrupt onset of emotional lability, obsessive-compulsive symptoms, and separation anxiety (e.g., refusing to be left alone outside in the backyard, needing to sleep in her parents' room at night, and calling her mother's work excessively). One to 4 weeks after the onset of the psychological symptoms, the chorea would manifest with motoric hyperactivity (squirming and fidgetiness), weakness (source of the diagnostic "milkmaid's grip"), and adventitious movements. The chorea would remain for 4–18 months (mean = 6 months) before gradually subsiding. With the important exceptions of the distractibility and inattentiveness (which were still apparent on follow-up at 12–18 months) (Casey et al. 1994a, 1994b), it appeared that the psychological symptoms followed a similar time course and resolved completely.

With regard to OCD, all children had been free of obsessive-compulsive symptoms until shortly before the onset of their chorea, when over 70% experienced the abrupt onset of obsessive thoughts and/or compulsive rituals (Swedo 1994; Swedo et al. 1993). In some cases, the symptoms were not of sufficient distress or interference to meet the DSM-III-R diagnostic criteria for OCD (American Psychiatric Association 1987), but they were of sufficient severity to be spontaneously reported by the children and their parents. The obsessive-compulsive symptoms were indistinguishable from those in classical childhood-onset OCD and included contamination fears and fear of harm coming to self or others, with resultant washing and checking compulsions, respectively; counting, symmetry concerns, and hoarding also occurred. The obsessions started 1–4 weeks before the chorea began, peaked in severity when the chorea was at its most severe level, and then slowly decreased over time. In two instances (10%), the obsessive-compulsive symptoms persisted even after the chorea had remitted, suggesting that chronic OCD could be a sequela of poststreptococcal autoimmunity, even in the absence of neurological abnormalities.

PANDAS

Clinical Presentation

Early in 1991, a young boy, whom we will call "Bobby," presented to the Child Psychiatry clinic with choreiform movements and the abrupt, dramatic onset of obsessive concerns about contamination (from germs, including AIDS) and safety, spitting compulsions, and extremely excessive hoarding (to such a degree that we had to clear all brochures out of the waiting room before his visit). Bobby's older brother had been diagnosed with Tourette's syndrome 3 years earlier and was also having a symptom exacerbation at the time of the patient's symptom onset. Of note, both boys had recently had documented streptococcal throat infections, and at presentation Bobby's antistreptococcal antibody titers were markedly elevated and antineuronal antibodies were also present in the serum (Kiessling et al. 1993b). Over the next several weeks, Bobby's OCD symptoms decreased in severity to a subclinical level and his antibody titers also fell. About 6 months later, following a second streptococcal infection, he had another dramatic symptom exacerbation, which was again associated with increased antibody titers. He was followed closely over the ensuing year. We observed that each time his symptoms worsened, the antistreptolysin-O and antineuronal antibody titers were elevated, and during periods of remission, the titers were in the normal range.

This patient was the first in a series of children with OCD and tic disorders whose clinical course appeared to be characterized by periods of dramatic and acute symptom exacerbations. Further, several of the children reported a close association between the symptom exacerbations and preceding streptococcal infections, as was being observed in the studies of Sydenham's chorea. The systematic evaluations also began to suggest that the syndrome might include additional psychopathology (i.e., symptoms of separation anxiety and ADHD) and neurological symptoms (i.e., tics and Tourette's syndrome). Further, it became clear that viral infections could trigger symptom exacerbations in some children (Allen et al. 1995) but that the immunogenic mechanism underlying the virally triggered symptoms was unlikely to be the same as that triggered by GABHS infections (Behar and Porcelli 1995). Thus, the subgroup of interest was limited to those with streptococcus-triggered exacerbations, and their condition was identified by the acronym PANDAS, for Pediatric Autoimmune Neuropsychiatric Disorders Associated with Streptococcal infections.

The presentation of this subgroup of patients is defined by the following criteria:

1. *Pediatric onset.* Symptoms of the disorder first become evident between 3 years of age and the beginning of puberty (as is true for Sydenham's chorea).

2. *Presence of OCD and/or tic disorder.* Although other symptoms (e.g., separation anxiety and ADHD) are present in PANDAS, the subgroup is defined by the presence of obsessions, compulsions, and/or tics.

3. *Abrupt onset and/or episodic course.* The clinical course is characterized by the abrupt onset of symptoms and/or an episodic course of symptom severity. Onset of a specific symptom exacerbation can often be assigned to a particular day of the week, when symptoms seemed to "explode" in severity. Of note, the episodic course seen in PANDAS is sawtooth (i.e., dramatic relapses followed by gradual decline in symptom severity), in contrast to the waxing and waning course typically seen in Tourette's syndrome and other tic disorders. Symptoms increase abruptly and then resolve completely between episodes or continue at lesser severity.

4. *Temporal relation between GABHS infections and symptom exacerbations.* Symptom exacerbations must be associated with a GABHS infection, either by history (if prior to initial evaluation) or by documentation of infection by positive results on a throat culture, positive streptococcal serological findings (e.g., antistreptolysin-O or antistreptococcal DNAase B), or a history of streptococcus-related illness (e.g., pharyngitis or scarlet fever). Because fever and other stresses of illness can independently increase symptom severity, the increased neuropsychiatric symptoms should not occur exclusively during the period of illness. Similarly, during periods of neuropsychiatric symptom remission, the child should be free of GABHS-triggered autoimmunity (i.e., findings for antistreptococcal titers should be negative when the child is free of symptoms).

5. *Choreiform movements present during symptom exacerbations.* Adventitious movements are present during exacerbations of OCD and tics, particularly during the early months of the illness.

Phenomenology: Is It a Unique Subgroup?

The clinical characteristics of the first 50 children meeting the diagnostic criteria for PANDAS are summarized in Table 5–1 (Swedo et al. 1998).

TABLE 5–1. *Demographic characteristics of 50 children with PANDAS*

Characteristic	Mean (SD)	
Age at baseline evaluation (years)	9.3 (2.6)	
Age at onset of obsessions/compulsions (years)	7.4 (2.7)	
Age at onset of tics (years)	6.3 (2.7)	
	n	%
DSM-III-R or DSM-IV diagnosis		
Subclinical OCD with tics or OCD and tics	32	64
Tics only	8	16
OCD only	10	20
OCD		
Meets DSM-IV criteria	28	56
Subclinical	14	28
None	8	16
Tics		
Tic disorder	40	80
None	10	20
Comorbidity		
ADHD	20	40
Oppositional defiant disorder	20	40
Conduct disorder	2	4
Major depression	18	36
Dysthymia	6	12
Mania	0	0
Separation anxiety	10	20
Avoidant disorder	4	8
Overanxious disorder	14	28
Specific phobia	8	16
Eating disorder	1	2
Enuresis	6	12
Encopresis	5	10
Somatization disorder	0	0
Psychoses	0	0

Note. PANDAS = Pediatric Autoimmune Neuropsychiatric Disorders Associated with Streptococcal infections; OCD = obsessive-compulsive disorder; ADHD = attention-deficit/hyperactivity disorder.

As shown in Table 5–2, the PANDAS subgroup differed from other pediatric samples in several respects: higher male:female ratio (2.6:1), which is closer to the gender ratio reported for tic disorders and may have been the result of the mixed population making up the cohort); high comorbidity of ADHD (40%) and separation anxiety (20%); and younger age at onset of symptoms and younger age at presentation to the NIMH clinic. (It should be noted that prepubertal symptom onset is a diagnostic requirement in PANDAS; see PANDAS criteria earlier in this section.)

It appears that this subgroup of patients is similar to cohorts within previously studied samples but differs from the sample as a whole in terms of gender distribution and family history of OCD (Figure 5–1).

The unique clinical characteristics of the PANDAS subgroup suggest that PANDAS may be a distinct phenotype of childhood-onset OCD. Patients in this subgroup differ from the typical OCD patient in that they are younger (by definition), more likely to be male, and more likely to have comorbid tics, separation anxiety, and ADHD. If PANDAS represents a different pathophysiology from other forms of OCD, then future investigations of OCD and tic disorders will need to address the issue of multiple etiologies in their research design. This will be particularly important for investigations of the genetics of these neuropsychiatric disorders, since the PANDAS phenotype might confound the results of these studies if it were confused with other familial forms of OCD and Tourette's syndrome.

What Can It Teach Us About Other Neuropsychiatric Disorders?

The PANDAS subgroup was defined by studies directed at determining the pathophysiology of OCD. Sydenham's chorea was chosen as a potential medical model for OCD because both disorders appear to involve pathology within the basal ganglia. In OCD, various brain imaging studies have demonstrated dysfunction within the caudate nucleus, anterior cingulate, and orbital frontal cortex (see, e.g., Baxter 1992). Pathology studies of Sydenham's chorea also demonstrated abnormalities in the cortex (albeit diffusely) and basal ganglia, particularly within the caudate nucleus (for review, see Marques-Dias et al. 1997). As noted

TABLE 5–2.   *Phenomenology of PANDAS subgroup and unselected cases of childhood-onset obsessive-compulsive disorder*

	PANDAS (n = 50)[a]	Childhood-onset OCD (n = 70)[b]
Mean age at onset	7.4 ± 2.7	13.7 ± 2.67
Male:female ratio	2.6:1	2.04:1
NIMH Obsessive-Compulsive Scale	5.9 ± 3.5	8.5 ± 1.3[c]
Most common obsessions	Contamination (67%)	Contamination (40%)
	Somatic (46%)	Harm to self or others (24%)
	Other (46%)	Scrupulosity (17%)
	Harm to others (42%)	
Most common compulsions	Washing, cleaning, spitting (63%)	Excessive washing, grooming (85%)
	Repeating (58%)	Repeating (51%)
	Checking (50%)	Checking (46%)
	Ordering, arranging, table setting (50%)	Rituals to remove contaminants (23%)
	Other (71%)	Touching (20%)
Comorbidity	ADHD (40%)	Major depression (33%)
	ODD (40%)	Simple phobia (17%)
	Major depression (36%)	Overanxious disorder (16%)
	Separation anxiety (20%)	
	Specific phobia (16%)	

Note. Percentage in parentheses is proportion of sample reporting the specified obsession, compulsion, or disorder. PANDAS = Pediatric Autoimmune Neuropsychiatric Disorders Associated with Streptococcal infections; ADHD = attention-deficit/hyperactivity disorder; OCD = obsessive-compulsive disorder. ODD = oppositional defiant disorder.
[a]Swedo et al. 1998.
[b]Swedo et al. 1989b.
[c]Leonard et al. 1989.

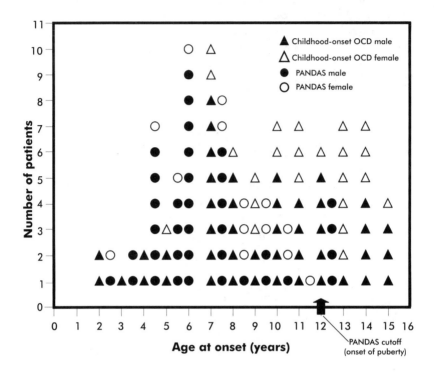

FIGURE 5–1.   *Gender distribution in PANDAS versus other childhood-onset obsessive-compulsive disorder.*
Source. Data from Swedo et al. 1989b, 1998.

earlier, it is postulated that Sydenham's chorea results when antibodies form in response to a streptococcal infection and then cross-react with neuronal cells (i.e., antineuronal antibodies), resulting in inflammation in the regions containing the neuronal cells, such as the basal ganglia. The inflammation causes dysfunction (and possibly, damage) in the basal ganglia that is manifested as behavior changes, obsessive-compulsive symptoms, and motoric disturbances, including choreiform movements and tics.

Husby et al. (1976) demonstrated the presence of antineuronal antibodies in the serum of children with Sydenham's chorea. Using a modification of Husby et al.'s methodology, Kiessling et al. (1993a, 1993b) obtained antineuronal antibody titers from 14 children with PANDAS. Nine (64%) had positive titers. The children were followed over time.

A strong correlation was found between the presence of antineuronal antibodies and symptom exacerbations, such that when the antibody titers were reduced, the symptoms were less problematic, and when the antibody titers were elevated, the symptoms were exacerbated (Swedo et al., unpublished data, 1993). In a related study, Kiessling et al. (1994) found increased rates of positive antineuronal antibody titers among children with episodic tic disorders, compared with children without tics, and a close temporal association between titer levels and symptom severity. It should be noted, however, that antineuronal antibodies are fairly nonspecific, with a significant proportion of healthy children (22% in a study reported by Kiessling et al. [1993b]) having positive titers.

If these antineuronal antibody titers are found to correlate with symptom severity, and it is possible to identify the epitope recognized by the antibody, then the antibodies may provide a means of identifying the origin of the obsessions, compulsions, and tics in PANDAS. Knowing the source and nature of the neuropsychiatric symptoms in PANDAS could help pinpoint the location of pathology in OCD and allow for more focused studies in other forms of the disorder. It should also provide new opportunities for treatment, including therapies targeting the underlying pathophysiology, such as immunomodulatory interventions (plasmapheresis and intravenous immunoglobulin) for PANDAS or endocrine interventions for hormonally mediated forms of OCD. Further, the identification of state markers of disease activity in PANDAS (e.g., antineuronal antibodies) would allow for more accurate assessments of treatment response and might allow for studies of disease prevention.

Finally, the similarities between PANDAS and rheumatic fever may allow the development of trait markers of disease susceptibility. Zabriskie and colleagues at Rockefeller University have developed a B-cell marker that identifies 95% of rheumatic fever patients and is positive in only 5%–10% of the general population (Zabriskie 1985). The marker, labeled D8/17, also appears to distinguish patients with PANDAS (Swedo et al. 1997) and those with childhood-onset OCD (Murphy et al. 1997) from the general population. If subsequent studies confirm its specificity, the marker may enable researchers to conduct large-scale epidemiological studies examining risk factors for disease onset and provide new opportunities for preventive efforts.

In PANDAS, the use of penicillin as prophylaxis against GABHS infections is being evaluated for its ability to decrease the frequency of symptom exacerbations. Preliminary results show that penicillin is effective in improving overall symptom severity; they also suggest that it may decrease tic or OCD symptom severity in some individuals, but for the group as a whole this effect did not reach significance (Garvey et al. 1999). If penicillin prophylaxis is effective in reducing symptom exacerbations (by preventing the manifestations of GABHS-triggered autoimmunity), it should also be effective in preventing the onset of symptoms in susceptible patients—if they can be identified and prophylaxis can be provided prior to GABHS exposure.

The availability of trait markers of susceptibility and an effective means of preventing symptom onset opens the door to the possibility that early-onset OCD and tic disorders will one day be eradicated, just as rheumatic fever has been rendered obsolete through effective prophylaxis and treatment interventions.

References

Allen AJ, Leonard HL, Swedo SE: Case study: a new infection-triggered, autoimmune subtype of pediatric OCD and Tourette's syndrome. J Am Acad Child Adolescent Psychiatry 34:307–311, 1995

American Psychiatric Association: Diagnostic and Statistical Manual of Mental Disorders, 3rd Edition, Revised. Washington, DC, American Psychiatric Association, 1987

Baxter LR Jr: Neuroimaging studies of obsessive compulsive disorder. Psychiatr Clin North Am 15:871–884, 1992

Behar SM, Porcelli SA: Mechanisms of autoimmune disease induction: the role of the immune response to microbial pathogens. Arthritis Rheum 4:458–476, 1995

Casey BJ, Vauss Y, Chused A, et al: Cognitive functioning in Sydenham's chorea, Part II: executive functioning. Developmental Neuropsychology 10:89–96, 1994a

Casey BJ, Vauss Y, Swedo S: Cognitive functioning in Sydenham's chorea, Part I: attentional processes. Developmental Neuropsychology 10:75–88, 1994b

Chapman AH, Pilkey L, Gibbons MJ: A psychosomatic study of eight children with Sydenham's chorea. Pediatrics 21:582–595, 1958

Denckla MB: Neurological examination, in Obsessive-Compulsive Disorder in Children and Adolescents. Edited by Rapoport JL. Washington, DC, American Psychiatric Press, 1989, pp 107–115

Diefendorf AR: Mental symptoms of acute chorea. J Nerv Ment Dis 39:161–173, 1912

Flament MF, Rapoport JL, Berg CJ, et al: Clomipramine: treatment of childhood obsessive disorder. Arch Gen Psychiatry 42:977–983, 1985

Freeman JM, Aron AM, Collard JE, et al: The emotional correlates of Sydenham's chorea. Pediatrics 35:42–49, 1965

Froud J, Gibofsky A, Buskirk DR, et al: Cross-reactivity between streptococcus and human tissue: a model of molecular mimicry and autoimmunity. Curr Top Microbiol Immunol 145:5–26, 1989

Garvey MA, Perlmutter SJ, Allen AJ, et al: Penicillin prophylaxis for PANDAS (Pediatric Autoimmune Neuropsychiatric Disorders Associated With Streptococcal Infections)—a double-blind placebo-controlled study. Biol Psychiatry 45:1564–1571, 1999

Giedd JN, Rapoport JL, Kruesi MJP, et al: Sydenham's chorea: magnetic resonance imaging of the basal ganglia. Neurology 45:2199–2202, 1995

Goldman S, Amrom D, Szliwowski HB, et al: Reversible striatal hypermetabolism in a case of Sydenham's chorea. Mov Disord 8:355–358, 1993

Grimshaw L: Obsessional disorder and neurological illness. J Neurol Neurosurg Psychiatry 27:229–231, 1964

Husby G, van de Rijn I, Zabriskie JB, et al: Antibodies reacting with cytoplasm of subthalamic and caudate nuclei neurons in chorea and acute rheumatic fever. J Exp Med 144:1094–1110, 1976

Insel TR: Toward a neuroanatomy of obsessive-compulsive disorder. Arch Gen Psychiatry 49:739–744, 1992

Kienzle GD, Breger RK, Chun RWM, et al: Sydenham chorea: MR manifestations in two cases. Am J Neuroradiol 12:73–76, 1991

Kiessling LS, Marcotte AC, Benson M, et al: Relationship between GABHS and childhood movement disorders. Poster presentation at the annual meeting of the Society for Pediatric Research, May 4, 1993a

Kiessling LS, Marcotte AC, Culpepper L: Antineuronal antibodies in movement disorders. Pediatrics 92:39–43, 1993b

Kiessling LS, Marcotte AC, Culpepper L: Antineuronal antibodies: tics and obsessive-compulsive symptoms. Dev Behav Pediatr 15:421–425, 1994

Leonard HL, Swedo SE, Rapoport JL, et al: Treatment of obsessive-compulsive disorder with clomipramine and desipramine in children and adolescents: a double-blind crossover comparison. Arch Gen Psychiatry 46:1088–1092, 1989

Leonard HL, Swedo SE, Lenane MC, et al: A 2- to 7-year follow-up study of 54 obsessive-compulsive children and adolescents. Arch Gen Psychiatry 50:429–439, 1993

Marques-Dias MJ, Mercadante MT, Tucker D, et al: Sydenham's chorea. Psychiatr Clin North Am 20:809–820, 1997

Modell J, Mountz J, Curtis G, et al: Neurophysiologic dysfunction in basal ganglia/limbic striatal and thalamocortical circuits as a pathogenetic mechanism of obsessive-compulsive disorder. J Neuropsychiatry Clin Neurosci 1:27–36, 1989

Murphy T, Goodman W, Fudge MW, et al: B lymphocyte antigen D8/17: a peripheral marker for childhood-onset obsessive-compulsive disorder and Tourette's syndrome? Am J Psychiatry 154:402–407, 1997

Nausieda PA, Grossman BJ, Koller WC, et al: Sydenham chorea: an update. Neurology 30:331–334, 1980

Osler W: On Chorea and Choreiform Affections. Philadelphia, PA, P Blakiston Son & Co, 1894, pp 33–35

Rapoport JL, Wise SP: Obsessive-compulsive disorder: evidence for basal ganglia dysfunction. Psychopharmacol Bull 24:380–384, 1989

Rettew DC, Swedo SE, Leonard HL, et al: Obsessions and compulsions across time in 79 children and adolescents with obsessive-compulsive disorder. J Am Acad Child Adolesc Psychiatry 31:1050–1056, 1992

Swedo SE: Grand Rounds at the Clinical Center of the National Institutes of Health. Sydenham's chorea: a model for childhood autoimmune neuropsychiatric disorders. JAMA 272:1788–1791, 1994

Swedo SE, Rapoport JL, Cheslow DL, et al: High prevalence of obsessive-compulsive symptoms in patients with Sydenham's chorea. Am J Psychiatry 146:246–249, 1989a

Swedo SE, Rapoport JL, Leonard HL, et al: Obsessive-compulsive disorder in children and adolescents: clinical phenomenology of 70 consecutive cases. Arch Gen Psychiatry 46:335–341, 1989b

Swedo SE, Leonard HL, Schapiro MB, et al: Sydenham's chorea: physical and psychological symptoms of St Vitus dance. Pediatrics 91:706–713, 1993

Swedo SE, Leonard HL, Kiessling L: Speculations on antineuronal antibody-mediated neuropsychiatric disorders of childhood. Pediatrics Commentaries 93:323–326, 1994

Swedo SE, Leonard HL, Mittleman BB, et al: Identification of children with Pediatric Autoimmune Neuropsychiatric Disorders Associated With Streptococcal Infections by a marker associated with rheumatic fever. Am J Psychiatry 154:110–112, 1997

Swedo SE, Leonard HL, Garvey M, et al: Pediatric Autoimmune Neuropsychiatric Disorders Associated With Streptococcal Infections: clinical description of the first 50 cases. Am J Psychiatry 155:264–271, 1998

Thiebaut F: Sydenham's chorea, in Handbook of Clinical Neurology. Edited by Vinken PJ, Bruyn GW. Amsterdam, North Holland, 1968, pp 409–434

Zabriskie JB: Rheumatic fever: the interplay between host, genetics and microbe. Circulation 71:1077–1086, 1985

6

Prenatal Antecedents of Neuropsychiatric Disorder Over the Life Course: Collaborative Studies of United States Birth Cohorts

Ezra Susser, M.D., Dr.P.H.

Alan Brown, M.D.

Tom Matte, M.D., M.P.H.

In this chapter we discuss the application of "life course" epidemiology to the study of neuropsychiatric disorders. First, we provide an introduction to life-course epidemiology. Then we consider research on

The collaborative work described here results from combined efforts with investigators at four sites in the United States. The key investigators were Steve Buka, Jill Goldstein, and Ming Tsuang (Providence and Boston National Collaborative Perinatal Project [NCPP] cohorts); Janet Hardy and Gerald Nestadt (Baltimore NCPP cohort); and Bea van den Berg, Barbara Cohn, and Cathy Schaefer (Oakland Child Health and Development Study cohort). This work was supported in part by grants from the National Institute of Mental Health (R01-MH53147-01A3), the National Alliance for Research on Schizophrenia and Depression, and The Theodore and Vada Stanley Foundation. The collaborative aspect of the work was sponsored by a grant from the New York Community Trust.

schizophrenia as a cutting-edge example, reviewing the neurodevelopmental paradigm of schizophrenia, epidemiological findings that support this paradigm, and ongoing research on schizophrenia in U.S. birth cohorts ideally suited to the life-course approach. Finally, we discuss opportunities for broadening inquiries within these same cohorts to examine the early life antecedents of a range of adult health and mental health outcomes.

Life-Course Epidemiology

The past 50 years has been an extremely productive era for the epidemiological approach that we often refer to as *risk factor epidemiology* (Rothman and Greenland 1998; M. Susser and Susser 1996a, 1996b). Many important determinants of the major causes of morbidity and mortality in developed countries have been revealed. In particular, epidemiological discoveries in this era have led to a far better understanding of the relation of adult behaviors to the risk of chronic disease. Epidemiologists can be credited with, for example, quantifying the increased risks of lung cancer, heart disease, and chronic obstructive pulmonary disease that are attributable to cigarette smoking. Study designs and statistical methods were developed and refined to study just such relationships.

Despite these accomplishments, some have begun to express frustration with the constraints of conventional risk factor epidemiology (M. Susser and Susser 1996a, 1996b). As the methods of risk factor epidemiology have become increasingly sophisticated, epidemiologists have tended to limit the questions they pose to those best suited to this approach. Much of the variation in health in our population remains unexplained, and, to some observers, we have reached a point of diminishing returns in conventional studies of risk factors for chronic disease.

Efforts are being made, therefore, to develop a more comprehensive schema that would subsume—though by no means dispense with—risk factor epidemiology (Schwartz et al. 1999). Ideally, epidemiological research should be able to broaden its focus from individual risk factors for chronic disease to take into account causes that operate as a chain of events or at multiple levels, causes that change over time, and reciprocal relationships among causes. An epidemiological framework should be readily applicable to the full range of health outcomes, including the infectious diseases that are the predominant causes of morbidity and mortality in most countries of the world.

The means to develop such a schema are not yet at hand. Nonetheless, the elements required are under development. This can be seen in the ways in which epidemiology is being extended in current research. For instance, epidemiologists have begun to collaborate with researchers from other disciplines in hopes of elucidating entire classes of causes that were, until recently, poorly understood. Investigators are reaching "upward" from the individual to consider social groups of individuals (Diez-Roux 1998) and "downward" to cells or molecules within individuals (Perera 1997; M. Susser and Susser, in press; Whyatt and Perera 1995), as seen in the growth of research on social determinants of health (Evans et al. 1994) and of genetic epidemiology (Khoury et al. 1993), respectively.

Another dimension in which epidemiology is being extended is that of time, through the development of what has been termed *life-course epidemiology* (Kuh and Ben Shlomo 1997). Of particular interest is the study of potential influences of the prenatal environment on adult health. The study of causes that operate over decades, rather than years, presents special methodological challenges. The difficulties are practical as well as scientific; causes that operate over long time spans cannot always be investigated within a single funding cycle. Hence, we know a great deal about, for example, the effects of maternal smoking on birth outcomes (Kline et al. 1989) and the effects of birth outcomes such as preterm birth on growth and development in childhood. We know much less, however, about how maternal smoking during pregnancy might affect the health of offspring in adulthood.

Studies of Prenatal Antecedents: Early Examples

It has long been recognized that the prenatal period is a time of rapid development during which the fetus is vulnerable to a range of infectious, toxic, metabolic, and nutritional insults that can have a manifest and lasting impact on the health of the newborn and child. Early exam-

ples were the recognized syndromes of congenital syphilis, rubella, and
hypothyroidism (Gregg 1944; Hetzel 1989; Kline et al. 1989). It is
remarkable that in the nineteenth century, before the advent of the germ
theory, Diday inferred that syphilis could be transmitted in utero from
mother to fetus and that the baby could be born apparently healthy but
with latent infection (Brandt 1985, pp. 10–11). (Discoveries about syphilis at the other end of the life course were no less remarkable; by the
early 1900s syphilis was recognized as a major cause of insanity in later
life arising from infection earlier in the life course. By some estimates,
syphilitic disease accounted for up to one-half of institutionalized
mental patients in the United States [Brandt 1985, p. 9].)

In the era of risk factor epidemiology, an especially dramatic
example was the discovery of thalidomide embryopathy (Lenz and
Knapp 1962). The thalidomide tragedy provided a strong stimulus for
the study of other medications as potential teratogens and, by extension,
for investigating the relation of a broad variety of prenatal experiences
to birth outcomes under the paradigm of risk factor epidemiology (Kline
et al. 1989). Although a birth outcome is a status at a certain point in
time rather than a chronic disease, the time interval between prenatal
exposure and the manifest outcome in the newborn is relatively short,
and risk factor epidemiology is readily adaptable to the study of birth
outcomes.

More challenging from an epidemiological point of view is the study
of connections between prenatal exposures and health outcomes that
may be manifest only when an individual is an adult. Yet, early models
for such a causal connection can be found. A notable example is the
link between prenatal exposure to diethylstilbestrol (DES) and vaginal
cancer in female offspring in their teens and twenties (Herbst et al. 1971).
The sudden increase in the incidence of a rare type of tumor caused
investigators to search for common exposures in the affected women.
DES was soon pinpointed as the culprit. Animal studies and a growing
body of human research reinforce the lessons of the DES episode:
prenatal exposures may produce health outcomes that are evident only
when an individual reaches maturity. Such latent effects of prenatal and
early childhood exposures have long been suspected, but it is just in the
last 10 years that compelling studies, some of which we consider in this
chapter, have begun to emerge (Marmot and Wadsworth 1997).

Public Health Implications

Research on prenatal antecedents has important public health implications. Chronic physical and mental illness in adults still constitutes an enormous public health burden, despite significant strides in identification of lifestyle risk factors and medical treatment. Interventions directed at pregnant women and children during critical developmental windows might prove to be simpler and more powerful methods than are currently available to improve the health of adults.

The Example of Schizophrenia

We now turn to schizophrenia to illustrate a current application of life-course epidemiology to a neuropsychiatric disorder in adulthood. Our understanding of schizophrenia has already been advanced in significant ways by the use of this approach. Indeed, as will be seen later in this section, schizophrenia researchers have been at the forefront in the use of life-course methods.

The Neurodevelopmental Paradigm

Findings from several areas of research on schizophrenia have converged to support the view that an early disruption in brain development is an antecedent in some cases of adult-onset schizophrenia (Waddington 1993; Weinberger 1987). The evidence includes an excess of minor physical anomalies that indicates in utero malformation (Green et al. 1989; Lane et al. 1997); cognitive abnormalities that are manifested in early childhood (e.g., Done et al. 1994; Jones et al. 1994); and structural brain abnormalities that are present by the time of onset of the disorder (Degreef et al. 1992; Ron and Harvey 1990). This perspective on the disorder, which traces the origins of the disorder as far back as fetal development, is sometimes termed the *neurodevelopmental paradigm* of schizophrenia.

The neurodevelopmental paradigm does not posit that the causes of schizophrenia are exclusively either genetic or epigenetic. (We use the term *epigenetic* rather than environmental in order to underscore that we have in mind factors that may influence the expression of genes and of genetically "programmed" neurodevelopment.) Indeed, for other neurodevelopmental disorders, a model of biological synergy between genes and environment has often proven most appropriate. Neural tube defects, for instance, have been related to a folate-sensitive genetic defect in homocysteine metabolism (Kingman 1995; Van der Put et al. 1995). It appears that in the presence of high maternal dietary folate, this genetic defect is less likely to lead to neural tube defect in the offspring.

Moreover, in neurodevelopmental schizophrenia, gene-environment interaction is likely to be more complex than in the example of neural tube defects just described. Some authors have proposed a nonlinear interaction of multiple genetic and environmental factors affecting brain development in schizophrenia (Bloom 1993; Cloninger 1994; Gottesman 1991). Bloom (1993), for instance, has postulated that multiple genes orchestrate the precise temporal pattern of neuronal migration and other aspects of neurodevelopment and that such genes might be switched on or off at abnormal times by a variety of adverse prenatal events. Such a schema introduces complexity by allowing multiple genes and environmental factors to play a role and by allowing environment to influence the expression of genes.

It is also important to note that the neurodevelopmental paradigm in no way precludes contributions from postnatal experience to the risk of schizophrenia. A disturbance in early brain development due to genetic or epigenetic factors may increase vulnerability and may result in cognitive deficits or other manifestations early in life. At the same time, some further postnatal insult may contribute to the later development of schizophrenia.

More Recent Research on Prenatal Antecedents

Over the past decade, motivated by the neurodevelopmental paradigm, investigators have launched an intense effort to identify prenatal exposures that might—perhaps in conjunction with genetic factors—disrupt brain development and thereby increase the risk of schizophrenia (E. Susser et al. 1998, 1999). It has proved extremely difficult, however, to investigate these hypothesized antecedents with any precision. One prohibitive factor involves obtaining valid measures of prenatal and perinatal exposures—as well as potential confounders—in large numbers of individuals who could then be comprehensively assessed for perinatal events and childhood manifestations and, ultimately, carefully diagnosed for adult schizophrenia. Another impediment is the modeling of gene-environment interaction (Malaspina et al. 1999); for the few samples with good data on early exposures, there has tended to be limited family history data and inadequate statistical power for such modeling. Nonetheless, using imaginative designs, researchers have produced several plausible candidates for fetal brain insult.

In the following subsections, we review the considerable progress that has been made in a short time in this field. Designs have evolved from relatively crude ecological approaches to individual-level studies with precise exposure and outcome data. For illustration, we select three of the more plausible early antecedents of schizophrenia, namely, prenatal influenza, prenatal nutritional deficiency, and prenatal rubella.

Early Ecological Designs

In an early landmark study of a birth cohort, Mednick et al. (1988) found an increased risk of schizophrenia with exposure to an influenza epidemic during midgestation. This ecological study demonstrated the potential, and also the limitations, of most research in this field. Hence, although the findings were intriguing, the study has been criticized for the lack of precision in the measurement of the exposure (at that time unavoidable, since no individual markers of influenza exposure were available) as well as in the outcome (ICD-9 chart diagnoses of schizophrenia were used) (Crow 1994). Some studies have replicated this association, but others have not. In our own studies in Holland and in Croatia, we found no association between prenatal influenza and the risk of developing schizophrenia (Erlenmeyer-Kimling et al. 1994; E. Susser et al. 1994).

Strengthened Ecological Designs

Following this precedent, subsequent studies with progressively stronger ecological designs have reported associations between prenatal exposures and schizophrenia. These studies are exemplified by our own study of schizophrenia after prenatal exposure to the Dutch Hunger Winter of 1944/45 (E. Susser et al. 1996, 1998). The Hunger Winter was precipitated by a Nazi embargo toward the end of World War II on transport in the region still under occupation, which included the six largest cities in the Netherlands, all of which are in the western part of the country. The famine began in October 1944 and progressively increased in severity. By February 1945, the daily ration fell to less than the equivalent of 1,000 kcal and consisted mainly of bread, potatoes, and sugar beets.

The famine reached its peak in the 8-week period preceding the liberation of the country by the Allied forces in early May 1945. The exposure to famine resulted in severe adverse effects in the population, including high frequencies of mortality due to malnutrition, stillbirths, and infant mortality. In addition, there was a notable increase in congenital anomalies of the central nervous system in the birth cohort conceived during the peak of the famine. Motivated by this finding, we tested whether the risk of schizophrenia, a presumed neurodevelopmental disorder, was also increased in this same birth cohort.

The study design afforded a unique opportunity to address this question. This famine affected the great majority of a well-demarcated segment of a national population, features that strengthened the ecological design. The famine was brief and of a clearly defined duration in a population that maintained excellent records on food rations before and during the famine. Thus, using dates of birth of exposed and unexposed individuals, we were able to precisely define the exposure during specific periods of gestation. With regard to outcome, we obtained access to the data of the Dutch National Psychiatric Registry, which afforded comprehensive ascertainment of hospitalization for schizophrenia in adulthood.

The study demonstrated that the birth cohort conceived during the peak of the famine exhibited a significant, twofold increased risk of schizophrenia, which occurred in the context of an otherwise stable incidence. This was the same birth cohort that had an excess of congenital CNS anomalies, as described earlier. In a further study of this cohort, we are now comparing brain structure and function, making use of brain imaging data, in individuals with schizophrenia exposed versus unexposed to prenatal famine (Hoek et al. 1998; E. Susser et al. 1998).

Individual-Level Studies

Most recently, this field has progressed from ecological studies to studies of individual prenatal exposure. One example is our follow-up of the

Rubella Birth Defects Evaluation Project (A. S. Brown, E. Susser, P. Cohen, et al., "Non-affective Psychosis After Prenatal Exposure to Rubella," manuscript under review for publication, 1999), a birth cohort prospectively documented to have been exposed to rubella in utero during the 1964 epidemic (Chess et al. 1971). The majority of individuals in this cohort had been gestationally exposed to rubella, as confirmed by IgM-specific antibody in the infants' sera. Over 25 years ago, Dr. Stella Chess assessed this cohort for psychiatric disorders in childhood and reported a markedly increased rate of autism and other behavioral problems (Chess et al. 1971). Further assessments were conducted during adolescence and young adulthood. In the last follow-up, at which time the cohort members were 21–23 years of age, a structured psychiatric interview was administered that covered all major psychiatric disorders in accordance with DSM-III-R. The risk of schizophrenia was assessed in the cohort exposed to rubella. For comparison, we used an unexposed, age-matched cohort administered the same diagnostic interview.

The rubella-exposed cohort, compared with the unexposed cohort, exhibited a nearly 12-fold increase in risk of schizophrenia, and substantial increases in most psychotic symptoms were also shown. The findings were not confounded by deafness or ethnicity differences and could not be accounted for by selection bias. Analysis of the occurrence of schizophrenia symptoms stratified by prenatal timing of exposure suggests that the third month may confer a particularly increased risk. Given the precision of documentation of the exposure, the large effect size, and a substantial literature on its teratogenic potential, rubella may serve as a model for other prenatal infections in the etiology of schizophrenia. We have recently initiated another follow-up study of this cohort, who are now aged 33–34, aimed at identifying new cases of schizophrenia, collecting family history information, and conducting neuroimaging studies.

Limitations

Ecological studies and individual-level studies, as well as other studies, of the past decade have contributed to an upsurge of interest in early antecedents of schizophrenia. No prenatal exposure has been definitively established, however, as a cause of schizophrenia. The absence of definitive results is related in part to continuing limitations in research design. It has still not been possible to study large samples in which precise individual data can be obtained. In order to be useful in elaborating causal pathways, these data need to include not only prenatal infection, prenatal nutritional deficiency, and a wide range of other potential sources of brain insult, but also potential confounders, mediators, and antecedents such as social class of origin and maternal health conditions.

The Emergent Era: Schizophrenia Research in Life-Course Cohorts

Recent advances in epidemiology have created a new and far more promising context for life-course research (Kuh and Ben-Shlomo 1997; Marmot and Wadsworth 1997; Paneth 1994). *Life-course cohorts* established by far-sighted investigators have now been carefully followed from early life over periods of 25–50 years and into the age at risk for adult diseases, including schizophrenia. This rich resource of prospectively collected exposure data has made possible studies that are more powerful and precise.

Prospectively followed birth cohorts came into being in the post–World War II era, initially in Britain and later in the United States, Western Europe, Israel, and other developed countries. The first veritable, large life-course cohort, the National Survey of Health and Development, established in Britain in 1946, has now been followed from birth into middle age at 5- to 10-year intervals (Wadsworth 1987, 1991). These birth cohorts are assuming an increasingly central role in epidemiology and are being used to investigate prenatal, perinatal, and childhood origins of a wide variety of adult diseases. The yield has already been significant, for instance, for cardiovascular disease, breast cancer, and diabetes (Kuh and Ben-Shlomo 1997; Marmot and Wadsworth 1997).

Life-course epidemiology has particular import for epidemiological research on schizophrenia. For the first time, the relation of well-defined prenatal events and childhood status to subsequent risk of schizophrenia can be examined while potential confounding factors are controlled.

TABLE 6–1. *Definition of terms for life-course cohorts in the study of schizophrenia*

Life-course cohort	A generic term that refers to any cohort that is followed from early life into at least the age at risk for schizophrenia
Birth cohort	An unselected life-course cohort based on a general population sample (e.g., all births in a given region in a given year)
Genetic high-risk cohort	A life-course cohort that was selected to be enriched for genetic etiologies of schizophrenia (e.g., offspring of parents with schizophrenia)
Epigenetic high-risk cohort	A life-course cohort that was selected to be enriched for a hypothesized prenatal environmental etiology of schizophrenia (e.g., a cohort with congenital rubella)

Thus, as the birth cohorts come of age for schizophrenia, the possibilities for research on antecedents of neurodevelopmental schizophrenia are greatly increased.

Types of Life-Course Cohorts

As this new era unfolds, three distinct types of life-course cohorts — population-based birth cohorts, genetic high-risk cohorts, and epigenetic high-risk cohorts — have already begun to be used to study fetal origins and early manifestations of schizophrenia (Table 6–1). Population-based birth cohorts are unselected for any specific etiology; genetic high-risk cohorts are selected so as to be enriched for genetic etiology, and epigenetic high-risk cohorts are selected so as to be enriched for environmental factors that can have an impact on genetically programmed neurodevelopment (e.g., prenatal brain insult).

For brevity, we limit our discussion in this chapter to the use of population-based birth cohorts in the United States. We illustrate the potential of these birth cohorts for schizophrenia research, first with an ongoing study in a single cohort and then with a collaborative initiative that will combine data from this and other cohorts that are being followed up for schizophrenia.

Prenatal Determinants of Schizophrenia Study

For purpose of illustration, we shall describe an ongoing follow-up study of schizophrenia based in the Child Health and Development Study (CHDS) cohort in Oakland, California. The CHDS birth cohort study was initiated by Dr. Jacob Yerushalmy, at the University of California, Berkeley, who directed it from 1959 to 1973 (Van den Berg 1984). A primary aim was to investigate the relation of events in pregnancy, labor, and delivery to the normal and abnormal development of offspring.

The CHDS was designed on the premise that the study of pregnancy must start with its inception, rather than its termination. This approach required contemporaneous and systematic documentation of prenatal and perinatal exposures and a longitudinal design in which the offspring were followed from the neonatal period through childhood and adolescence. It also required a large number of enrolled mothers and children. In fact, the CHDS sample comprised 20,530 pregnancies during 1959–1966, which resulted in 19,044 liveborn children, of whom 18,751 survived the neonatal period. The majority of the mothers began prenatal care in early pregnancy; for 59%, the first contact with the study was during the first trimester.

The mothers delivered in the Oakland hospital of the Kaiser Foundation Health Plan (KFHP), a prepaid medical care program, and were members of KFHP. Consequently, all cohort members were also born as KFHP members. At that time, approximately one-third of the population of Oakland belonged to KFHP. Subsequent studies of the KFHP membership showed that it was socioeconomically broad-based and that it was reasonably representative of the population of the Oakland region (Krieger 1992), except that individuals from extremely high and extremely low social strata were somewhat underrepresented.

Data on antecedents were originally obtained from three sources: 1) abstraction of maternal and infant medical records, including records of prenatal care, as well as labor and delivery records; 2) a maternal interview conducted during early pregnancy; and 3) analysis of maternal and fetal blood samples. In addition, blood samples were drawn throughout pregnancy and the postpartum period, and stored sera are available for the great majority of cohort members. These sera will be used to generate new exposure data for factors that have only more recently emerged as potential risk factors for schizophrenia.

The schizophrenia follow-up based in the CHDS cohort is referred to as the Prenatal Determinants of Schizophrenia Study. The at-risk cohort for the follow-up study on schizophrenia comprises the 12,094 cohort members who remained in the KFHP prepaid health plan on or after 1981. At that time, KFHP computerized the databases required for ascertainment of cohort members with a psychiatric treatment history. By 1981, the cohort members (born 1960–1967) were aged 13–20 years.

The Prenatal Determinants of Schizophrenia Study is a *continuous follow-up study*, a design that is powerful but not often used because stringent conditions must be met. The three crucial conditions for a continuous follow-up study are 1) the population at risk at any give time can be precisely specified, 2) cases among cohort members can be identified at or near the onset of disorder, and 3) each identified case among cohort members can be compared with the population at risk at the time of identification. The Prenatal Determinants of Schizophrenia Study has been able to apply this design because all three conditions are approximately met. First, KFHP maintains a membership registry to define the population at risk at any given time. Second, KFHP also maintains a hospitalization registry and outpatient registries so that members of this cohort who receive psychiatric treatment can generally be ascertained at first treatment contact. Third, these registries can be linked to one another and to the CHDS study data through KFHP medical record numbers assigned to individuals at birth so that each identified case cohort member can be compared with the appropriate population at risk.

Using these registries, we ascertained *potential* schizophrenia and schizophrenia spectrum disorder cases—that is, cohort members who have been hospitalized or received outpatient care for a psychiatric disorder. Using a three-step screening procedure, we targeted a subset of these potential cases for a full diagnostic interview and finally diagnosed 71 cases of schizophrenia spectrum disorder (66 psychotic and 5 nonpsychotic spectrum cases).

In combination, the remarkable range and precision of the prenatal data, including stored sera, and the thorough diagnostic screening of cases represent a qualitative improvement on the designs of the previous decade. The Prenatal Determinants of Schizophrenia Study and similar ongoing studies offer the possibility of a leap forward in research on the contribution of prenatal experience to the development of schizo-phrenia. It is our hope that in the coming decade, the pace of research in this field will continue to accelerate.

Collaborative Initiative

Yet, from a scientific viewpoint, the present use of data from a single birth cohort in schizophrenia research is unnecessarily restricted. Because of limitations of statistical power in single birth cohorts, researchers must focus on hypothesized antecedents that are common in the general population. However, many of the factors of interest are rare. To illustrate, consider the relation of moderate to severe low birthweight (<2,000 g) to the risk of schizophrenia. If we assume a 0.75% risk of schizophrenia and a 2% prevalence of moderate to severe low birthweight, in a cohort of 5,000 live births, the power to detect a sixfold relative risk is less than 80%; in a cohort of 30,000 live births, by contrast, the power to detect a threefold relative risk is close to 90%. Thus, a comprehensive study with adequate statistical power requires an extremely large cohort, of a size only achievable with formal multisite collaboration.

Nowhere is the potential yield of collaborative birth cohort research as great as in the United States. During 1959–1966, the National Institutes of Health established the 12 cohorts of the National Collaborative Perinatal Project (NCPP) (involving approximately 58,000 individuals across sites) (Broman 1984) as well as the large single cohort of the CHDS described above (Van den Berg 1984). Compared with previous birth cohort investigations, these U.S. studies collected far more extensive data on all types of antecedents: prenatal and perinatal exposures, childhood neurodevelopmental status, and potential confounding factors and mediating variables. They also collected prenatal sera, which were frozen and stored and can now be analyzed for new measures of prenatal exposures. Moreover, in 3 of the 12 NCPP cohorts (Baltimore, Providence, Boston) and in the CHDS cohort (4 cohorts to be combined; see Table 6–2), follow-up studies of schizophrenia involving face-to-face interviews are now under way.

We described earlier the follow-up of one of these cohorts, the CHDS, in relation to schizophrenia. The other cohorts also have notable

TABLE 6–2. *Ongoing schizophrenia follow-up studies in U.S. birth cohorts*

Birth cohort[a]	Description[b]	Selection of potential cases for diagnostic interview	Diagnostic protocol	
			Instrument[c]	Final diagnosis
CHDS (Oakland) (N = 12,094)	The CHDS sample included 19,044 live births during 1959–1966. All of the mothers were members of the KHFP.	Cohort members with evidence of psychotic symptoms in psychiatric records were selected for interview; psychiatric records were abstracted/rated by two diagnosticians.	DIGS	Case material was reviewed by two psychiatrists and interviewer; consensus DSM-IV diagnosis was made.
Spectrum cases	The study was based on potential cases ascertained from the 12,094 members of KFHP during 1981–1997. This is the period for which KFHP registries were available so that cohort members who received psychiatric treatment could be ascertained.			

TABLE 6–2.   Ongoing schizophrenia follow-up studies in U.S. birth cohorts (continued)

Birth cohort[a]	Description[b]	Selection of potential cases for diagnostic interview	Diagnostic protocol	
			Instrument[c]	Final diagnosis
NCPP–Providence (N = 4,140)	The Providence site of the NCPP enrolled 4,140 pregnancies during 1959–1966. In a subsequent study of psychiatric disorder at ages 18–27 years, the DIS was completed for a subsample of the cohort.	Cohort members with chart diagnosis of a psychotic disorder were selected for interview. (For those identified in previous follow-up assessment, cohort members with DIS diagnosis of a psychotic disorder were selected for interview.)	SCID-IV	Case material was reviewed by senior investigator; best-estimate DSM-IV diagnosis was made.
Projected spectrum cases: 20–30	The present study is based on potential cases ascertained through 1) linkage of the Rhode Island Department of Mental Health patient files with NCPP–Providence files, and 2) previous follow-up assessments with DIS at ages 18–27 years.			

TABLE 6–2.   *Ongoing schizophrenia follow-up studies in U.S. birth cohorts* (continued)

Birth cohort[a]	Description[b]	Selection of potential cases for diagnostic interview	Diagnostic protocol	
			Instrument[c]	Final diagnosis
NCPP–Boston (N = 12,193)	The Boston site of the NCPP enrolled 12,193 pregnancies during 1959–1966.	Cohort members with chart diagnosis of a psychotic disorder were selected for interview.	SCID-IV	Case material was reviewed by senior investigator; best-estimate DSM-IV diagnosis was made.
Projected spectrum cases: 60–90	The present study is based on potential cases ascertained through linkage of the Massachusetts Department of Mental Health patient files with NCPP–Boston files.			

TABLE 6–2.   *Ongoing schizophrenia follow-up studies in U.S. birth cohorts* (continued)

Birth cohort[a]	Description[b]	Selection of potential cases for diagnostic interview	Diagnostic protocol	
			Instrument[c]	Final diagnosis
NCPP–Baltimore (N = 2,694)	The Baltimore site of the NCPP enrolled 3,549 pregnancies during 1959–1965. The Pathways to Adulthood Project, conducted during 1992–1994, followed up a subsample (N = 2,694) of the original cohort.	All cohort members with a history of psychiatric treatment were selected for interview.	DIGS	Case material was reviewed by two psychiatrists and interviewer; consensus DSM-IV diagnosis was made.
Projected spectrum cases: 20–30	The present study is based on potential cases ascertained through cohort member's having reported a history of psychiatric treatment in the Pathways to Adulthood Project.			

Note. CHDS = Child Health and Development Study; KHFP = Kaiser Foundation Health Plan; DIGS = Diagnostic Interview for Genetic Studies; NCPP = National Collaborative Perinatal Project; DIS = Diagnostic Interview Schedule; SCID-IV = Structured Clinical Interview for DSM-IV.

[a]For this table, spectrum cases include only schizophrenia spectrum psychoses (i.e., schizophrenia, schizoaffective disorder, schizophreniform disorder, delusional disorder, and psychotic disorder not otherwise specified). In the CHDS, 5 cases of schizotypal personality were also diagnosed.

[b]Potential cases refer to individuals with a history of psychiatric treatment.

[c]All diagnostic interviews administered by experienced, trained master's-level clinical interviewers.

features. For instance, the Baltimore and Providence NCPP cohorts were previously followed up in adulthood, and this has increased the quality and comprehensiveness of the data for the schizophrenia follow-up. The Boston NCPP cohort data allow for identification of parents with schizophrenia, so that a nested high-risk genetic study can be conducted.

The comparability of all these U.S. birth cohorts and the quality of their data create the potential for an extremely productive collaboration. The combining of birth cohorts enables the evaluation of a wide range of antecedents that are too rare to be well studied within a single cohort and permits careful control of confounding factors. We have therefore initiated a collaborative study aimed at integrating selected antecedent data and all outcome data in order to examine the relation of rare hypothesized antecedents to risk of schizophrenia.

Beyond Schizophrenia

The initial long-term follow-up studies of the birth cohorts described in the previous section often focused on psychiatric disorders that can be manifest in young adults. As the cohorts enter middle age, the opportunity to examine possible early origins of other important chronic health conditions is presented. Prior research suggests a broad range of possible health endpoints influenced by early life exposures. We consider two areas—cognitive-behavioral function and cardiovascular disease risk—to illustrate the kinds of questions that can be addressed within the NCPP and CHDS populations.

Cognitive-Behavioral Function

A major motivation for establishing the NCPP and CHDS cohorts was to examine the pre- and perinatal determinants of neurodevelopment in children. Thus, the key outcomes measured at childhood follow-ups included cognitive ability and hearing, speech, and language development. Although these studies were not originally designed to follow subjects into adulthood, the rationale for the studies included concerns that neurodevelopmental impairment in children would influence their ability to lead full and productive lives.

Potential early influences on neurodevelopment are manifold; here we consider as an example restricted fetal growth indicated by low birth weight and/or preterm birth. The adverse influence of low birth weight and preterm birth on cognitive function and behavior in children is a major public health concern. Data from these cohorts and other, more recent studies have identified low birth weight and preterm birth as possibly important determinants of childhood impairments in cognitive performance (Breslau et al. 1996b) and attentiveness (Breslau et al. 1996a) and even of frank attention-deficit/hyperactivity disorder (Lou 1996).

To provide a basis for public health intervention, however, we need a better understanding of these effects. The relative importance of gestational age at birth and intrauterine growth retardation on childhood health and mental health, and the underlying brain insult that mediates their effect (Whittaker et al. 1997), are only beginning to be understood. In addition, the potential influence on cognitive development of variation in birth weight within the normal range is unclear (Breslau et al. 1996b; Broman et al. 1975). Of most relevance to the present discussion, we know little about the implications for adult life. Studies following children who were born preterm through adolescence suggest that effects on cognitive function persist (Paz et al. 1995; Rose and Feldman 1996). However, the effects of low birth weight and preterm birth on adult abilities and achievement have not been studied prospectively. The NCPP and CHDS cohorts now provide the opportunity to examine the impact of these factors on adult cognitive ability and behavior and the implications for social and economic position.

Cardiovascular Disease Risk

Perhaps the most extensive body of evidence on the possible influence of fetal growth on adult health is that concerning cardiovascular disease risk. This field of investigation was launched in a series of ecological studies led by Dr. David Barker (Barker 1992). An example was an analysis showing a correlation between infant mortality rates in three towns in the north of England early in this century and cardiovascular disease mortality some 60 years later. Barker and his colleagues inferred that higher infant mortality rates were a proxy for poor prenatal maternal health and nutrition, which in turn predisposed individuals to cardio-vascular disease as adults. Subsequent studies have suggested a link between low birth weight and increased blood pressure, lipid levels, glucose intolerance, and cardiovascular disease risk. Animal studies of prenatal maternal starvation support the hypothesis that impaired fetal nutrition may "program" the fetus toward a metabolism predisposed to cardiovascular disease. Recently, further support for the fetal program-ming hypothesis was provided by the observation of impaired glucose tolerance among adults exposed to prenatal maternal starvation during the Dutch famine (Ravelli et al. 1998).

Until now, however, research in this area has been limited by the lack of one or more of the following: prospectively measured prenatal factors, individual exposure data, and control for familial environmental or genetic factors that might confound the relation between low birth weight and cardiovascular disease risk. The NCPP and CHDS cohorts have the potential to address these limitations. For the investigation of antecedents of cardiovascular disease risk, these cohorts provide prospec-tively collected, individual-level prenatal data on exposures as well as potential confounders; geographic and demographic diversity; and the availability of frozen banked serum for additional assessment of prenatal nutritional, metabolic, and environmental factors.

Potential of Collaborative Research

We have earlier noted the potential of collaborative research in using the NCPP and CHDS birth cohorts to understand the causes of schizo-phrenia. The usefulness of collaboration is not limited to infrequent outcomes such as schizophrenia. The same principle is applicable to a broader range of outcomes, including cognitive/behavioral function and cardiovascular disease risk.

Again, this applicability can be exemplified by the NCPP and CHDS cohorts. The combined cohorts include several thousand sibling pairs. Even with fairly strict selection criteria, such as same-sex siblings discordant for low birth weight, an informative number of sibling pairs is potentially available. A cohort study based on such a sample can address some of the major criticisms of previous work in this area because it allows for tight control of familial factors that may be related to antecedents such as birth weight and outcomes such as IQ. Assembling such highly selected members of these cohorts for follow-up as adults, however, requires collaboration among investigators at multiple sites. As a basis of just such a study, two of the authors (E.S., T.M.) have initiated a collaborative partnership among investigators who have been studying the CHDS (Oakland) and selected NCPP (Boston and Providence) cohorts.

Conclusion

As epidemiologists explore new methods and new classes of determinants, one promising development is the renewed interest in the early antecedents of adult health. In particular, the study of prenatal factors and latent effects that emerge in adulthood has led to provocative findings that point to a neurodevelopmental origin for many cases of schizophrenia. Large U.S. birth cohorts, established more than three decades ago, are now enabling the further exploration of the neurodevelopmental paradigm. In addition, these cohorts will make possible powerful new studies of the early antecedents of a range of important adult health conditions. Life-course epidemiology holds the promise of identifying new opportunities for preventing ill health based on interventions targeted at critical developmental periods.

References

Barker DJP: Fetal and Infant Origins of Adult Disease. London, British Medical Journal Monographs, 1992

Bloom FE: Advancing a neurodevelopmental origin for schizophrenia. Arch Gen Psychiatry 50:224–227, 1993

Brandt A: No Magic Bullet. New York, Oxford University Press, 1985

Breslau N, Brown GG, DelDotto JE, et al: Psychiatric sequelae of low birth weight at 6 years of age. J Abnorm Child Psychol 24:385–400, 1996a

Breslau N, Chilcoat H, DelDotto JE, et al: Low birth weight and neurocognitive status at six years of age. Biol Psychiatry 40:389–397, 1996b

Broman SH: The Collaborative Perinatal Project: an overview, in Handbook of Longitudinal Research, Vol 1. Edited by Mednick SA, Harway Finello KM. New York, Praeger, 1984, pp 166–179

Broman SH, Nichols PL, Kennedy WA: Preschool IQ: Prenatal and Early Developmental Correlates. Hillsdale, NJ, Lawrence Erlbaum, 1975

Chess S, Korn SJ, Fernandez P: Psychiatric Disorders of Children With Congenital Rubella. New York, Brunner/Mazel, 1971

Cloninger RL. Turning point in the design of linkage studies in schizophrenia. Am J Med Gen 5:83–92, 1994

Crow TJ: Prenatal exposure to influenza as a cause of schizophrenia. There are inconsistencies and contradictions in the evidence. Br J Psychiatry 164:588–592, 1994

Degreef G, Ashtari M, Bogerts B, et al: Volumes of ventricular system subdivisions measured from magnetic resonance images in first-episode schizophrenic patients. Arch Gen Psychiatry 49:531–537, 1992

Diez-Roux A: Bringing context back into epidemiology: variables and fallacies in multilevel analysis. Am J Public Health 88:216–222, 1998

Done DJ, Crow TJ, Johnstone EV, et al: Childhood antecedents of schizophrenia and affective illness: social adjustment at ages 7 and 11. BMJ 309:699–703, 1994

Erlenmeyer-Kimling N, Solmegovic Z, Hraabak-Zerjavic V, et al: Schizophrenia and prenatal exposure to the 1957 A2 influenza epidemic in Croatia. Am J Psychiatry 151:1496–1498, 1994

Evans RG, Barer ML, Marmor TR (eds): Why Are Some People Healthy and Others Not? The Determinants of Health in Populations. New York, Aldine De Gruyter, 1994

Gottesman II: Schizophrenia Genesis: The Origins of Madness. New York, WH Freeman, 1991

Green MF, Satz P, Gaier DJ, et al: Minor physical anomalies in schizophrenia: a family affair. Schizophr Bull 15:91–99, 1989

Gregg NM: Further observations on congenital defects in infants following maternal rubella. Trans Opthalmol Soc 4:119–131, 1944

Herbst A, Ulfelder H, Poskanzer D: Adenocarcinoma of the vagina: association of maternal stilbesterol therapy and tumor appearance in young women. N Engl J Med 284:878–881, 1971

Hetzel BS: The Story of Iodine Deficiency. Oxford, UK, Oxford University Press, 1989

Hoek WH, Brown AS, Susser E: The Dutch famine and schizophrenia spectrum disorders. Soc Psychiatry Psychiatr Epidemiol 33:373–379, 1998

Jones P, Rogers B, Murray R, et al: Child developmental risk factors for adult in the British 1946 birth cohort. Lancet 344:1398–1402, 1994

Khoury MJ, Beaty TH, Cohen BH: Fundamentals of Genetic Epidemiology (Monographs in Epidemiology and Biostatistics, Vol 22). Oxford, UK, Oxford University Press, 1993

Kingman S: Why does folic acid prevent neural tube defects? Journal of NIH Research 7:44–46, 1995

Kline J, Stein Z, Susser M: Conception to Birth: Epidemiology of Prenatal Development. New York, Oxford University Press, 1989

Krieger N: Overcoming the absence of socioeconomic data in medical records: validation and application of census-based methodology. Am J Public Health 82:703–710, 1992

Kuh DL, Ben Shlomo Y: A Life Course Approach to Adult Disease. Oxford, UK, Oxford University Press, 1997

Lane A. Kinsella A, Murphy P, et al: The anthropometric assessment of dysmorphic features in schizophrenia as an index of its developmental origins. Psychol Med 27:1155–1164, 1997

Lenz W, Knapp K: Thalidomide embryopathy. Arch Environ Health 5:100–105, 1962

Lou HC: Etiology and pathogenesis of attention-deficit hyperactivity disorder (ADHD): significance of prematurity and perinatal hypoxic-haemodynamic encephalopathy. Acta Paediatr 85:1266–1271, 1996

Malaspina D, Sohler NL, Susser ES: Integration of genes and prenatal exposures in schizophrenia, in Prenatal Exposures in Schizophrenia. Edited by Susser ES, Brown AS, Gorman JM. Washington, DC, American Psychiatric Press, 1999, pp 35–59

Marmot M, Wadsworth M (eds): Fetal and Early Childhood Environment: Long-Term Health Implications. British Medical Bulletin 53:1–227, 1997

McCarton CM, Wallace IF, Divon M, et al: Cognitive and neurologic development of the premature, small for gestational age infant through age 6: comparison by birth weight and gestational age. Pediatrics 98:1167–1178, 1996

Mednick SA, Machon RA, Muttunen MO, et al: Adult schizophrenia following prenatal exposure to an influenza epidemic. Arch Gen Psychiatry 45:189–192, 1988

Paneth N: The impressionable fetus? Fetal life and adult health. Am J Public Health 84:1372–1373, 1994

Paz I, Gale R, Laor A, et al: The cognitive outcome of full term small for gestational age infants at late adolescence. Obstet Gynecol 85:452–456, 1995

Perera FP: Environment and cancer: who are susceptible? Science 278:1068–1073, 1997

Ravelli ACJ, van der Meulen JHP, Michels RPJ, et al: Glucose tolerance in adults after prenatal exposure to famine. Lancet 351:173–177, 1998

Ron MA, Harvey I: The brain in schizophrenia. J Neurol Neurosurg Psychiatry 53:725–726, 1990

Rose SA, Feldman JF: Memory and processing speed in preterm children at eleven years: a comparison with full-terms. Child Dev 67:2005–2021, 1996

Rothman KJ, Greenland S: Modern Epidemiology, 2nd Edition. Philadelphia, PA, Lippincott-Raven, 1998

Schwartz S, Susser E, Susser M: The future of epidemiology. Annu Rev Public Health 20:15–33, 1999

Susser E, Lin S, Brown A, et al: No increase in schizophrenia after prenatal exposure to A2 influenza. Am J Psychiatry 151:922–924, 1994

Susser E, Neugebauer R, Hoek HW, et al: Schizophrenia after prenatal famine: further evidence. Arch Gen Psychiatry 53:25–31, 1996

Susser E, Hoek HW, Brown AS: Neurodevelopmental disorders after prenatal famine: the story of the Dutch Famine Study. Am J Epidemiol 147:213–216, 1998

Susser E, Brown A, Gorman J (eds): Prenatal Exposures in Schizophrenia. Washington, DC, American Psychiatric Press, 1999

Susser M, Susser E: Choosing a future for epidemiology, I: eras and paradigms. Am J Public Health 86:668–673, 1996a

Susser M, Susser E: Choosing a future for epidemiology, II: from black boxes to Chinese boxes and eco-epidemiology. Am J Public Health 86:674–677, 1996b

Susser M, Susser E: Comment on Ambrosone and Kadlubar letter. Am J Epidemiol (in press)

Van den Berg BJ: The California Child Health and Development Studies, in Handbook of Longitudinal Research, Vol 1. Edited by Mednick SA, Harway M, Finello KM. New York, Praeger, 1984, pp 166–179

Van der Put NMJ, Steegers-Theunissen RPM, Frosst P, et al: Mutated methylenetetrahydrofolate reductase as a risk factor for spina bifida. Lancet 346:1070–1071, 1995

Waddington JL: Schizophrenia: developmental neuroscience and pathobiology. Lancet 341:531–536, 1993

Wadsworth MEJ: Follow-up of the First National Birth Cohort: findings from the Medical Research Council National Survey of Health and Development. Paediatr Perinat Epidemiol 1:95–117, 1987

Wadsworth MEJ: The Imprint of Time: Childhood, History and Adult Life. Oxford, UK, Oxford University Press, 1991

Weinberger DR: Implications of normal brain development for the pathogenesis of schizophrenia. Arch Gen Psychiatry 44:660–669, 1987

Whittaker AH, Van Rossem R, Feldman JF, et al: Psychiatric outcomes in low-birth-weight children at age 6 years: relation to neonatal cranial ultrasound abnormalities. Arch Gen Psychiatry 54:847–856, 1997

Whyatt RM, Perera FP: Application of biologic markers to studies of environmental risks in children and the developing fetus. Environ Health Perspect 103 (suppl 6):105–110, 1995

Schizophrenia:
Specific Disorders

CHAPTER 7

Late-Onset Schizophrenia: New Insights Into Disease Etiology

Lisa T. Eyler Zorrilla, Ph.D.

Dilip V. Jeste, M.D.

The notion that schizophrenia can manifest for the first time later in life has been controversial, especially in the United States. Kraepelin's original conceptualization of schizophrenia as *dementia praecox* required onset during adolescence or early adulthood with progressive personality deterioration (Kraepelin 1919/1971). Patients with later onset of illness and paranoid symptoms were classified as having *paraphrenia* (Kraepelin 1919/1971), a term that has been used since then by researchers in the United Kingdom and other parts of Europe (Harris and Jeste 1988). M. Bleuler, using his father's term *schizophrenia*, expressed the belief that the disorder could begin in later life (M. Bleuler 1943). In the United States, however, the idea of late-onset schizophrenia has been slow to gain acceptance. As recently as the era of DSM-III (American Psychiatric Association 1980), late-onset schizo-

This work was supported, in part, by the National Institute of Mental Health (grants MH49671, MH45131, MH43693, and MH19934) and the Department of Veterans Affairs.

phrenia was explicitly excluded by criteria that restricted the age at onset of schizophrenia to 45 years or younger. The revised edition, known as DSM-III-R (American Psychiatric Association 1987), contained no requirements regarding age at onset and created a separate diagnostic category of late-onset schizophrenia for patients whose symptoms began after age 45. In DSM-IV (American Psychiatric Association 1994), there are no age-at-onset specifications for schizophrenia.

Despite the fact that the existence of late-onset schizophrenia is no longer precluded by diagnostic criteria, questions remain about the nature of this disorder. First, do patients meeting the criteria for schizophrenia with onset after age 45 years have the same disorder as those meeting the criteria at an earlier age? That is, do patients diagnosed with late-onset schizophrenia have schizophrenia per se? Second, to the extent that late-onset schizophrenia differs from early-onset schizophrenia, what implications does this distinction have for understanding the etiology of late-onset schizophrenia in particular and schizophrenia in general?

Two issues make these questions difficult to answer. The first challenge is that there is disagreement as to what constitutes schizophrenia. Although strict diagnostic schemes emphasize a unified view of the disorder, the criteria are broad enough that the clinical presentations of two patients with schizophrenia can be very different (e.g., a patient with predominantly negative symptoms and somatic delusions vs. a highly disorganized patient with command hallucinations and formal thought disorder). Schizophrenia, as defined by such diagnostic schemes, could therefore be the result of a common etiology or the final common pathway of multiple pathologies. Others would argue that the heterogeneity of clinical presentation reflects the fact that there is not one entity called schizophrenia, but rather a cluster of disorders, the "schizophrenias," that resemble one another but are the product of varied causal factors (E. Bleuler 1911/1950). These theoretical disagreements about the nature of schizophrenia complicate an exploration of the similarities and differences between late-onset schizophrenia and early-onset schizophrenia. A second challenge to research in this area is the problem of defining age at onset of schizophrenia. Possible definitions include onset of prodromal symptoms, onset of positive symptoms, first contact with a mental health professional, and first hospitalization. Each of these definitions has limitations in terms of reliability and/or validity (Maurer and Hafner 1995).

At the University of California, San Diego (UCSD) Center for the Study of Late-Life Psychoses, we have sought answers to questions about late-onset schizophrenia while addressing the issues that pose challenges in this area of research. We have studied middle-aged and elderly patients who meet the DSM-III-R criteria for schizophrenia (as determined by the Structured Clinical Interview for DSM-III-R, Patient Version [SCID-P; Spitzer et al. 1990]), as well as a set of further inclusion and exclusion criteria designed to minimize false positive results (Jeste et al. 1995b). These criteria include ability to participate in assessments, availability of corroboration of history from records or other informants, and exclusion of diagnosed dementia, seizure disorder, head injury with more than 30-minute loss of consciousness, and substance abuse of a severity that might have led to psychosis. Late-onset schizophrenia patients were defined as those having no history of prodromal symptoms, psychiatric hospitalization, or functional decline before the age 45. Also excluded from the late-onset schizophrenia group were those with severe premorbid schizoid, schizotypal, or paranoid personality or those treated with neuroleptics, antidepressants, or lithium for more than 1 month prior to the age of 45.

We addressed the difficulty of defining schizophrenia by comparing two groups of carefully diagnosed patients with onset of illness before versus after age 45. We compared the groups at several levels: clinical, psychosocial, neuropsychological, psychophysiological, and neuroanatomic. In this way, we relied less on any particular theory of the nature of schizophrenia. In order to address difficulties in reliably determining age at onset, we examined empirically the reliability of our estimation of age at onset of prodromal symptoms by determining age at onset at baseline and at 2-year follow-up in 53 patients with late-onset schizophrenia or early-onset schizophrenia who were middle-aged or elderly. Our determinations were highly reliable; the intraclass correlation coefficient between initial and follow-up ratings was 0.96 ($P < 0.001$) (Jeste et al. 1997).

In this chapter, we review the findings from our studies of the clinical, psychosocial, neuropsychological, psychophysiological, and neuroanatomic similarities and differences between late-onset schizophrenia and early-onset schizophrenia. Then, we examine the implications of these findings for the question of whether what is diagnosed as late-onset schizophrenia is truly schizophrenia. Finally, we present our theories about the origin of differences between late-onset and early-onset schizophrenia and how further investigation can illuminate the pathophysiology of the former.

Clinical Characteristics

We have studied several hundred subjects, including patients with late-onset schizophrenia, older patients with early-onset schizophrenia, younger patients with early-onset schizophrenia, and healthy comparison subjects over the age of 45. (It should be noted that not all of the evaluations could be performed in the group of younger patients with early-onset schizophrenia.) The methods for clinical, psychosocial, neuropsychological, psychophysiological, and brain imaging assessment have been detailed elsewhere (Corey-Bloom et al. 1995; Jeste et al. 1995b; Olichney et al. 1997). Clinical evaluations were made every 6 months, and diagnostic evaluation and neuropsychological testing were repeated annually. Psychophysiological assessment and brain magnetic resonance imaging (MRI) were performed for a subset of patients who consented to and were eligible for these protocols.

No group differences in the overall severity of global psychopathology, as rated by the Brief Psychiatric Rating Scale (BPRS; Overall and Gorham 1962), or positive symptoms, as assessed by the Scale for the Assessment of Positive Symptoms (SAPS; Andreasen and Olsen 1982), were found. However, negative symptoms, as rated by the Scale for Assessment of Negative Symptoms (SANS; Andreasen 1982), were less severe in the patients with late-onset schizophrenia than in either early-onset schizophrenia group. In addition, daily neuroleptic dose was significantly lower for late-onset schizophrenia patients than for both the older patients with early-onset schizophrenia and the younger early-onset schizophrenia patients. It may be that the dosage in the older early-onset schizophrenia patients was escalated in an attempt to treat persistent negative symptoms, or, conversely, the greater dosage of neuroleptics could have produced secondary negative symptoms of akinesia and psychomotor retardation in this group. Caution should be exercised, however, in interpreting the dose-related findings, because the study was not dose-controlled.

Family history of schizophrenia was assessed with interviews of every available source of information (e.g., patient, family, friends, referring physician). Contrary to some other investigators (Harris and Jeste 1988), we found no differences in the percentages of late-onset schizophrenia and early-onset schizophrenia patients having a first-degree relative with schizophrenia (10%–15% in both groups).

The late-onset and early-onset schizophrenia groups were found to have comparable numbers of minor physical anomalies, with both groups having a significantly greater number than the healthy control subjects or the patients with Alzheimer's disease (Lohr et al. 1997). Such anomalies are usually congenital and suggest developmental defects.

Premorbid adjustment, as assessed by the scale developed by Gittelman-Klein and Klein (1969), was poor in both late-onset and older early-onset patients during childhood years compared with the healthy control subjects. The late-onset schizophrenia patients, however, fared much better than their counterparts with early-onset schizophrenia during early adulthood, though they were still rated as having poorer adjustment than the healthy control group. Patients with late-onset schizophrenia were more likely to have been married at one time than patients in either group of early-onset schizophrenia.

Some investigators have suggested that late-onset schizophrenia is related to sensory deficits (Cooper et al. 1974). We found no differences in visual or auditory impairment among late-onset schizophrenia patients, older early-onset schizophrenia patients, and healthy control subjects when their vision and hearing were tested without correction (i.e., without eyeglasses or hearing aids) (Prager and Jeste 1993). Patients in the late-onset schizophrenia and older early-onset schizophrenia groups, however, performed more poorly than the healthy control group when patients with correction devices used those devices. This suggests that poorly corrected sensory deficits were a characteristic of older schizophrenia patients regardless of age at onset of the schizophrenia — a discrepancy that may be the result of poor access to optimal health care.

In terms of quality of life, we found that the late-onset and early-onset schizophrenia groups had a similar degree of impairment compared with the healthy control subjects as assessed on the Quality of Well-Being Scale (Patterson et al. 1996).

We also examined annual mortality rates over a 4-year period and found a 200%–300% increase in mortality among patients with late-onset schizophrenia and older patients with early-onset schizophrenia compared with the healthy control subjects, the elderly U.S. population, and even patients with other late-onset psychotic disorders (Jeste et al. 1995a). This finding highlights another similarity between late- and early-onset schizophrenia and emphasizes the seriousness of both as public health concerns.

Neuropsychological Performance

Using an expanded version of the Halstead-Reitan Neuropsychological Test Battery (Heaton et al. 1994), we compared the cognitive deficit scores of late-onset and early-onset patients. The scores were corrected for age, gender, and education. The overall pattern of neuropsychological impairment was similar in the late-onset and early-onset schizophrenia groups (Heaton et al. 1994; Jeste et al. 1995b), with both schizophrenia groups being intermediate between the healthy control group and a group of outpatients with Alzheimer's disease (Heaton et al. 1994). In the arena of learning and memory, both schizophrenia groups showed difficulty with learning information but no deficits in retention over a delay (Paulsen et al. 1995). Their performance contrasted with that of the patients with Alzheimer's disease, who showed deficits in both learning and retention. In addition, patients with late-onset schizophrenia differed somewhat from patients with early-onset schizophrenia on learning measures, in that the learning deficits were less severe in the late-onset group. Furthermore, later age at onset of schizophrenia predicted better total recall across learning trials and better effortful retrieval of information. Integrity of semantic memory also distinguished between patients with late-onset schizophrenia and older patients with early-onset schizophrenia (Paulsen et al. 1996). Organization of semantic memory in the patients with late-onset schizophrenia closely mirrored that of the healthy control subjects, but semantic memory was highly disorganized in the older patients with early-onset schizophrenia. Finally, the late-onset schizophrenia patients were less impaired than the older early-onset schizophrenia patients on measures of abstraction and flexibility of thinking (Jeste et al. 1995b). There was no evidence that the deficits seen in either group of older patients with schizophrenia reflected progressive decline. Repeated neuropsychological evaluation of patients with late-onset schizophrenia and older patients with early-onset schizophrenia over a period ranging from 2 to 8 years has revealed no deterioration in function in any cognitive domain (Heaton 1998).

Psychophysiology

In young adults, there is a language-related negative brain potential approximately 400 msec after stimulus onset (called N400) that is much larger in amplitude when a word is presented that is semantically incongruous with its context (Kutas and Hillyard 1982, 1984). The magnitude of difference in the potential between semantically congruous and incongruous words is referred to as the N400 *congruity effect*. Studies of younger patients with early-onset schizophrenia have shown reduced amplitude and longer latency of the congruity effect (Andrews et al. 1993; Bloom 1993). We found that the peak latency of the N400 congruity effect was significantly delayed in the late-onset schizophrenia patients compared with the healthy control subjects (and the older early-onset schizophrenia patients) (Olichney et al. 1997), whereas there were no significant differences in latencies between the older early-onset schizophrenia patients and the healthy control subjects.

We have also studied the P300 brain potential that is evoked in response to unexpected task-relevant events (Olichney et al. 1998). Much as with younger patients with schizophrenia (Ford et al. 1992), we found that the older patients with early-onset schizophrenia had significantly smaller auditory oddball P300 amplitudes than the healthy control subjects. The late-onset schizophrenia group, in contrast, did not differ significantly from the healthy control group in terms of P300; 11 of 12 of the late-onset schizophrenia patients had P300 amplitudes in the normal range.

Structural Brain Imaging

We found no differences among the late-onset schizophrenia patients, older early-onset schizophrenia patients, and healthy control subjects in terms of the presence of clinically relevant structural brain abnormalities (e.g., strokes, tumors, cysts, other obvious lesions) (Symonds et al. 1997). (We should clarify that the late-onset schizophrenia patients with a history or physical examination consistent with stroke or tumor had been excluded from our subject pool, as we believe that these individuals would be more properly classified as having psychosis not otherwise specified or psychosis due to a general medical condition.) Quantitative, morphometric analyses (Jernigan et al. 1990) of the MRI scans of a smaller subset of subjects revealed significant differences among the late-onset schizophrenia patients, older early-onset schizophrenia patients, and healthy control subjects only for ventricular and thalamic volumes (Corey-Bloom et al. 1995). The patients with late-onset schizophrenia had significantly larger ventricles than the healthy control subjects, with the older early-onset schizophrenia patients showing intermediate values. Ventricular volume was not significantly different between the late-onset and older early-onset groups. Thalamic volume was largest in the late-onset schizophrenia patients, smallest in the older early-onset schizophrenia patients, and intermediate in the healthy control subjects. The difference in thalamic volume between the late-onset and older early-onset patients was significant. Although our finding of nonsignificantly smaller thalamic volume in the older patients with early-onset schizophrenia compared with the healthy control subjects is consistent with prior MRI (Andreasen et al. 1990, 1994; Baumer 1954; Pakkenberg 1990, 1992; Treff and Hempel 1958) and positron-emission tomography (Buchsbaum et al. 1996) studies of early-onset schizophrenia showing thalamic deficits, the larger thalamic volume in the late-onset schizophrenia patients is a new result that needs replication in view of the relatively small sample sizes on which these data are based.

Discussion

The results of the studies conducted at the UCSD Center for the Study of Late-Life Psychoses suggest that late-onset schizophrenia shares a number of characteristics with early-onset schizophrenia and thus should be classified as schizophrenia. Specifically, age-comparable groups of patients with late-onset and early-onset schizophrenia are similar in overall degree of psychopathology, severity of positive symptoms, increased mortality, and presence of constitutional sensory deficits (Table 7–1). Also, family history of schizophrenia is similarly elevated in both groups, and each group shows evidence of poor childhood psychosocial adjustment. In addition, the quality of well-being and the overall pattern of cognitive deficits and nonspecific structural brain abnormalities are similar in late-onset and early-onset schizophrenia.

As seen in Table 7–1, we found a number of differences between late-onset schizophrenia and early-onset schizophrenia. Specifically, the late-onset schizophrenia group included more women and more patients with paranoid subtype than the early-onset schizophrenia group, and the late-onset patients had less severe negative symptoms and better premorbid adjustment. Neuropsychological impairment was milder in the realms of learning, abstraction, and semantic organization. Finally, the late-onset schizophrenia patients appeared to have more normal P300 amplitude but longer latency of the N400 brain potential and probably larger thalami on MRI than did the comparably aged early-onset schizophrenia patients.

What implications do these findings have for understanding the relationship of late-onset schizophrenia to early-onset schizophrenia? Some investigators have characterized late-onset schizophrenia as a neurodegenerative disorder (Castle and Murray 1993) that results from specific structural brain lesions (Feinberg 1982; Miller et al. 1991) and/ or is secondary to sensory deficits (Cooper et al. 1974). Our results provide little evidence for the view that late-onset schizophrenia is a neurodegenerative disease. The overall level of neuropsychological deficits seen in the late-onset schizophrenia patients was similar to that seen in older patients with early-onset schizophrenia. Further, when differences were seen, the late-onset schizophrenia patients exhibited milder deficits than the older early-onset schizophrenia patients, especially in areas known to be sensitive to neurodegeneration (i.e., learning, retrieval, and abstraction). In addition, the deficits seen in the late-onset schizophrenia patients did not progress over the follow-up period.

Our results also do not support the idea that late-onset schizophrenia is the result of specific structural brain lesions such as strokes or tumors. There was no increase in qualitative MRI abnormalities in the late-onset schizophrenia group, and quantitatively determined ventricular

TABLE 7–1. *Late-onset schizophrenia: similarities with and differences from early-onset schizophrenia*

Similarities	Differences
Clinical/Psychosocial	
Overall degree of psychopathology	Preponderance of women
Severity of positive symptoms	Less severe negative symptoms
Family history of schizophrenia	Disorganized subtype rare
Qualitative response to neuro-leptics	Lower daily neuroleptic doses
Early childhood maladjustment	Better psychosocial functioning in early adulthood
Constitutional (uncorrected) sensory impairment	
Quality of well-being	
Minor physical anomalies	
Increased mortality	
Neuropsychological	
Overall pattern of neuropsycho-logical impairment	Milder impairment in learning, retrieval, and abstraction/cognitive flexibility
	Less disturbance of semantic network
Psychophysiological	
	Longer latency of N400 congruity effect[a]
	Normal P300 amplitude
Neuroanatomic	
Degree of nonspecific structural brain abnormalities (ventricular enlargement, white matter hyper-intensities)	Larger thalamus

[a]This finding was based on comparison of patients with late-onset schizophrenia and older patients with early-onset schizophrenia but is similar to results reported in literature for younger early-onset schizophrenia patients.

enlargement was similarly present in both the late-onset and early-onset groups. In a preliminary study, the unique structural brain feature found in the late-onset schizophrenia group was an enlarged thalamus—a finding that argues against neurodegeneration. As for sensory deficits, we found similar visual and auditory impairments in both the late-onset and early-onset schizophrenia patients when testing was done without the use of any correcting devices.

Thus, in contrast to traditional views, we believe that our results support a neurodevelopmental concept of late-onset schizophrenia. Equivalent degrees of childhood maladjustment were seen in the late-onset and early-onset patients, and this suggests that some liability for the disorder exists early in life. In addition, there were increased rates of schizophrenia among first-degree relatives of both the late-onset and early-onset patients, and this points to similar degrees of genetic loading in these two groups. Furthermore, equivalent degrees of minor physical anomalies in the late-onset and early-onset patients suggest the presence of developmental defects in both groups.

At the same time, if late-onset schizophrenia has a neurodevelopmental basis, how do we explain the delayed onset? One possibility is that late-onset schizophrenia is a less severe form of the disorder and, as such, is less likely to manifest early in life. Our results indicate that in several arenas, late-onset schizophrenia deficits are milder than those of early-onset schizophrenia. For example, neuropsychological impairments in learning, retrieval, abstraction, and semantic memory, as well as P300 abnormalities, are less severe. Also, negative symptoms are less pronounced and neuroleptic doses are considerably lower in late-onset schizophrenia patients.

The etiology and onset of early-onset schizophrenia are often explained by a diathesis-stress model in which there is a genetic vulnerability in combination with an environmental insult, such as obstetric complications, with onset triggered by maturational changes or life events that stress a developmentally damaged brain (Feinberg 1983; Weinberger 1987; Wyatt 1996). In such a "multiple hit" model, patients with late-onset schizophrenia might have had fewer "hits" and thus had a delayed onset of the illness. As discussed earlier, genetic loading for schizophrenia is probably similar in late-onset and early-onset schizophrenia, though some investigators have found a weaker family history in late-onset schizophrenia patients (Castle and Howard 1992; Castle et al. 1997; Rokhlina 1975).

An alternative or complementary explanation for the delayed onset in late-onset schizophrenia is that patients with this illness share protective features that cushion the blow of any additional "hits." For instance, the larger thalamus in late-onset schizophrenia patients (if this finding is replicated), in contrast to the abnormally small thalamus in patients with early-onset schizophrenia, could conceivably protect the integrity of brain circuits and thereby contribute to a delayed onset of the disorder. In support of this hypothesis, we found that age at onset was positively correlated with thalamic volume in a mixed group of younger and older patients with schizophrenia (Jeste et al. 1998). In addition, the preponderance of postmenopausal women among late-onset schizophrenia patients has led some investigators to speculate that estrogen might have played a protective role in those women (Ellis et al. 1998; Lindamer et al. 1997; Seeman and Lang 1990).

The view of late-onset schizophrenia as a less severe form of schizophrenia in which the delayed onset results from fewer detrimental "hits" or the presence of protective factors suggests a continuous relationship between age at onset and severity of liability. An alternative view is that late-onset schizophrenia is a distinct neurobiological subtype of schizophrenia. The consistent sex difference and the preponderance of the paranoid subtype support this view. In addition, the finding of an enlarged thalamus (if confirmed with larger samples) suggests a distinct underlying pathology. Furthermore, other investigators have reported a bimodal distribution of age at onset (Castle and Murray 1993), which could be consistent with two subtypes.

Additional research is needed to determine whether differences between late-onset schizophrenia and early-onset schizophrenia are best explained by a subtype model or by a continuous distribution of age at onset resulting from continuous differences in degree of liability. However, to the extent that a subtype model fits the available data, we propose that neurobiological differences between late-onset and early-onset schizophrenia may be related to differential involvement of cortico-striato-pallido-thalamic (CSPT) circuits. The three nonmotor CSPT circuits—orbitofrontal, dorsolateral-prefrontal, and anterior cingulate—are reported to subserve cognitive and emotional behaviors

(Cummings 1993; Mega and Cummings 1994). Lesions of the dorso-lateral-prefrontal circuit putatively lead to disruption of executive functions, damage to the orbitofrontal circuit may result in behavioral disinhibition, and lesions of the anterior cingulate circuit are believed to lead to motivational deficits. It can be argued that impairments in executive functions seen in schizophrenia may be related to dorsolateral-prefrontal dysfunction, positive symptoms might result from orbitofrontal deficits, and negative symptoms might be related to dysfunction of the anterior cingulate circuit (Jeste et al. 1997). We therefore hypothesize that patients with late-onset schizophrenia share orbitofrontal dysfunction with early-onset schizophrenia patients but have relatively less involvement of the anterior cingulate circuit. Dorsolateral-prefrontal dysfunction could be expected in both groups but would be expected to a greater degree in early-onset schizophrenia patients.

Future studies at our center are planned to test this model. For example, we would predict that late-onset schizophrenia patients would be less impaired on cognitive tasks that involve the anterior cingulate, such as the Stroop Interference Test (Larrue et al. 1994; Pardo et al. 1990; Stroop 1935). In addition, the model can be tested with functional neuroimaging tasks that preferentially activate different CSPT cognitive circuits. We have developed a version of the Stroop task suitable for use with functional MRI and have shown that it activates anterior cingulate cortex in healthy individuals (Jeste et al. 1998). Similarly, we have developed a test of memory for temporal order that reliably activates dorsolateral prefrontal cortex in healthy volunteers (Eyler Zorrilla et al. 1996). These tasks could be used to examine the integrity of each of the relevant CSPT circuits in late-onset and early-onset schizophrenia patients. Other directions for future study include continued longitudinal follow-up of late-onset and early-onset schizophrenia patients in order to characterize more completely the clinical, psychosocial, psychophysiological, and neuroanatomic features of these groups. Further genetic, neurochemical, and postmortem studies would also advance our understanding of late-onset schizophrenia.

In summary, we have found that late-onset and early-onset schizophrenia share many features in common but also differ in important respects. Thus, we conclude that late-onset schizophrenia is indeed schizophrenia but is probably a distinct neurobiological subtype of the disorder. We speculate that differences between late-onset and early-onset schizophrenia may be related to differential involvement of CSPT circuitry. Further investigation of the interactions among age at onset, clinical presentation, and neural circuitry is likely to advance our knowledge of schizophrenia in general.

References

American Psychiatric Association: Diagnostic and Statistical Manual of Mental Disorders, 3rd Edition. Washington, DC, American Psychiatric Association, 1980

American Psychiatric Association: Diagnostic and Statistical Manual of Mental Disorders, 3rd Edition, Revised. Washington, DC, American Psychiatric Association, 1987

American Psychiatric Association: Diagnostic and Statistical Manual of Mental Disorders, 4th Edition. Washington, DC, American Psychiatric Association, 1994

Andreasen NC: Negative symptoms in schizophrenia: definition and reliability. Arch Gen Psychiatry 39:784–788, 1982

Andreasen NC, Olsen S: Negative vs positive schizophrenia: definition and validation. Arch Gen Psychiatry 39:789–794, 1982

Andreasen NC, Ehrhardt JC, Swayze VW, et al: Magnetic resonance imaging of the brain in schizophrenia. Arch Gen Psychiatry 47:35–44, 1990

Andreasen NC, Arndt S, Swayze VW, et al: Thalamic abnormalities in schizophrenia visualized through magnetic resonance image averaging. Science 266:294–298, 1994

Andrews S, Shelley AM, Ward PB, et al: Event-related potential indices of semantic processing in schizophrenia. Biol Psychiatry 34:443–458, 1993

Baumer H: Veränderungen des Thalamus bei Schizophrenie. J Hirnforsch 1:157–172, 1954

Bleuler E: Dementia Praecox or the Group of Schizophrenias (1911). Translated by Zinken J. New York, International Universities Press, 1950

Bleuler M: Late schizophrenic clinical pictures. Fortschr Neurol Psychiatr 15:259–290, 1943

Bloom F: Advancing a neurodevelopmental origin for schizophrenia. Arch Gen Psychiatry 50:224–227, 1993

Buchsbaum MS, Someya T, Teng CY, et al: PET and MRI of the thalamus in never-medicated patients with schizophrenia. Am J Psychiatry 153:191–199, 1996

Castle DJ, Howard R: What do we know about the aetiology of late-onset schizophrenia. European Psychiatry 7:99–108, 1992

Castle DJ, Murray RM: The epidemiology of late-onset schizophrenia. Schizophr Bull 19:691–700, 1993

Castle DJ, Wessely S, Howard R, et al: Schizophrenia with onset at the extremes of adult life. Int J Geriatr Psychiatry 12:712–717, 1997

Cooper AF, Curry AR, Kay DWK, et al: Hearing loss in paranoid and affective psychoses of the elderly. Lancet 2:851–854, 1974

Corey-Bloom J, Jernigan T, Archibald S, et al: Quantitative magnetic resonance imaging in late-life schizophrenia. Am J Psychiatry 152:447–449, 1995

Cummings JL: Frontal-subcortical circuits and human behavior. Arch Neurol 50:873–880, 1993

Ellis RJ, Jan K, Kawas C, et al: Diagnostic validity of the Dementia Questionnaire for Alzheimer Disease. Arch Neurol 55:360–365, 1998

Eyler Zorrilla LT, Aquirre GK, Zarahn E, et al: Activation of the prefrontal cortex during judgments of recency: a functional MRI study. NeuroReport 7:15–17, 1996

Feinberg I: Schizophrenia and late maturational brain changes in man. Psychopharmacol Bull 18:29–31, 1982

Feinberg I: Schizophrenia: caused by a fault in programmed synaptic elimination during adolescence? J Psychiatr Res 17:319–334, 1983

Ford J, Roth W, Pfefferbaum A, et al: P3 and schizophrenia, inPsychophysiology and Experimental Psychopathology: A Tribute to Samuel Sutton. Edited by Friedman D, Bruder G. New York, New York Academy of Sciences, 1992, pp 146–162

Gittelman-Klein R, Klein DF: Premorbid asocial adjustment and prognosis in schizophrenia. J Psychiatr Res 7:35–53, 1969

Harris MJ, Jeste DV: Late-onset schizophrenia: an overview. Schizophr Bull 14:39–55, 1988

Heaton R: Schizophrenia in late-life: reliability and stability of neuropsychological functioning. Paper presented at the 11th annual meeting of the American Association for Geriatric Psychiatry, San Diego, CA, March 1998

Heaton R, Paulsen J, McAdams LA, et al: Neuropsychological deficits in schizophrenia: relationship to age, chronicity, and dementia. Arch Gen Psychiatry 51:469–476, 1994

Jernigan TL, Press GA, Hesselink JR: Methods for measuring brain morphologic features on magnetic resonance images: validation and normal aging. Arch Neurol 47:27–32, 1990

Jeste DV, Halpain MC, Nemiroff B, et al: Do patients with late-onset schizophrenia develop dementia? (abstract). Society for Neuroscience Abstracts 21:745, 1995a

Jeste DV, Harris MJ, Krull A, et al: Clinical and neuropsychological characteristics of patients with late-onset schizophrenia. Am J Psychiatry 152:722–730, 1995b

Jeste DV, Symonds LL, Harris MJ, et al: Non-dementia non-praecox dementia praecox?: late-onset schizophrenia. Am J Geriatr Psychiatry 5:302–317, 1997

Jeste DV, McAdams LA, Palmer BW, et al: Relationship of neuropsychological and MRI measures to age of onset of schizophrenia. Acta Psychiatr Scand 98:156–164, 1998

Kraepelin E: Dementia Praecox and Paraphrenia (1919). Translated by Barclay RM. Edited by Robertson GM. Huntington, NY, Krieger, 1971

Kutas M, Hillyard SA: The lateral distribution of event-related potentials during sentence processing. Neuropsychologia 20:579–590, 1982

Kutas M, Hillyard SA: Brain potentials during reading reflect word expectancy and semantic association. Nature 307:161–163, 1984

Larrue V, Celsis P, Bes A: The functional anatomy of attention in humans: cerebral blood flow changes induced by reading, naming, and the Stroop effect. J Cereb Blood Flow Metab 14:958–962, 1994

Lindamer LA, Lohr JB, Harris MJ, et al: Gender, estrogen, and schizophrenia. Psychopharmacol Bull 33:221–228, 1997

Lohr JB, Alder M, Flynn K, et al: Minor physical anomalies in older patients with late-onset schizophrenia, early-onset schizophrenia, depression, and Alzheimer's disease. Am J Geriatr Psychiatry 5:318–323, 1997

Maurer K, Hafner H. Methodological aspects of onset assessment in schizophrenia. Schizophr Res 15:265–276, 1995

Mega MS, Cummings JL: Frontal-subcortical circuits and neuropsychiatric disorders. J Neuropsychiatry Clin Neurosci 6:358–370, 1994

Miller BL, Lesser IM, Boone KB, et al: Brain lesions and cognitive function in late-life psychosis. Br J Psychiatry 158:76–82, 1991

Olichney JM, Iragui VJ, Nowacki R, et al: N400 abnormalities in late-life schizophrenia and related psychoses. Biol Psychiatry 42:13–23, 1997

Olichney JM, Iragui VJ, Kutas M, et al: Relationship between auditory P300 amplitude and age at onset of schizophrenia in older patients. Psychiatry Res 79:241–254, 1998

Overall JE, Gorham DR: The Brief Psychiatric Rating Scale. Psychol Rep 10:799–812, 1962

Pakkenberg B: Pronounced reduction of total neuron number in mediodorsal thalamic nucleus and nucleus accumbens in schizophrenia. Arch Gen Psychiatry 47:1023–1028, 1990

Pakkenberg B: The volume of the mediodorsal thalamic nucleus in treated and untreated schizophrenics. Schizophr Res 7:95–100, 1992

Pardo J, Pardo PJ, Janer KW: The anterior cingulate cortex mediates processing selection in the Stroop attentional conflict paradigm. Proc Natl Acad Sci U S A 87:256–259, 1990

Patterson TL, Kaplan RM, Grant I, et al: Quality of well-being in late-life psychosis. Psychiatry Res 63:169–181, 1996

Paulsen JS, Heaton RK, Sadek JR, et al: The nature of learning and memory impairments in schizophrenia. Journal of the International Neuropsychological Society 1:88–99, 1995

Paulsen JS, Romero R, Chan A, et al: Impairment of the semantic network in schizophrenia. Psychiatry Res 63:109–121, 1996

Prager S, Jeste DV: Sensory impairment in late-life schizophrenia. Schizophr Bull 19:755–772, 1993

Rokhlina ML: A comparative clinico-genetic study of attack-like schizophrenia with late and early manifestations with regard to age (in Russian). Zh Nevrol Psikhiatr 75:417–424, 1975

Seeman MV, Lang M: The role of estrogens in schizophrenia gender differences. Schizophr Bull 16:185–194, 1990

Spitzer RL, Williams JBW, Gibbon M, et al: User's Guide for the Structured Clinical Interview for DSM-III-R. Washington, DC, American Psychiatric Press, 1990

Stroop JR: Studies of interference in serial verbal reactions. J Exp Psychol 18:643–662, 1935

Symonds LL, Olichney JM, Jernigan TL, et al: Lack of clinically significant structural abnormalities in MRIs of older patients with schizophrenia and related psychoses. J Neuropsychiatry Clin Neurosci 9:251–258, 1997

Treff WM, Hempel KJ: Die Zelldichte bei Schizophrenen und klinisch Gesunden. J Hirnforsch 4:314–369, 1958

Weinberger DR: Implications of normal brain development for the pathogenesis of schizophrenia. Arch Gen Psychiatry 44:660–669, 1987

Wyatt RJ: Neurodevelopmental abnormalities and schizophrenia: a family affair. Arch Gen Psychiatry 53:11–15, 1996

CHAPTER 8

Childhood-Onset Schizophrenia: What Can It Teach Us?

Rob Nicolson, M.D.

Judith L. Rapoport, M.D.

Age at onset of illness has been an important approach to the under-standing of disease across all of medicine. Few have discussed this approach as eloquently as Dr. Barton Childs, whose exposition is presented in Chapter 2 of this volume. Earlier papers by Dr. Childs played a significant role in the inspiration of our studies of early-onset obsessive-compulsive disorder (OCD) and, more recently, childhood-onset schizophrenia. In his reviews, Dr. Childs points out how earlier onset of illness often has greater genetic and environmental influence, and he presents supporting evidence for this across all of pediatric medi-cine (Childs and Scriver 1986). In some cases, the early-onset disorder may be physiologically and etiologically different from the later-onset illness. For example, the study of early-onset disease led to a description of different and important mechanisms of illness in insulin-dependent (type I) diabetes mellitus, for which allelic variations in the major histo-compatibility complex in the human histocompatibility leukocyte antigen (HLA) area on chromosome 6 have been described. Although 45% of Caucasians in the United States have HLA-DR3 or HLA-DR4 genotypes, 95% of patients with insulin-dependent diabetes mellitus have at least one of these HLA-DR antigens. Susceptibility is also increased by HLA-DR1, HLA-DR8, and HLA-DR16 but decreased by HLA-DR11 and HLA-DR15 (Weiss 1993). More generally, molecular genetic discoveries in human diseases have often been tied to a particular age at onset for illnesses as diverse as breast cancer and Alzheimer's disease, with this wide applicability attesting to the importance of the present topic.

While most cases of schizophrenia have their onset in late adolescence and early adulthood (Hafner et al. 1993), the disorder has been identified in children since early in the 20th century (Asarnow 1994). Despite this, the nosological status of schizophrenia in children was controversial for many years, and the DSM-II category of *childhood schizophrenia* included all psychotic disorders in children in addition to autistic disorder (American Psychiatric Association 1968), a feature that limited the usefulness of early studies that relied on this diagnostic scheme. However, the landmark studies by Kolvin and colleagues (Kolvin 1971) clearly differentiated schizophrenia of childhood onset and autistic disorder.

The study of children with schizophrenia was neglected for long periods, in part because of the nosological difficulties just described as well as the rarity of the disorder in this population. Although the treated prevalence has been reported to be 2% of the prevalence of adult-onset schizophrenia (Beitchman 1985), this is almost certainly an overestimation, given the high number of false positive diagnoses found by our group (McKenna et al. 1994a). Recently, there has been a renewed interest in children with schizophrenia, spurred on in large part by the possibility that this may be a group with a more severe and homogenous illness, less confounded by long-term antipsychotic treatment, chronic institutionalization, or substance use (Asarnow 1994). As Kallmann and Roth (1956) pointed out, "[T]here must be an important factor or group of factors which in some cases leads to clinically recognizable symptoms at an unusually young age" (p. 599). Elucidation of these factors may provide important insights into the etiology and pathophysiology of schizophrenia.

Since 1990, a study of childhood-onset schizophrenia has been ongoing at the National Institute of Mental Health (NIMH) (Gordon et al. 1994a). The study addressed first the continuity of childhood- and adult-onset schizophrenia. It is now examining the association between the early-onset form of the disorder and risk or etiological factors. In this chapter, we review the results of the first part of this study and then present preliminary data from the second part that suggest salient risk factors. In addition, some data indicating that childhood-onset schizophrenia may be a more progressive form of the illness are presented. These results form the basis of a model of very-early-onset illness as a function of both more potent genetic risk and more general vulnerability in this very young group of patients with this rare form of the disorder.

Is Childhood-Onset Schizophrenia Continuous With Adult-Onset Schizophrenia?

The question of continuity between early- and later-onset schizophrenia is fundamental to the other aspects of our research. If childhood-onset schizophrenia is the same as that seen in patients with the disorder of later onset, it may provide important clues about the etiology of schizophrenia. If continuity cannot be demonstrated, then any findings from studies of childhood-onset schizophrenia would have limited generalizability.

The NIMH study addressed the continuity question comprehensively (Gordon et al. 1994a; Jacobsen and Rapoport 1998; McKenna et al. 1994b). Examination of the phenomenology, neuropsychology, and biology of these patients has provided strong evidence that childhood-onset schizophrenia is clinically and biologically continuous with later-onset forms of the disorder. Since the data supporting continuity have been reviewed elsewhere (Jacobsen and Rapoport 1998), we limit ourselves here to a brief overview of the studies whose results are summarized in Table 8–1.

Clinical Features

Although early studies of children with schizophrenia were plagued by problems of diagnostic heterogeneity (Werry 1996), recent studies, including the NIMH study, have demonstrated that schizophrenia can

TABLE 8–1.   *Childhood-onset schizophrenia: continuity with adult-onset schizophrenia*

Measure	Continuity	Resemblance to adult onset with poor outcome	Reference(s)
Clinical presentation	+ (by definition)	+	Gordon et al. 1994a; McKenna et al. 1994
Premorbid functioning	+	+	Alaghband-Rad et al. 1995; Hollis 1995
Neuropsychology	+	+	R. F. Asarnow et al. 1994; Kumra et al., in press
Autonomic functioning	+	+	Zahn et al. 1997
SPEM abnormalities	+	+	Jacobsen et al. 1996b; Kumra et al. 1998a
Anatomic brain MRI	+	+	Frazier et al. 1996; Jacobsen et al. 1996a, 1997a, 1997b, 1997c
PET	+	–	Jacobsen et al. 1997d
MRS	+	?	Bertolino et al. 1998

Note. MRI = magnetic resonance imaging; MRS = magnetic resonance spectroscopy; PET = positron-emission tomography; SPEM = smooth pursuit eye movements.

be reliably diagnosed in children on the basis of the same criteria as those used for adults (Gordon et al. 1994a; Green et al. 1992; Russell 1994; Spencer and Campbell 1994). Males and females were equally represented in the NIMH group, and although few, if any, sex differences in clinical or biological parameters were found, there were some striking premorbid sex differences (discussed below). There was no excess of undifferentiated and disorganized subtypes, and the paranoid subtype was diagnosed at a similar frequency as in adult disorders. Because patients in the NIMH study all had treatment-refractory schizophrenia, it is not surprising that they resembled adult patients with poor outcomes in various ways. However, others have also found that childhood-onset schizophrenia, even in unselected series, is a severe disorder with a poor outcome (J. R. Asarnow et al. 1994).

A subject of related interest is the question of how narrow the diagnostic band should be. A group of children who do not meet the criteria for schizophrenia but have histories of transient psychotic symptoms in addition to disruptive behavior and learning deficits have been studied in parallel with children with schizophrenia to determine whether their conditions are a possible forme fruste of childhood-onset schizophrenia. This group, whose conditions are not properly described by any current DSM diagnosis, have been described by our group as "multidimensionally impaired." The pattern of developmental disturbances in these children is similar to that in children with schizophrenia, and the two groups resemble each other in a number of biological parameters (Kumra et al. 1998b). Because "multidimensionally impaired" children are probably more numerous than children with narrowly defined childhood-onset schizophrenia, more ambitious genetic studies may be possible.

Premorbid Course

Patients with schizophrenia have been shown to have poor premorbid development (Cannon-Spoor et al. 1982), particularly in the areas of language and social development (Done et al. 1994; Jones et al. 1994), and a poor outcome in schizophrenia is correlated with more deviant premorbid development (Gupta et al. 1995). Patients with a very early onset of schizophrenia have been shown to have similar but more exaggerated abnormalities (Alaghband-Rad et al. 1995; Hollis 1995). Hollis (1995) reported that patients with an onset of schizophrenia before age 13 years had significantly more premorbid social, language, and motor delays and difficulties than did patients with onset later in adolescence. An earlier analysis of the first 23 patients in the NIMH childhood-onset study had revealed similar results (Alaghband-Rad et al. 1995). The NIMH patients showed delays in motor and language milestones, and over half had either failed a grade or been placed in special education. In addition, a number of patients showed transient, premorbid autistic symptoms such as handflapping, social isolation, and odd speech.

An updated analysis of the prepsychotic developmental data from 46 patients with childhood-onset schizophrenia has confirmed and extended these findings. In our sample, 48% of the patients had social abnormalities, 48% had language abnormalities, and 54% had motor abnormalities years prior to the onset of psychotic symptoms. About 50% had transient premorbid behavioral and language symptoms resembling those seen in patients with autistic disorder. One of the most striking findings was the high rate of special-education placement and failed grades. Twenty-nine (63%) either failed a grade or required placement in a special education setting prior to the onset of their illness.

Some important sex differences were found in relation to premorbid developmental history. Males had had more motor abnormalities, including delayed milestones, abnormal movements, and clumsiness (20 of the 28 males, but only 5 of the 18 females; $P = 0.003$). In addition, 7 females, but only 4 males, did not have an insidious onset of their illness. Thus, males had a more blatantly disrupted early development.

These findings, because they appear more striking than those found for adult-onset schizophrenia, argue for a more severe early disruption of brain development in childhood-onset schizophrenia. This more severe disruption could be due to greater environmental or genetic liability of a specific or nonspecific nature.

Because the patients in the NIMH study were selected for a poor treatment response, a comparison with unselected patients with adult-onset schizophrenia may not be entirely appropriate, and ongoing studies are addressing this issue. Similarly, retrospective adult data cannot be strictly compared with the data from our study because of a lack of blinding and different age of the historical material (i.e., adults having to recall information from many years earlier).

Neuropsychology

Adults with schizophrenia have particularly poor neuropsychological functioning in the areas of attention, working memory, and executive function (Goldberg and Gold 1995). Several studies in patients with childhood-onset schizophrenia (R. F. Asarnow et al. 1994), including studies with our NIMH sample (Kumra et al., in press), have found similar deficits.

Brain Morphology

Magnetic resonance imaging abnormalities of brain morphology have repeatedly been observed in adults with schizophrenia (Shenton et al.

1997), and individuals with childhood-onset schizophrenia have similar abnormalities (Frazier et al. 1996; Jacobsen et al. 1997a, 1997b). Analysis of the scans of 35 patients and 57 matched control subjects (Table 8–2) showed the expected increase in lateral ventricular volume with decreased cerebellar volume and midsagittal thalamic area. It is of interest, however, that reductions in the volumes of the anterior frontal lobes and medial temporal lobes (Frazier et al. 1996; Jacobsen et al. 1996a, 1997c) were not found. The changes in the ventricular volume were more pronounced in the early-onset patients than have been found in imaging studies of adults with schizophrenia. Similarly, the decrease in total gray volume was also more striking than that usually reported for adult patients.

Functional Brain Imaging

Although studies of resting brain metabolism in adults with schizophrenia have produced conflicting results, studies of cerebral metabolism during activation tasks have revealed frontal hypometabolism (Swanson et al. 1997). Patients with childhood-onset schizophrenia were noted to have similar abnormalities in a positron-emission tomography (PET) study. Although interpretation of hypofrontality in these patients is limited, since they could not adequately perform the activation task, it seems likely that hypofrontality was not more salient for these patients with early-onset schizophrenia (Jacobsen et al. 1997d).

A magnetic resonance spectroscopy study of patients with childhood-onset schizophrenia revealed decreases in the NAA:creatine ratio (a putative marker of neuronal density) in the prefrontal cortex and hippocampus (Bertolino et al. 1998). These results are similar in direction and extent to those seen in adult patients (Keshavan and Pettegrew 1997).

Autonomic Functioning

Abnormalities in peripheral indicators of autonomic activity, such as skin conductance and heart rate, have been noted in adult-onset schizophrenia. A study of autonomic functioning in patients with childhood-onset schizophrenia (Zahn et al. 1997) found abnormalities in measures of autonomic functioning similar to those found in adults with chronic schizophrenia with poor outcome.

TABLE 8–2. *MRI brain anatomy in childhood-onset schizophrenia*

	ANOVA		ANCOVA[a]		
Measure	F	P	F	P	Comment[b]
Total cerebral volume	1.53	0.13			
White matter	0.00	0.98	29.00	0.0001	COS > Control
Gray matter	9.98	0.002	45.00	0.0001	COS < Control
Prefrontal cortex	4.42	0.04	2.65	0.11	
Corpus callosum	1.36	0.25	5.02	0.03	COS > Control
Lateral ventricles	8.47	0.004	9.33	0.003	COS > Control
Ventricle: brain ratio	3.23	0.002			COS > Control
Temporal lobe	0.19	0.66	0.20	0.66	Subdivisions also not significantly different
					Planum temporale asymmetry in COS and Control not different
Hippocampus	3.74	0.056	2.10	0.15	Control: R > L COS: R = L
Amygdala	2.86	0.09	0.77	0.38	Control: R > L COS: R >> L
Cerebellum	9.71	0.003	7.56	0.008	COS < Control COS: Decreased midsagittal vermal area and inferior posterior lobe (VIII–X)
Thalamus (area)	4.81	0.0001	16.50	0.0001	COS < Control

[a]ANCOVA covaried for total brain volume; all P values 2-tailed.
[b]COS = patients with childhood-onset schizophrenia ($n = 35$); Control = healthy control subjects ($n = 57$).

Smooth Pursuit Eye Movements

From 40% to 80% of patients with adult-onset schizophrenia have abnormalities in smooth pursuit eye movements, and the finding of similar abnormalities in their relatives suggests that such abnormalities may be a genetic marker of vulnerability to the illness (Levy et al. 1993). Patients with childhood-onset schizophrenia have abnormalities similar to those reported in adult patients: decreased gain (i.e., ratio of eye speed to target speed), increased RMSE (i.e., global level of aberrant tracking), and increased anticipatory saccades (Jacobsen et al. 1996b; Kumra et al. 1998a).

Summary

Findings from the NIMH study strongly support clinical and biological continuity between childhood-onset and adult-onset schizophrenia. As expected, this group of patients with treatment-refractory childhood-onset schizophrenia resembled chronically ill adult patients with treatment-refractory schizophrenia. The clear evidence for continuity allows us to turn to the more intriguing and potentially more important question of why these children develop schizophrenia at such an early age.

Is Childhood-Onset Schizophrenia Associated With More Salient Risk Factors?

Virtually all models of schizophrenia include genetic and environmental components. The earlier onset of schizophrenia in childhood-onset cases may result from a "heavier load" of genetic factors, a more potent environmental insult, or a combination of both.

A number of environmental factors, including prenatal maternal infections and perinatal complications, have been implicated in the pathogenesis of schizophrenia. A greater frequency or severity of these factors could result in an earlier onset of schizophrenia, and indeed, at least for patients with adult-onset schizophrenia, obstetric complications have been associated with an earlier age at onset (O'Callaghan et al. 1993; Verdoux et al. 1997).

Alternatively, the earlier age at onset may be related to a greater genetic load. As discussed previously, increased familiality has been observed in a number of early-onset disorders (Childs and Scriver 1986), although the genetic loading reported for patients with childhood-onset schizophrenia was not higher than that reported for adult patients with adult-onset schizophrenia (Kallmann and Roth 1956; Kolvin 1971). Thus, Kallmann and Roth (1956) noted that the earlier age at onset in this group "would seem to be connected with variable constellations of secondary factors lowering constitutional resistance" (p. 605). Risk factors potentially associated with the earlier age at onset in childhood-onset schizophrenia are discussed below.

Obstetric Risk

A number of studies have found an excess of prenatal and perinatal complications in patients with schizophrenia. Patients with adult-onset schizophrenia have been reported to have an increased rate of obstetric complications when compared with their siblings (Eagles et al. 1990; Gunther-Genta et al. 1994) or healthy control groups (O'Callaghan et al. 1993), although not all studies have found such an increase (Done et al. 1991). Two meta-analyses have also demonstrated an increased rate of obstetric complications in patients with adult-onset schizophrenia (Geddes and Lawrie 1995; Verdoux et al. 1997), with one of these finding that complications were consistently greater in patients with an earlier onset of illness (Verdoux et al. 1997).

Blinded scoring of the birth records of 31 patients with childhood-onset schizophrenia and 27 sibling control subjects found no significant differences between the groups (Nicolson et al., in press). Moreover, the rate of complications in the early-onset patients in the NIMH sample was similar to that seen in adult-onset patients (Table 8–3). These preliminary results suggest that although obstetric complications may play a role in the development of schizophrenia in some patients, they are not, as previously hypothesized (Lewis et al. 1989), more salient in childhood-onset cases.

Prenatal viral infections have also been implicated in the pathogenesis of schizophrenia (Yolken and Torrey 1995). Studies are currently in progress to determine if patients with childhood-onset schizophrenia

TABLE 8–3. *Prenatal and perinatal events in childhood-onset schizophrenia*

	Prevalence of prenatal and perinatal events					
	COS patients (n = 31)		Siblings (n = 27)		AOS patients[a]	Healthy control subjects[a]	References
Measure	n	Rate	n	Rate			
Buka Scale	8	26%	12	44%	50%–67%	43%–54%	Buka et al. 1993; Jones et al. 1998
Lewis Scale (definite complications)	11	35%	5	19%	22%–32%	9%–22%	O'Callaghan et al. 1993; Verdoux et al. 1997

Note. No significant differences were found between the patients with childhood-onset schizophrenia and siblings on any scale. AOS = adult-onset schizophrenia; COS = childhood-onset schizophrenia.
[a]Data from studies of adults with schizophrenia (see references).

have a greater rate of exposure to prenatal viruses.

Other environmental factors, such as socioeconomic status and unusual psychological trauma, do not appear to account for the earlier age at onset on a clinical basis. Similarly, there is no evidence that the earlier age at onset is due to an earlier age at puberty (Frazier et al. 1997).

In summary, investigation of nongenetic factors in the very-early-onset cohort in the NIMH study has not revealed more salient features than those found in studies of adult-onset schizophrenia. Indirectly, this suggests that the earlier age at onset may be related to genetic factors, a topic to which we now turn.

Genetic Factors

Genetic factors are believed to play a significant role in the pathogenesis of schizophrenia (Kendler and Diehl 1993), and the notion that such factors may be more salient in very-early-onset cases has fuelled two classic studies (Kallmann and Roth 1956; Kolvin 1971).

Age at onset in schizophrenia has a lower correlation between affected siblings (approximately 0.26) and concordant dizygotic twins (approximately 0.30) than between concordant monozygotic twins (mean = 0.68) (Kendler et al. 1987), and this suggests that there are genetic influences on age at onset. However, the lack of relationship between pedigree density and age at onset in most studies (Kendler et al. 1987, 1996) suggests that age at onset is influenced by genetic factors that are unrelated to the disease liability. Additionally, the correlation of less than 1.0 in monozygotic twins suggests a role for nongenetic factors in determining age at onset. Like most studies, those reviewed by Kendler and colleagues (1987, 1996) did not include childhood-onset populations. Thus, it is still possible that very-early-onset cases may reveal more unique or potent genetic factors.

Schizophrenia and schizophrenia spectrum disorders (schizoaffective disorder and schizotypal and paranoid personality disorders) are more prevalent in the relatives of patients with schizophrenia (Kendler et al. 1993a, 1993b, 1993c), and adoption studies (Kendler et al. 1994) have documented the genetic basis for these spectrum disorders. First-degree relatives of the NIMH cohort under age 18 years were administered the Diagnostic Interview for Children and Adolescents (Reich et al. 1995), and relatives 18 years and older were administered the Schedule for Affective Disorders and Schizophrenia (SADS; Fyer et al. 1985) and the Structured Interview for DSM-IV Personality Disorders (SID-P; Pfohl et al. 1995). The results of these interviews are summarized in Table 8–4. Three first-degree relatives were determined to have schizophrenia, and another was diagnosed with schizoaffective disorder. In addition, 21% of the available first-degree relatives had either paranoid or schizotypal personality disorder, and 41% of the probands had at least one relative with a spectrum disorder (Lenane et al. 1999).

Although the rates of schizophrenia and schizoaffective disorder in relatives of the childhood-onset patients are similar to those seen in relatives of adult-onset patients, there appears to be an excess of schizotypal and paranoid personality disorders in the former. These results, however, must be interpreted with great caution, since the interviews were not administered blindly. These preliminary data nonetheless suggest a striking and perhaps causative role for genetic factors in patients with very-early-onset schizophrenia.

Spectrum disorders in first-degree relatives were powerfully related to premorbid abnormalities in the patients with childhood-onset schizophrenia in our study: 13 (72%) of the patients with relatives with schizo-

TABLE 8–4. *Rates of schizophrenia spectrum disorders in first-degree relatives of patients with childhood-onset schizophrenia*

Diagnosis	Relatives of COS patients	Relatives of AOS patients[a]	Relatives of healthy control subjects[a]
Schizophrenia	3.3% (3/92)	6.5%	0.5%
Schizoaffective disorder	1.1% (1/89)	2.3%	0.7%
Schizotypal personality disorder	11.1% (10/90)	6.9%	1.4%
Paranoid personality disorder	11.3% (9/80)	1.4%	0.4%
Schizophrenia spectrum disorder	25.0% (23/92)	16.1%	

Note. Rates determined with hierarchical method (Kendler 1988). AOS = adult-onset schizophrenia. COS = childhood-onset schizophrenia.
[a]Kendler et al. 1993a, 1993b, 1993c.

phrenia or spectrum disorders had premorbid language abnormalities, whereas only 9 (35%) without a similar family history had early language difficulties ($P = 0.01$) (Nicolson et al. 1998).

Another indirect measure of genetic risk for schizophrenia is smooth pursuit eye movements, which have been proposed as a marker of liability to schizophrenia in unaffected relatives of probands (Levy et al. 1993). To date, 71 relatives of the probands in our sample have been examined and, with qualitative ratings, 21% were determined to have abnormal eye tracking, whereas only 5% of the control subjects had similar results ($P = 0.006$). The frequency of these abnormalities appears to be similar to that seen in the relatives of patients with adult-onset schizophrenia. The data from these analyses are summarized in Table 8–5.

Other Genetic Studies

A few candidate abnormalities were examined in childhood-onset schizophrenia, and the results are summarized in Table 8–6. An increased rate of sex chromosome abnormalities has been reported in

TABLE 8–5. *Smooth pursuit eye movements in the relatives of patients with childhood-onset schizophrenia*

Measure	Relatives of COS patients (n = 71)	Control subjects (n = 62)	t	df	P	Comment	References
Gain	0.80 ± 0.15	0.84 ± 0.12	2.01	131	0.05	Effect size similar to that for relatives of patients with adult-onset schizophrenia	Litman et al. 1997; Clementz et al. 1992; Keefe et al. 1997
RMSE	3.18 ± 1.7	2.40 ± 0.9	3.23	131	0.002	Effect size similar to that in most studies of patients with adult-onset schizophrenia	Clementz et al. 1992; Grove et al. 1992

Note. COS = childhood-onset schizophrenia; RMSE = root mean square error.

TABLE 8–6. *Childhood-onset schizophrenia: association with genetic risk factors*

Measure	Abnormality relative to control subjects	Salience relative to AOS patients	References
Cytogenetic anomalies[a]	+	+	DeLisi et al. 1994[b] Gordon et al. 1994b; Kumra et al. 1998b; Yan et al. 1998
Candidate genes			
HLA	–	NA	Jacobsen et al. 1998b
Trinucleotide repeats	–	NA	Sidransky et al. 1998
Apo E4	–	NA	Fernandez et al. 1998

Note. AOS = adult-onset schizophrenia; Apo = apolipoprotein; HLA = histocompatibility leukocyte antigen; NA = not applicable.
[a]Sex chromosome aneuploidy, chromosomal translocations, deletions.
[b]NIMH data support findings of DeLisi et al.'s study.

adult-onset schizophrenia (DeLisi et al. 1994), and other chromosomal abnormalities have also been found (Bassett 1992; Karayiorgou and Gogos 1997). To date, 5 of the 46 patients with childhood-onset schizophrenia in our sample have been found to have cytogenetic abnormalities (a female with Turner's syndrome, a boy and two girls with velocardiofacial syndrome, and a boy with a balanced translocation of chromosomes 1 and 7) (Gordon et al. 1994b; Yan et al. 1998), and an additional three sex chromosome abnormalities (two Klinefelter's syndrome [XXY] and one XYY) occurred in the 28 multidimensionally impaired patients (Kumra et al. 1998c). Additional cytogenetic studies of these childhood-onset patients are in progress.

Trinucleotide repeats, HLA, and apolipoprotein (Apo) E4 have been investigated as possible etiological factors in adult-onset schizophrenia, and the results have been conflicting (Karayiorgou and Gogos 1997). Among the childhood-onset patients in the NIMH study, no associations were found for Apo E4 (Fernandez et al. 1998), HLA (Jacobsen et al. 1998b), or trinucleotide repeats (Sidransky et al. 1998). Thus, although these factors might play a role in schizophrenia (and the literature generally does not support this), they are not more salient in patients with childhood-onset schizophrenia.

The possibility remains that some more general protective or liability factors unrelated to the illness itself will be found to be most important in childhood-onset cases. Several examples exist of "protective" genes affecting the expression or inheritance of disorders, including AIDS (Picchio et al. 1997), Alzheimer's disease (Corder et al. 1994), and diabetes (Wicker et al. 1994). Recently, Ginns et al. (1998) have reported protective genes in bipolar disorder that seem to prevent or modify the clinical manifestations of the disorder.

Summary

Patients with childhood-onset schizophrenia have more significant premorbid abnormalities than do patients with adult-onset schizophrenia and may also have a greater history of schizophrenia spectrum disorders in their first-degree relatives. Although eye movement abnormalities are also seen in the families, it is not clear whether the rates are higher than those for relatives of patients with adult-onset schizophrenia. Additionally, there seems to be a greater rate of cytogenetic abnormalities in patients with childhood-onset schizophrenia and the multidimensionally impaired group. However, the earlier age at onset does not seem to be associated with a greater rate of obstetric complications. These findings, summarized in Table 8–7, point toward a range of genetic factors accounting for the early age at onset in childhood-onset schizophrenia.

Is Childhood-Onset Schizophrenia More Progressive Than Adult-Onset Schizophrenia?

The question of whether childhood-onset schizophrenia is more progressive than adult-onset schizophrenia is distinct from the first two discussed in the pervious sections. The accrual of a cohort for a study of childhood-onset schizophrenia permitted a study of the probands and, potentially, their siblings during early and midadolescence. Because

TABLE 8–7. *Childhood-onset schizophrenia: association with risk and etiological factors*

Measure	Abnormality relative to control subjects	More striking than in AOS patients	Comment	Reference
Cytogenetic abnormalities	+	+		Kumra et al. 1998b
Birth complications	–	–		Nicolson et al., in press
Early language and motor abnormalities	+	++	Significant association with schizophrenia spectrum disorders in relatives	Nicolson et al. 1998
Pubertal timing	–	–		Frazier et al. 1997
Schizophrenia and spectrum disorders in relatives	+	+ (?)	Possible ascertainment bias; data not examined in blinded fashion	Lenane et al. 1999
SPEM abnormalities in relatives	+	– (?)		Nicolson et al. 1999

Note. AOS = adult-onset schizophrenia; SPEM = smooth pursuit eye movements.

such studies are extremely difficult, and probably impossible, to carry out for adult-onset illness, similar data on most adult patients during adolescence remain unavailable in cases of later-onset schizophrenia.

It is known that the human brain undergoes significant changes during adolescence (Huttenlocher 1979), and these changes have been suggested as fundamental to the development of schizophrenia (Feinberg 1982–1983). A prospective, longitudinal study of anatomic brain changes as measured by MRI scans has been an integral component of the NIMH study of childhood-onset schizophrenia. In contrast, anatomic brain development of healthy children does not demonstrate a unique ventricular expansion in adolescence, but rather a very subtle linear progressive change starting in the first decade. Thus, the normal slight increase in ventricular volume is not tightly linked to puberty and therefore is not typically accelerating during the years before the usual onset of schizophrenia.

Although progressive changes in the brains of patients with schizophrenia have been reported (DeLisi et al. 1995; Gur et al. 1998; Lieberman et al. 1996), patients with childhood-onset schizophrenia appear to have a differential enlargement of the lateral ventricles that is more marked and consistent than has been reported for patients with adult-onset schizophrenia (Rapoport et al. 1997). Although brain changes have been noted after treatment with atypical antipsychotics (Chakos et al. 1995; Frazier et al. 1996), the differential progression in these patients is not accounted for by such confounds. Despite the progressive ventricular enlargement in patients with childhood-onset schizophrenia, there is no evidence of cognitive deterioration.

Temporal lobe developmental progression may have a similar late component. In a small number of healthy adolescents, there is a growing asymmetry of the temporal lobes that is not seen in patients with childhood-onset schizophrenia during early adolescence. Pilot data indicate a differential progression, with normal asymmetry increasing in the healthy control subjects but decreasing in the patients with very-early-onset schizophrenia (Jacobsen et al. 1998a).

These developmental changes in adolescence focus attention on putative genetic markers. Most nerve growth factors, for example, have different biologic effects at different stages of development and maturation. EGF and TGF-α can be either mitogens or differentiation factors depending on when cells are exposed to them. Neurotrophins seem to have different effects that are developmental stage–dependent as well.

For example, Levitt and co-workers (Burrows 1997) have identified a mouse (Wa-1) that has a mutation at the TGF-α locus. This mouse has a near-normal level of the growth factor at birth, but by 45 days postnatally this level is reduced by 90%. Concomitant with this decrease is a 15% increase in ventricular size that reaches a plateau by 90 days.

Other factors controlling early brain development of hippocampus, entorhinal and frontal cortices, thalamus, and regulators of glutamate and developmental proteins could be examined for both early and late developmental patterns, and candidate genes could be derived from such studies. These numerous candidate factors should account for both early and late effects and for variability in expression across patient groups.

Neurodevelopmental models of schizophrenia (Murray and Lewis 1987; Weinberger 1987) must be able to account for the disorders of both early and late brain development observed in childhood-onset schizophrenia. DeLisi (1997), for example, has proposed that the underlying basis for the neuropathology of schizophrenia is the periodic activation of a gene or genes that determine the rate of cerebral growth. Such a process could cause cortical maldevelopment prenatally and be activated during pruning of neurons in adolescence and again during the gradual aging process in the brain throughout adulthood.

Summary

The initial phase of the NIMH childhood-onset schizophrenia study has yielded convincing evidence for clinical and biological continuity between the very-early-onset and adult-onset forms of the disorder. This has allowed us to turn to the potentially more important question of why these children have an earlier age at onset of the disorder. In investigating potential causes, we have found that our subjects have more severe premorbid abnormalities, more cytogenetic abnormalities, and potentially greater family histories. They do not, however, have a greater rate of obstetric complications or abnormalities of candidate genes.

Although these data are limited by several factors, including possibly selection and ascertainment bias, the pattern of our findings is suggestive of a greater genetic vulnerability in our patients that may result in the earlier development of symptoms.

The association of spectrum disorders in relatives with premorbid speech and language abnormalities in our patients is of great interest. The British birth cohort studies (Jones and Done 1997) found speech and motor development in infancy and speech difficulties and word pronunciation at ages 7 and 11 years to be predictive of later onset of schizophrenia. Our finding of an association with spectrum disorders in relatives could support a model in which a specific disease-related factor (spectrum disorders) interacts with a more general liability; alternatively, it could indicate a more specific association between speech and language difficulties and the spectrum disorders themselves. Further language studies are indicated in adults with spectrum disorders to untangle these possibilities.

The cytogenetic and clinical findings suggest that even more intense screening of chromosome 7 and the X chromosome would be relevant given the relatively low IQ and autistic-like features in a significant proportion of our cohort. Such studies are ongoing.

Future studies of our cohort will be devoted to exploring and determining the genetic basis for the earlier age at onset in childhood-onset schizophrenia. It is anticipated that the cell lives immortalized from our cohort will be of great value as molecular and cytogenetic methods evolve for mapping and scanning the human genome.

References

Alaghband-Rad J, McKenna K, Gordon CT, et al: Childhood-onset schizophrenia: the severity of premorbid course. J Am Acad Child Adolesc Psychiatry 34:1273–1283, 1995

American Psychiatric Association: Diagnostic and Statistical Manual of Mental Disorders, 2nd Edition. Washington, DC, American Psychiatric Association, 1968

Asarnow JR: Annotation: childhood-onset schizophrenia. J Child Psychol Psychiatry 35:1345–1371, 1994

Asarnow JR, Tompson MC, Goldstein MJ: Childhood-onset schizophrenia: a followup study. Schizophr Bull 20:599–617, 1994

Asarnow RF, Asamen J, Granholm E, et al: Cognitive/neuropsychological studies of children with a schizophrenic disorder. Schizophr Bull 20:647–669, 1994

Bassett AS: Chromosomal aberrations and schizophrenia. Autosomes. Br J Psychiatry 161:323–334, 1992

Beitchman JH: Childhood schizophrenia. A review and comparison with adult-onset schizophrenia. Psychiatr Clin North Am 8:793–814, 1985

Bertolino A, Kumra S, Callicott J, et al: Proton magnetic resonance spectroscopic imaging in childhood-onset schizophrenia. Am J Psychiatry 155:1376–1383, 1998

Buka SL, Tsuang MT, Lipsitt LP: Pregnancy/delivery complications and psychiatric diagnosis: a prospective study. Arch Gen Psychiatry 50:151–156, 1993

Burrows R: The role of epidermal growth factor receptor mediated signaling in cortical and striatal development and its ligand transforming growth factor alpha, in the maintenance of mature cws. Doctoral thesis, Rutgers University and Robert Wood Johnson Medical School, October 1997

Cannon-Spoor HE, Potkin SG, Wyatt RJ: Measurement of premorbid adjustment in chronic schizophrenia. Schizophr Bull 8:470–484, 1982

Chakos MH, Lieberman JA, Alvir J, et al: Caudate nuclei volumes in schizophrenic patients treated with typical antipsychotics or clozapine. Lancet 345:456–457, 1995

Childs B, Scriver CR: Age at onset and causes of disease. Perspect Biol Med 29:437–460, 1986

Clementz BA, Grove WM, Iacono WG, et al: Smooth-pursuit eye movement dysfunction and liability for schizophrenia: implications for genetic modeling. J Abnorm Psychol 101:117–129, 1992

Corder EH, Saunders AM, Risch NJ, et al: Protective effect of apolipoprotein E type 2 allele for late onset Alzheimer disease. Nat Genet 7:180–184, 1994

DeLisi LE: Is schizophrenia a lifetime disorder of brain plasticity, growth and aging? Schizophr Res 23:119–129, 1997

DeLisi LE, Friedrich U, Wahlstrom J, et al: Schizophrenia and sex chromosome anomalies. Schizophr Bull 20:495–505, 1994

DeLisi LE, Tew W, Xie S, et al: A prospective follow-up study of brain morphology and cognition in first-episode schizophrenic patients: preliminary findings. Biol Psychiatry 38:349–360, 1995

Done DJ, Johnstone EC, Frith CD, et al: Complications of pregnancy and delivery in relation to psychosis in adult life: data from the British Perinatal Mortality Survey Sample. BMJ 302:1576–1580, 1991

Done DJ, Crow TJ, Johnstone EC, et al: Childhood antecedents of schizophrenia and affective illness: social adjustment at ages 7 and 11. BMJ 309:699–703, 1994

Eagles JM, Gibson I, Bremner MH, et al: Obstetric complications in DSM-III schizophrenics and their siblings. Lancet 335:1139–1141, 1990

Feinberg I: Schizophrenia: caused by a fault in programmed synaptic elimination during adolescence? J Psychiatr Res 17:319–334, 1982–1983

Fernandez T, Yan WL, Saunders AM, et al: Apolipoprotein E alleles in childhood-onset schizophrenia. Am J Med Genet 88:211–213, 1999

Frazier JA, Giedd JN, Hamburger SD, et al: Brain anatomic magnetic resonance imaging in childhood-onset schizophrenia. Arch Gen Psychiatry 53:617–624, 1996

Frazier JA, Alaghband-Rad J, Jacobsen L, et al: Pubertal development and onset of psychosis in childhood onset schizophrenia. Psychiatry Res 70:1–7, 1997

Fyer AJ, Endicott J, Mannuzza S, et al: Schedule for Affective Disorders and Schizophrenia—Lifetime Anxiety Version (SADS-LA). New York, Anxiety Disorders Clinic, New York State Psychiatric Institute, 1985

Geddes JR, Lawrie SM: Obstetric complications and schizophrenia: a meta-analysis. Br J Psychiatry 167:786–793, 1995

Ginns EI, St Jean P, Philibert RA, et al: A genome-wide search for chromosomal loci linked to mental health wellness in relatives at high risk for bipolar disorder among the Old Order Amish. Proc Natl Acad Sci U S A 95:15531–15536, 1998

Goldberg TE, Gold JM: Neurocognitive functioning in patients with schizophrenia: an overview, in Psychopharmacology: The Fourth Generation of Progress. Edited by Bloom FE, Kupfer DJ. New York, Raven, 1995, pp 1245–1257

Gordon CT, Frazier JA, McKenna K, et al: Childhood-onset schizophrenia: an NIMH study in progress. Schizophr Bull 20:697–712, 1994a

Gordon CT, Krasnewich D, White B, et al: Brief report: translocation involving chromosomes 1 and 7 in a boy with childhood-onset schizophrenia. J Autism Dev Disord 24:537–545, 1994b

Green WH, Padron-Gayol M, Hardesty AS, et al: Schizophrenia with childhood onset: a phenomenological study of 38 cases. J Am Acad Child Adolesc Psychiatry 31:968–976, 1992

Grove WM, Clementz BA, Iacono WG, et al: Smooth pursuit ocular motor dysfunction in schizophrenia: evidence for a major gene. Am J Psychiatry 149:1362–1368, 1992

Gunther-Genta F, Bovet P, Hohlfeld P: Obstetric complications and schizophrenia. A case-control study. Br J Psychiatry 164:165–170, 1994

Gupta S, Rajaprabhakaran R, Arndt S, et al: Premorbid adjustment as a predictor of phenomenological and neurobiological indices in schizophrenia. Schizophr Res 16:189–197, 1995

Gur RE, Cowell P, Turetsky BI, et al: A follow-up magnetic resonance imaging study of schizophrenia: relationship of neuroanatomical changes to clinical and neurobehavioral measures. Arch Gen Psychiatry 55:145–152, 1998

Hafner H, Maurer K, Loffler W, et al: The influence of age and sex on the onset and early course of schizophrenia. Br J Psychiatry 162:80–86, 1993

Hollis C: Child and adolescent (juvenile onset) schizophrenia: a case control study of premorbid developmental impairments. Br J Psychiatry 166:489–495, 1995

Huttenlocher PR: Synaptic density in human frontal cortex—developmental changes and effects of aging. Brain Res 163:195–205, 1979

Jacobsen LK, Rapoport JL: Childhood-onset schizophrenia: implications of clinical and neurobiological research. J Child Psychol Psychiatry 38:697–712, 1998

Jacobsen LK, Giedd JN, Vaituzis AC, et al: Temporal lobe morphology in childhood-onset schizophrenia. Am J Psychiatry 153:355–361, 1996a

Jacobsen LK, Hong WL, Hommer DW, et al: Smooth pursuit eye movements in childhood-onset schizophrenia: comparison with attention-deficit hyperactivity disorder and normal controls. Biol Psychiatry 40:1144–1154, 1996b

Jacobsen LK, Giedd JN, Berquin PC, et al: Quantitative morphology of the cerebellum and fourth ventricle in childhood-onset schizophrenia. Am J Psychiatry 154:1663–1669, 1997a

Jacobsen LK, Giedd JN, Rajapakse JC, et al: Quantitative magnetic resonance imaging of the corpus callosum in childhood onset schizophrenia. Psychiatry Res 68:77–86, 1997b

Jacobsen LK, Giedd JN, Tanrikut C, et al: Three-dimensional cortical morphometry of the planum temporale in childhood-onset schizophrenia. Am J Psychiatry 154:685–687, 1997c

Jacobsen LK, Hamburger SD, Van Horn JD, et al: Cerebral glucose metabolism in childhood onset schizophrenia. Psychiatry Res 75:131–144, 1997d

Jacobsen LK, Giedd JN, Vaituzis AC, et al: Progressive reduction of temporal lobe structures in childhood-onset schizophrenia. Am J Psychiatry 155:678–685, 1998a

Jacobsen LK, Mittleman BB, Kumra S, et al: HLA antigens in childhood onset schizophrenia. Psychiatry Res 78:123–132, 1998b

Jones PB, Done J: From birth to onset: a developmental perspective in two national birth cohorts, in Neurodevelopment and Adult Psychopathology. Edited by Keshavan MS, Murray RM. New York, Cambridge University Press, 1997, pp 119-136.

Jones P, Rodgers B, Murray R, et al: Child development risk factors for schizophrenia in the British 1946 Birth Cohort. Lancet 344:1398–1402, 1994

Jones PB, Rantakallio P, Hartikainen AL, et al: Schizophrenia as a long-term outcome of pregnancy, delivery, and perinatal complications: a 28-year follow-up of the 1966 North Finland General Population Birth Cohort. Am J Psychiatry 155:355–364, 1998

Kallmann FJ, Roth B: Genetic aspects of preadolescent schizophrenia. Am J Psychiatry 112:599–606, 1956

Karayiorgou M, Gogos JA: A turning point in schizophrenia genetics. Neuron 19:967–979, 1997

Keefe RS, Silverman JM, Mohs RC, et al: Eye tracking, attention, and schizotypal symptoms in nonpsychotic relatives of patients with schizophrenia. Arch Gen Psychiatry 54:169–176, 1997

Kendler KS: The impact of diagnostic hierarchies on prevalence estimates for psychiatric disorders. Compr Psychiatry 29:218–227, 1988

Kendler KS, Diehl SR: The genetics of schizophrenia: a current, genetic-epidemiologic perspective. Schizophr Bull 19:261–285, 1993

Kendler KS, Tsuang MT, Hays P: Age at onset in schizophrenia: a familial perspective. Arch Gen Psychiatry 44:881–890, 1987

Kendler KS, McGuire M, Gruenberg AM, et al: The Roscommon Family Study, I: methods, diagnosis of probands, and risk of schizophrenia in relatives. Arch Gen Psychiatry 50:527–540, 1993a

Kendler KS, McGuire M, Gruenberg AM, et al: The Roscommon Family Study, II: the risk of nonschizophrenic nonaffective psychoses in relatives. Arch Gen Psychiatry 50:645–652, 1993b

Kendler KS, McGuire M, Gruenberg AM, et al: The Roscommon Family Study, III: schizophrenia-related personality disorders in relatives. Arch Gen Psychiatry 50:781–788, 1993c

Kendler KS, Gruenberg AM, Kinney DK: Independent diagnoses of adoptees and relatives as defined by DSM-III in the provincial and national samples of the Danish Adoption Study of Schizophrenia. Arch Gen Psychiatry 51:456–468, 1994

Kendler KS, Karkowski-Shuman L, Walsh D: Age at onset in schizophrenia and risk of illness in relatives. Results from the Roscommon Family Study. Br J Psychiatry 169:213–218, 1996

Keshavan MS, Pettegrew JW: Magnetic resonance spectroscopy in schizophrenia and psychotic disorders, in Brain Imaging in Clinical Psychiatry. Edited by Krishnan KRR, Doraiswamy PM. New York, Marcel Dekker, 1997, pp 382–400

Kolvin I: Studies in the childhood psychoses, I: diagnostic criteria and classification. Br J Psychiatry 118:381–384, 1971

Kumra S, Bedwell J, Hommer D, et al: Comparison of smooth pursuit eye movements in pediatric patients with childhood-onset schizophrenia and "multidimensionally impaired syndrome." Biol Psychiatry 43:685, 1998a

Kumra S, Jacobsen LK, Lenane M, et al: "Multidimensionally impaired disorder": is it a variant of very early-onset schizophrenia? J Am Acad Child Adolesc Psychiatry 37:91–99, 1998b

Kumra S, Wiggs E, Krasnewich D, et al: Brief report: association of sex chromosome anomalies with childhood-onset psychotic disorders. J Am Acad Child Adolesc Psychiatry 37:292–296, 1998c

Kumra S, Wiggs E, Bedwell J, et al: Neuropsychological deficits in childhood-onset schizophrenia and "multi-dimensionally impaired syndrome." Schizophr Res (in press)

Lenane MC, Nicolson R, Bedwell J, et al: Schizophrenia spectrum disorders in the relatives of patients with childhood-onset schizophrenia. Schizophr Res 36:92, 1999

Levy DL, Holzman PS, Matthysse S, et al: Eye tracking dysfunction and schizophrenia: a critical perspective. Schizophr Bull 19:461–536, 1993

Lewis SW, Owen MJ, Murray RM: Obstetric complications and schizophrenia: methodology and mechanisms, in Schizophrenia: Scientific Progress. Edited by Schulz SC, Tamminga CA. New York, Oxford University Press, 1989, pp 56–68

Lieberman JA, Alvir JM, Koreen A, et al: Psychobiologic correlates of treatment response in schizophrenia. Neuropsychopharmacology 14(3, suppl):13S–21S, 1996

Litman RE, Torrey EF, Hommer DW, et al: A quantitative analysis of smooth pursuit eye tracking in monozygotic twins discordant for schizophrenia. Arch Gen Psychiatry 54:417–426, 1997

McKenna K, Gordon CT, Lenane M, et al: Looking for childhood-onset schizophrenia: the first 71 cases screened. J Am Acad Child Adolesc Psychiatry 33:636–644, 1994a

McKenna K, Gordon CT, Rapoport JL: Childhood-onset schizophrenia: timely neurobiological research. J Am Acad Child Adolesc Psychiatry 33:771–781, 1994b

Murray RM, Lewis SW: Is schizophrenia a neurodevelopmental disorder? BMJ 295:681–682, 1987

Nicolson R, Hommer D, Thaker G, et al: Smooth pursuit eye movements in the relatives of patients with childhood-onset schizophrenia. Schizophr Res 36:93, 1999

Nicolson R, Malaspina D, Giedd JN, et al: Obstetrical complications in childhood-onset schizophrenia. Am J Psychiatry (in press)

Nicolson R, Singaracharlu S, Lenane MC, et al: Premorbid language and motor abnormalities in childhood-onset schizophrenia: association with genetic risk factors. Presentation at the annual meeting of the American College of Neuropsychopharmacology, 1998

O'Callaghan E, Gibson T, Colohan HA, et al: Risk of schizophrenia in adults born after obstetric complications and their association with early onset of illness: a controlled study. BMJ 305:1256–1259, 1993

Picchio GR, Gulizia RJ, Mosier DE: Chemokine receptor CCR5 genotype influences the kinetics of human immunodeficiency virus type 1 infection in human PBL-SCID mice. J Virol 71:7124–7127, 1997

Rapoport JL, Giedd J, Kumra S, et al: Childhood-onset schizophrenia: progressive ventricular change during adolescence. Arch Gen Psychiatry 54:897–903, 1997

Russell AT: The clinical presentation of childhood-onset schizophrenia. Schizophr Bull 20:631–646, 1994

Shenton ME, Wible CG, McCarley RW: A review of magnetic resonance imaging studies of brain abnormalities in schizophrenia, in Brain Imaging in Clinical Psychiatry. Edited by Krishnan KRR, Doraiswamy PM. New York, Marcel Dekker, 1997, pp 297–380

Sidransky E, Burgess C, Ikeuchi T, et al: A polymorphic long trinucleotide repeat on 17q accounts for most CAG/CTG expansions detected by the Repeat Expansion Detection (RED) technique. Am J Hum Genet 62:1548–1551, 1998

Spencer EK, Campbell M: Children with schizophrenia: diagnosis, phenomenology, and pharmacotherapy. Schizophr Bull 20:713–725, 1994

Swanson CL, Mozley LMH, Gur RE: Positron emission tomography studies of cerebral metabolism and blood flow in schizophrenia, in Brain Imaging in Clinical Psychiatry. Edited by Krishnan KRR, Doraiswamy PM. New York, Marcel Dekker, 1997, pp 401–424

Verdoux H, Geddes JR, Takei N, et al: Obstetric complications and age at onset in schizophrenia: an international collaborative meta-analysis of individual patient data. Am J Psychiatry 154:1220–1227, 1997

Weinberger DR: Implications of normal brain development for the pathogenesis of schizophrenia. Arch Gen Psychiatry 44:660–669, 1987

Weiss KM: Genetic Variation and Human Disease: Principles and Evolutionary Approaches. New York, Cambridge University Press, 1993

Werry JS: Childhood schizophrenia, in Psychoses and Pervasive Developmental Disorders in Childhood and Adolescence. Edited by Volkmar FR. Washington, DC, American Psychiatric Press, 1996, pp 1–48

Wicker LS, Todd JA, Prins JB, et al: Resistance alleles at two non–major histocompatibility complex–linked insulin-dependent diabetes loci on chromosome 3, Idd3 and Idd10, protect nonobese diabetic mice from diabetes. J Exp Med 180:1705–1713, 1994

Yan WL, Jacobsen LK, Krasnewich DM, et al: Chromosome 22q11.2 interstitial deletions among childhood-onset schizophrenics and "multidimensionally impaired." Am J Med Genet 81:41–43, 1998

Yolken RH, Torrey EF: Viruses, schizophrenia, and bipolar disorder. Clin Microbiol Rev 8:131–145, 1995

Zahn TP, Jacobsen LK, Gordon CT, et al: Autonomic nervous system markers of psychopathology in childhood-onset schizophrenia. Arch Gen Psychiatry 54:904–912, 1997

CHAPTER 9

Neurodevelopmental Hypothesis of Schizophrenia 12 Years On: Data and Doubts

Colm McDonald, M.B., M.R.C.Psych.

Paul Fearon, M.B., M.R.C.Psych.

Robin M. Murray, D.Sc., F.R.C.Psych.

In the early (Feinberg 1982–1983; Randall 1983) and mid-1980s (Murray et al. 1985, 1988; Schulsinger et al. 1984; Weinberger 1987), several research groups began to suggest that schizophrenia might have a significant developmental component. In 1987, these ideas were summarized in an editorial in the *British Medical Journal* entitled "Is Schizophrenia a Neurodevelopmental Disorder?" (Murray and Lewis 1987). Over the ensuing decade, what came to be known as the "neurodevelopmental hypothesis" gained momentum to the point where it now appears to be the dominant paradigm in schizophrenia research. Indeed, authors frequently refer to schizophrenia as a neurodevelopmental disease as if this were an established fact. It seems timely, therefore, to reexamine the evidence put forward in the mid-1980s in support of the neurodevelopmental hypothesis to assess whether it has received subsequent support and whether additional information not available at that time bolsters or undermines the hypothesis.

Has the Evidence Originally Proposed Stood Up to Subsequent Challenge?

The modern era of schizophrenia research began with the demonstration by Johnstone et al. (1976) of increased ventricular size in schizophrenia as evidenced on computed tomography (CT) scans. This finding, and its later confirmations (Chua and McKenna 1995; Lewis 1990; Woodruff and Murray 1994), were initially interpreted as evidence of neurodegeneration (Johnstone et al. 1978). However, as Lewis (1997) noted, "[i]t was the change of interpretation of these findings in the mid-1980s that was one of the founding observations which fuelled the emergence of the neurodevelopmental hypothesis of schizophrenia" (p. 178).

What Caused the Reinterpretation of Structural Brain Changes?

What determined the change in interpretation of structural brain changes in schizophrenia from a neurodegenerative to a neurodevelopmental hypothesis? Factors in this shift included the evidence that ventricular enlargement occurred in patients with first-onset schizophrenia (DeLisi et al. 1991; Turner et al. 1986) and that the ventricular enlargement demonstrated with CT did not progress over prolonged periods (Illowski et al. 1988; Nasrallah et al. 1986). Such observations suggested that the structural brain abnormalities found in schizophrenia are not degenerative, but they did not, of course, prove these abnormalities to be developmental in origin.

Was there in early imaging studies evidence of abnormal brain development in persons with schizophrenia? Importantly, Lewis (1990) pointed out that developmental brain lesions, such as aqueduct stenosis, arachnoid and septal cysts, and agenesis of the corpus callosum (Lewis and Murray 1987; O'Callaghan et al. 1992a; Owens et al. 1980), occur with excess frequency in schizophrenia. Although such lesions were noted in only a small minority of cases, the case was made that these were the visible manifestations of a much more common process of early developmental deviance. This, of course, was supposition, not evidence.

However, Weinberger et al. (1980) had noted an association between changes on CT and poor premorbid functioning in schizophrenia, an association later confirmed with magnetic resonance imaging (MRI) by Harvey et al. (1993). Subsequently, Walker et al. (1996) related MRI findings to observations made of childhood video recordings of patients with schizophrenia prior to the onset of the disorder and their healthy siblings; early childhood neuromotor defects and negative affect were associated with greater ventricular size in adult life.

Postmortem studies confirmed the evidence of ventricular enlargement in schizophrenia as well as reduced brain weight and length (Bruton et al. 1990; Johnstone et al. 1994; Pakkenberg 1987), particularly in patients who had an early onset of illness and poor premorbid functioning (Johnstone et al. 1989).

Is the Evidence Concerning Cytoarchitecture Robust?

Two reports of microscopic abnormalities in the brains of schizophrenic patients at postmortem were particularly influential in the formulation of the developmental hypothesis. In the first report, Kovelman and Scheibel (1984) claimed to find pyramidal cell disorientation in the CA1-prosubiculum, CA1-CA2, and CA2-CA3 interface zones of the hippocampus, and the authors argued that this disorientation could only have resulted from a developmental failure. Unfortunately, these findings have not been consistently replicated (Arnold et al. 1995; Benes et al. 1991b; Christison et al. 1989; Cotter et al. 1997).

In the second report, Jakob and Beckmann (1986) claimed to find displaced pre-alpha cells in the parahippocampal cortex in schizophrenia and concluded that this was due to impaired neuronal migration during the second trimester of pregnancy. Again, however, these findings have never been adequately replicated (Akil and Lewis 1997; Krimer et al. 1997).

Argument over the presence or absence of gliosis, a marker of brain injury, in postmortem schizophrenic brains also aroused much interest a decade ago (Falkai and Bogerts 1986; Roberts et al. 1987; Stevens et al. 1988). Since fetal brain tissue is incapable of a glial reaction until the sixth month (Larroche 1984), the absence of gliosis has been frequently cited in support of a developmental origin for schizophrenia. In truth, it simply indicates the absence of a degenerative process.

How Secure Is the Evidence of Exposure to Early Environmental Hazards?

Studies showing an excess of obstetric complications in schizophrenic patients compared with control subjects strongly influenced European groups toward a developmental view of schizophrenia in the 1980s (McNeil and Kaij 1978; Parnas et al. 1982; Murray and Lewis 1987; Murray et al. 1988). Initially controversial, this evidence is now overwhelming (Geddes et al., in press; Lewis and Murray 1987; McGrath and Murray 1995; McNeil 1995; O'Callaghan et al. 1992b).

Three recent studies have been particularly convincing. In a study from Sweden, Hultman et al. (1999) compared antenatal and delivery records for each of 167 schizophrenic patients with those for 5 matched control subjects; the schizophrenic patients, particularly males, were significantly more likely to have had an excess of pre- and perinatal complications.

Jones et al. (1998), who carried out a large birth cohort study in northern Finland, found that the 76 individuals who developed schizophrenia were seven times more likely to have had perinatal brain damage and six times more likely to have been born prematurely than the remainder of the cohort. Finally, Geddes et al. (in press) carried out a meta-analysis of 11 studies involving 700 patients with schizophrenia and 835 control subjects that had used the scale of Lewis et al. (1989) to assess obstetric complications. The obstetric complications particularly implicated included low birthweight, prematurity, required rescucitation, placement in an incubator, and premature rupture of membranes. A common factor underlying these complications may be hypoxic-ischemic brain damage (Fearon et al., in press; McNeil 1988; McNeil and Kaij 1978).

Are Delivery Complications Secondary to Earlier Abnormality?

The association of detectable obstetric complications with schizophrenia does not prove causality, since complications late in pregnancy may be a consequence of earlier fetal abnormality. Suggestions of earlier impairment of fetal brain growth come from reports that schizophrenia is associated with smaller head circumference at birth (Hultman et al. 1997; Kunugi et al. 1996; McNeil et al. 1993; Rifkin et al. 1994).

The small excess of late winter/early spring births among patients with schizophrenia (Hare 1988) has been repeatedly confirmed (Torrey et al. 1997), particularly among schizophrenic patients born in urban rather than rural settings (Machon et al. 1983; O'Callaghan et al. 1995; Takei et al. 1995; Verdoux et al. 1997b). A possible explanation for both the season-of-birth effect and decreased brain growth is prenatal exposure to an infection facilitated by winter and by urban crowding.

The epidemiology of influenza conforms to such a pattern, and some (e.g., Mednick et al. 1988; O'Callaghan et al. 1991b; Sham et al. 1992), but by no means all (e.g., Crow and Done 1992; Torrey et al. 1988), studies have reported an increase in births of schizophrenic individuals in the 4–5 months following influenza epidemics (for review, see McGrath and Murray 1995). The possibility that such infections may cause later obstetric complications was suggested by P. Wright et al. (1995), who demonstrated that schizophrenic individuals whose mothers recalled having influenza during the second trimester of gestation were of lower birthweight and had more perinatal complications than schizophrenic individuals whose mothers reported having no infections during pregnancy.

Recently, Brown et al. (1998) suggested that prenatal exposure to rubella is also a risk factor for later schizophrenia. The same group reported that persons exposed to severe malnutrition during the first trimester due to wartime famine in Holland were at increased risk of developing schizophrenia in adult life (Susser and Lin 1992; Susser et al. 1996). Neither of these studies has yet been replicated.

Finally, several recent studies have noted elevated rates of diabetes mellitus in mothers of schizophrenic patients (S. Buka, personal communication, 1998; A. Fishleigh-Eaton, personal communication, 1998; Hultman et al. 1999; P. Wright et al. 1996). The offspring of diabetic mothers are well known to be at increased risk of abortion, perinatal death, and congenital malformations (see Casson et al. 1997).

Do Early Hazards Contribute to Structural Brain Abnormalities?

Reports (Reveley et al. 1984; Schulsinger et al. 1984) of an association between increased VBR and obstetric complications played an important formative role in the neurodevelopmental hypothesis. For example, Murray et al. (1985) cited evidence that preterm infants are at risk of hypoxia-ischemia with resultant intra- and periventricular hemorrhage. Many subsequent studies (Kempley et al. 1996; Paneth et al. 1993; Penrice et al. 1996) have demonstrated that the long-term consequences of such hemorrhage include ventricular enlargement and cortical and corpus callosal abnormalities (Leviton and Gilles 1996; Stewart and Kirkbride 1996; Stewart et al. 1999).

Although a number of studies of patients with schizophrenia have found a relationship between obstetric complications and lateral ventricular enlargement, others have not (for review, see McGrath and Murray 1995). Consequently, the question of whether obstetric complications contribute to ventricular enlargement in schizophrenia remains unresolved, although in our view several of the negative studies are invalidated by their use of poor-quality obstetric data.

What about other structural abnormalities? Stefanis et al. (in press) tested the hypothesis that hippocampal volume decrement is secondary to perinatal hypoxia-ischemia by carrying out MRI scans on schizophrenic patients without a history of obstetric complications who came from multiply affected families (a group in whom genetic factors play an overwhelming role) and patients with nonfamilial schizophrenia who had a history of severe obstetric complications (i.e., a group enriched for early environmental insult). The familial group showed no decrement in hippocampal volume compared with the control subjects, but the group with obstetric complications did have significantly smaller hippocampi, especially on the left. Thus, hippocampal volume reduction in schizophrenia appears to be associated with hypoxic-ischemic damage. The fact that only a minority of schizophrenic patients have suffered such damage provides one explanation as to why reduction in hippocampal volume has not been found in some series (see Altshuler et al. 1990; Benes et al. 1991b; Bruton et al. 1990; Heckers et al. 1990).

What Does a Reassessment of the Original Evidence Tell Us?

The macroscopic findings in schizophrenia reported a decade ago—increased cerebrospinal fluid spaces and decreased brain volume—have generally been replicated. There is little convincing evidence of change after the onset of illness, and the abnormalities appear most marked in patients who had shown dysfunction in childhood. However, it has not been conclusively proven that the abnormalities occur in fetal or neonatal life. An alternative explanation is that that they occur during, or shortly before, adolescence (Feinberg 1997; Keshavan 1997). Furthermore, the findings in the two articles most frequently cited as providing incontrovertible evidence of early neurodevelopmental abnormality (Jakob and Beckmann 1986; Kovelman and Scheibel 1984) have not been substantiated.

However, evidence for an association between obstetric complications and schizophrenia has steadily accumulated, and this association must now be regarded as well established. Whether hypoxic-ischemic damage is the primary mediating factor or only one of a number of prenatal and perinatal risk factors is uncertain. The evidence concerning prenatal viral exposure and maternal diabetes is suggestive but not definitive, and the findings concerning malnutrition are tentative.

Furthermore, prenatal and perinatal risk factors are noted in only a minority of cases of schizophrenia, and the proportion of cases of schizophrenia that can be attributed to detectable early environmental hazards is reportedly less than 20%. Such factors, therefore, cannot explain all of the brain changes found in schizophrenia, though they may well be responsible for the hippocampal volume decrement found in some patients and probably make a contribution to increased ventricular volume.

What Have Subsequent Studies Contributed to the Neurodevelopmental Hypothesis?

It is clear that the evidence originally proposed in support of the neurodevelopmental hypothesis has proved untrustworthy in some respects.

However, other information not available in the 1980s has come from subsequent investigations. Such information concerns physical and childhood development in schizophrenia; it also comes from studies relating the nature of structural brain abnormalities to their time of origin and from new theories concerning aberrant neural networks in schizophrenia.

Is There Evidence of Deviant Physical and Psychological Development?

Dermatoglyphic patterns are formed in the late first and second trimesters and remain unchanged thereafter. Abnormality in these patterns, as well as minor physical abnormalities, can be regarded as "fossilized" evidence of disturbed development at the time that the brain, another ectodermally derived structure, was undergoing its most extensive period of growth.

Dermatoglyphic abnormalities are found in excess in schizophrenia (Davis and Bracha 1996; Fañanas et al. 1996), as are minor physical anomalies (Clouston 1891, 1892; Fañanas et al. 1996; Green et al. 1994; Griffiths et al. 1998; Lane et al. 1997; McGrath et al. 1995; Mellor 1992; O'Callaghan et al. 1991a). Furthermore, if MRI changes are secondary to disruption of fetal development, then they should be found particularly in schizophrenic patients who show dermatoglyphic abnormalities. Van Os et al. (1997b) found such a relationship between reduced total a-b ridge count and both frontal cerebrospinal fluid and third-ventricle volume and between total finger ridge count and both total cerebral and temporal lobe volume.

Fish (1977) pointed out that the increased prevalence of "soft" neurological signs in the offspring of individuals with schizophrenia was consistent with an "inherited neurointegrative deficit." Such findings attracted little interest until the advent of the neurodevelopmental hypothesis. Walker (1993), who examined home movies of individuals with schizophrenia as children prior to development of the disorder, noted more postural and upper-limb movement abnormalities than in their well siblings. These abnormalities were most noticeable in the first 2 years of life and ameliorated thereafter (Walker et al. 1996), a course that raises the possibility of ongoing recovery from an early lesion. The evidence concerning dermatoglyphic patterns and minor physical anomalies, and the findings that children who go on to develop schizophrenia tend to have abnormal neurological, social, and cognitive functioning (Foerster 1991a, 1991b; Jones et al. 1994; Walker 1993), are described in greater detail elsewhere in this volume (see Chapter 4).

Can the Nature of the Structural Abnormalities Be Used to Help Time Their Origin?

Murray and Lewis (1987) cited abnormalities of handedness in schizophrenia in support of the developmental hypothesis a decade ago. Subsequent studies have confirmed that mixed handedness occurs with increased frequency in schizophrenia, and two British cohort studies (Cannon et al. 1997; Crow et al. 1996) have shown an excess of mixed hand and eye dominance in children who went on to develop schizophrenia.

Might the above characteristics be related to loss of the normal brain asymmetry that has been reported in patients with schizophrenia (Bilder et al. 1994; Bullmore et al. 1995; Crow et al. 1989)? The normal brain is typically asymmetrical, with the right hemisphere being greater than the left in anterior regions and the left hemisphere being greater than the right in posterior regions. Brain asymmetry is usually complete by the middle of the third trimester of gestation. The reduced brain asymmetry found in individuals with schizophrenia must therefore originate during fetal life.

Furthermore, Sharma et al. (1998, in press) have shown that in families with several schizophrenic members, those unaffected parents who appear to be transmitting the disorder ("presumed obligate carriers") have not only enlarged lateral ventricles but also loss of frontal and occipitoparietal asymmetries. That is, these families are transmitting a liability to deviant fetal brain development.

Further evidence implicating deviant fetal development in schizophrenia comes from examination of the relationship between different brain structures. Woodruff et al. (1997b) demonstrated significant positive correlations between the volumes of regions of the frontal and temporal lobes in psychiatrically healthy subjects. However, these correlations were significantly reduced in a group of male patients with chronic schizophrenia, a finding that suggests a loss of early correlated development.

Do Dysplastic Neural Networks Underlie Loss of Normal Functional Connectivity

How does early brain abnormality increase the risk of later psychotic symptoms? One step toward an explanation has come from the formulation of theories postulating that symptoms of schizophrenia result from loss of functional connectivity between cortical networks involved in the performance of complex mental functions. For instance, psychiatrically healthy subjects performing a word generation task show increased regional cerebral blood flow (rCBF) in left dorsolateral prefrontal cortex but decreased rCBF in temporal regions (Frith et al. 1991a); this pattern of inverse correlation between frontal and temporal rCBF changes is lost in patients with schizophrenia (Friston 1994). Indeed, such patients fail to show the normal deactivation of temporal auditory processing areas when they generate inner speech. McGuire et al. (1993, 1995) suggest that this deficit leads the patients to mislabel their own internal speech as external voices.

Might there be a structural basis to this disruption of frontotemporal network integrity? I. C. Wright et al. (1999) reported that the maximal decrements in cortical volume between schizophrenic patients and control subjects were in frontotemporal areas. Furthermore, the previously noted finding of reduced volume correlations between frontal and temporal structures suggests a loss of the normal coordinated development of these regions (Bullmore et al. 1997; Woodruff et al. 1997b).

Woodruff et al. (1997a) also noted that schizophrenic patients showed a loss of the normal pattern of left-greater-than-right activation of temporal areas during processing of external speech. Is it possible that the loss of this activation pattern may be related to the loss of the normal asymmetry of brain structure seen on MRI in schizophrenia noted earlier?

The possibility that abnormal network connectivity in adult schizophrenia may be determined in part by dysplastic axonal projection in fetal or neonatal life is in accord with what we know concerning the plasticity of the immature brain in response to lesions. Thus, Karmiloff-Smith (1997) points out that an individual with early brain abnormality cannot be viewed as having a normal brain with some functions intact and others impaired; rather such a brain develops differently from the very outset. Indeed, Galaburda (1997) attributes dyslexia to the effect of such early compensatory plasticity in producing "abnormally connected neuronal groups" in response to cortical microgyria. Perhaps the preschizophrenic brain also develops unusual neuronal networks that, although largely functional, are nevertheless prone to dysfunction.

The idea of the early development of aberrant neuronal networks in schizophrenia gained support from the work of Benes and her colleagues, who demonstrated altered arrangement of neurons in the anterior cingulate (Benes and Bird 1987; Benes et al. 1986) and the prefrontal cortex (Anderson et al. 1996; Benes et al. 1991a) in schizo-phrenia. Benes (1997) implied that such abnormalities may be secondary to perinatal complications or prenatal stress.

Akbarian et al. (1993a, 1993b, 1996) have reported abnormal distribution of NADPH-d neurons in the frontal and temporal cortex of patients with schizophrenia; this distribution is consistent with a disturbance of either the normal pattern of programmed cell death or the orderly migration of neurons during the second or third trimesters. It may be relevant to the latter that decreased expression of the embryonic form of the neural cell adhesion molecule (NCAM) family, an essential trophic factor during neuronal migration and development, has been reported in schizophrenia (Barbeau et al. 1995).

The possibility that abnormal connectivity underlies schizophrenia is also given credence by recent studies investigating dendrites and synapses. Golgi studies have demonstrated a decrease in dendritic spines in schizophrenic subjects (Glantz and Lewis 1995), an alteration that has been confirmed by ultrastructural studies showing abnormal dendritic spine clustering (Ong et al. 1993). Likewise, the synaptic markers GAP 43 (Perrone-Bizzozero et al. 1996), synaptophysin and SNAP-35 (Eastwood et al. 1995a; Glantz and Lewis 1994), synapsin (Browning 1993), and the encoding mRNA for synaptophysin (Eastwood et al. 1995b) are reduced in schizophrenia.

What Does the Neurodevelopmental Hypothesis Fail to Explain?

Onset in Adolescence or Early Adult Life

A crucial difficulty for the neurodevelopmental hypothesis is the lack of a convincing explanation as to why abnormal neuronal networks present since fetal life do not cause psychosis until decades later. A variety of speculative explanations for this delay have been put forward, largely on the basis of the evidence that the normal processes of brain maturation continue until after adolescence (Clouston 1892; Benes 1989; Feinberg 1982–1983; Lipska and Weinberger 1993; Lipska et al. 1993; Olney and Farber 1995; Weinberger and Lipska 1995).

What factors influence the onset of psychosis? Although there are wide variations (Castle et al. 1998), indicators of aberrant neurodevelopment, such as cognitive deficits, minor physical anomalies, and larger cerebral ventricles, are associated with an earlier age at onset (Aylward et al. 1984; DeLisi et al. 1991; Green et al. 1987; Johnstone et al. 1989).

Furthermore, the age at onset of schizophrenia in males is earlier than in females (Angermeyer and Kuhn 1988; Castle et al. 1993, 1998). Is this sex difference genetically or environmentally determined? Walsh et al. (1996) compared patients from families with two or more schizophrenic members with patients from an epidemiological sample unselected for family history. The age at onset was earlier in the familial group, but, in contrast to the epidemiological sample, there was no difference between males and females. This lack of gender difference in such genetically loaded groups of patients with a family history of schizophrenia has been consistently reported (DeLisi et al. 1987; Leboyer et al. 1992; Wolyniec et al. 1992) and implies that the earlier age at onset in males must be environmentally determined.

How can this be explained? Schizophrenic patients exposed to obstetric complications develop the disorder earlier than those without such a history (Lewis et al. 1989; O'Callaghan et al. 1992b; Verdoux et al. 1997a), and some studies suggest that male schizophrenic individuals are more likely to have suffered obstetric complications than their female counterparts (Castle and Murray 1991; Hultman et al. 1999). Kirov et al. (1996) reported that male schizophrenic patients with a history of obstetric complications had an earlier age at onset than those without such a history but that their female equivalents did not; when patients with a history of obstetric complications were not considered in the comparison, the gender difference in age at onset disappeared.

Thus, it appears that obstetric complications are responsible for the earlier age at onset in male schizophrenic individuals. Males with schizophrenia are also more likely to have had premorbid cognitive deficits and poor social adjustment (Foerster et al. 1991b). Rifkin et al. (1994) found an association between obstetric complications and childhood dysfunction in male, but not female, schizophrenic patients. Neurological soft signs have also been reported in schizophrenic patients, especially in male patients with a history of obstetric complications (Lane et al. 1996).

Occurrence of Late-Onset Psychosis

From the foregoing it can be seen that known risk factors (family history and obstetric complications) are more common in early- than late-onset schizophrenia. Moreover, the very fact that schizophrenia can have onset later in life poses a problem for neurodevelopmental theorists (Castle et al. 1998). Most late-onset patients (those with onset after age 45 years) functioned reasonably well early in life (Castle et al. 1998), and their relatives have a lower morbid risk of schizophrenia, implying that in such cases less genetic loading for schizophrenia is carried. Indeed, we have found that the relatives of patients with late-onset schizophrenia have an increased risk of affective disorder (Howard et al. 1997). Thus, one possible explanation for cases of late-onset schizophrenia is that the patients may have an illness that is related to affective disorder. A second possibility is that brain abnormality of a degenerative type is involved (Murray et al. 1992).

Progression of Abnormality

Some reports have suggested progression of certain structural brain changes in patients with earlier-onset schizophrenia (Rapoport et al. 1997). For example, DeLisi et al. (1997) compared the rate of change in the size of certain brain structures in a 4-year follow-up of individuals with first-episode schizophrenia and age-matched control subjects. There were no differences in the rate of change for the volumes of the caudate nucleus, temporal lobes, or hippocampus, but there were differences in the overall volumes of the left and right hemispheres and the right cerebellum and in the area of the isthmus of the corpus callosum. The authors suggested that a subtle active brain process exists in the first few years of an illness related to schizophrenia.

A more common view is that there is a decline in IQ following the onset of schizophrenia. However, several such reports have used the National Adult Reading Test to estimate premorbid IQ for comparison with tests of current functioning (Crawford et al. 1992; Frith et al. 1991b). Russell and her colleagues (in press) have found that the National Adult Reading Test overestimates premorbid IQ in individuals with schizophrenia and that, therefore, researchers are misled into concluding that IQ has declined. Russell et al. (1997), in a follow-up study of schizophrenic patients who had been tested at a child guidance clinic some 20 years earlier, prior to the development of the disorder, found no significant decline in IQ.

Thus, there is no consensus on whether there are progressive changes in both cerebral structure and neuropsychological performance in schizophrenia. Although progression is not considered an alternative explanation to the developmental hypothesis of the etiology of schizophrenia, controversy remains over whether both developmental factors and progressive factors play a role.

Subtle and Relatively Nonspecific Abnormalities

The cerebral structural abnormalities found in schizophrenia are far from gross, and some neuroimaging studies have failed to find such differences in comparisons of patients with schizophrenia and control subjects (Chua and McKenna 1995). Similarly, the childhood abnormalities are minor in degree compared with the major dysfunction evidenced in frank psychosis; indeed, many individuals who develop schizophrenia perform at or above average levels in childhood. Do these "normal" children have neurodevelopmental impairment too subtle for us to detect, or does neurodevelopmental abnormality play no role in their condition?

The notion that schizophrenia is a neurodevelopmental disorder implies that schizophrenia is a discrete entity. However, the major psychoses display considerable overlap not only in phenomenology but also in outcome and risk factors (J. Van Os and R. M. Murray, "Neurodevelopmental and Social Risk Factors Across the Continuum of Psychosis," submitted; Van Os et al. 1996). Thus, obstetric complications are also found in excess in patients with early-onset affective disorder (Guth et al. 1993; Hultman et al. 1999), as are minor physical anomalies (Lohr and Flynn 1993; McGrath et al. 1995), though they are less common than among patients with schizophrenia. Furthermore, chronically depressed patients, particularly those who present for treatment early in life, tend to have childhood abnormalities similar to, though less severe than, those seen in schizophrenic patients (Van Os et al. 1997a). (See Chapter 4, this volume, for a fuller discussion of these issues.)

In addition, cerebral ventricle and sulcal enlargements are also found in affective psychosis, although the effect size is larger for schizophrenia (Elkis et al. 1995). On the other hand, at least some patients with schizophrenia, particularly female patients and patients with acute onset of the illness, appear to share both the familial predisposition of affective disorder and the excess of adverse life events that is found among patients with affective psychosis (Murray et al. 1992; J. Van Os and R. M. Murray, "Neurodevelopmental and Social Risk Factors Across the Continuum of Psychosis," submitted).

Where Is the Search for a Plausible Model Taking Us?

Does the evidence we have reviewed prove that there is a single or simple developmental origin for all of what we conventionally term schizophrenia? The short answer is no! The more plausible versions of the neurodevelopmental hypothesis, therefore, propose that a proportion, but only a proportion, of variance in liability to schizophrenia can be attributed to impairment of brain growth resulting from the inheritance of abnormal genes, some form of fetal or neonatal adversity, or a combination of these factors.

To address these issues, Murray et al. (1992) proposed a classification of schizophrenia consisting of two main forms: a congenital (or neurodevelopmental) type and an adult-onset type with much in common with affective psychosis. These authors also raised the possibility of a less common, late-onset degenerative form. Such a classification has as much genetic validity as the traditional Kraepelinian dichotomy of psychosis (Corrigall and Murray 1994), but it encounters as much difficulty as the latter when cases on the borders between the categories are being considered.

To overcome this problem, Van Os and Murray ("Neurodevelopmental and Social Risk Factors Across the Continuum of Psychosis," submitted) proposed a dimensional version of the model in which there exists a spectrum of psychosis that is under the influence of two major classes of risk factor. The first is a "neurodevelopmental" factor that operates across forms of psychosis but has the most effect in cases of chronic psychosis with early onset and poor outcome. Such individuals tend to have a history of a family member with schizophrenia or of obstetric complications; they are more likely to be male and to have shown poor premorbid functioning as well as negative symptoms and structural brain abnormality.

The second is a "social reactive" factor that reflects genetic predisposition to react to social adversity by developing psychotic symptoms; its effect is maximal at the acute onset–good outcome end of the psychosis spectrum. Such individuals characteristically have affective symptoms or a relative with affective disorder. They are more likely to be female and generally have good premorbid function, and their symptoms run a relapsing and remitting course.

Thus, 12 years after the modern reformulation of the neurodevelopmental hypothesis, it remains unclear exactly how neurodevelopment contributes to psychosis and how much of the variance in liability to psychosis developmental factors can explain. What is clear, however, is that the role of neurodevelopmental impairment can no longer be ignored as it was for almost a century.

References

Akbarian S, Bunney WE, Potkin SJ, et al: Altered distribution of nicotinamide-adenine dinucleotide phosphate-diaphorase cells in frontal lobe of schizophrenics implies disturbances of cortical development. Arch Gen Psychiatry 50:169–177, 1993a

Akbarian S, Vinuela A, Kim JJ, et al: Distorted distribution of nicotinamide-adenine dinucleotide phosphate-diaphorase cells in temporal lobe of schizophrenics implies anomalous cortical development. Arch Gen Psychiatry 50:178–187, 1993b

Akbarian S, Kim JJ, Potkin SG, et al: Maldistribution of interstitial neurones in prefrontal white matter of the brains of schizophrenic patients. Arch Gen Psychiatry 53:425–436, 1996

Akil M, Lewis DA: Cytoarchitecture of the entorhinal cortex in schizophrenia. Am J Psychiatry 154:1010–1012, 1997

Altshuler LL, Casanova MF, Goldberg TE, et al: The hippocampus and parahippocampus in schizophrenia, suicide and control brains. Arch Gen Psychiatry 47:1029–1034, 1990

Anderson S, Volk D, Lewis DA: Increased density of microtubule associated protein immunoreactive neurones in the prefrontal white matter of schizophrenic subjects. Schizophr Res 19:1211–1219, 1996

Angermeyer MC, Kuhn L: Gender differences in age of onset of schizophrenia: an overview. Eur Arch Psychiatry Neurol Sci 237:351–364, 1988

Arnold SE, Franz BR, Gur RC, et al: Smaller interneuron size in schizophrenia in hippocampal subfields that mediate cortical-hippocampal interactions. Am J Psychiatry 152:738–748, 1995

Aylward E, Walker E, Bettes B: Intelligence in schizophrenia. Schizophr Bull 10:430–459, 1984

Barbeau D, Liang JJ, Robitaille Y, et al: Decreased expression of the embryonic form of neural cell adhesion molecule in schizophrenic brains. Proc Natl Acad Sci U S A 92:2785–2789, 1995

Benes F: Myelination of cortical-hippocampal relays during late adolescence. Schizophr Bull 15:585–594, 1989

Benes F: The role of stress and dopamine-GABA interactions in the vulnerability for schizophrenia. J Psychiatr Res 31:257–275, 1997

Benes FM, Bird ED: An analysis of the arrangement of neurons in the cingulate cortex of schizophrenic patients. Arch Gen Psychiatry 44:608–616, 1987

Benes FM, Davidson J, Bird ED: Quantitative cytoarchitectural studies of the cerebral cortex of schizophrenics. Arch Gen Psychiatry 43:31–35, 1986

Benes FM, McSparren J, Bird ED, et al: Deficits in small interneurons in prefrontal and cingulate cortices of schizophrenic and schizoaffective patients. Arch Gen Psychiatry 48:996–1001, 1991a

Benes FM, Sorenson I, Bird ED: Reduced neuronal size in posterior hippocampus of schizophrenic patients. Schizophr Bull 17:597–608, 1991b

Bilder RM, Wu H, Bogerts B, et al: Absence of regional hemisphere volume asymmetries in first episode schizophrenia. Am J Psychiatry 151:1437–1447, 1994

Brown AS, Susser E, Cohen P, et al: Schizophrenia following prenatal rubella exposure: gestational timing and diagnostic specificity (abstract). Schizophr Res 229:17–18, 1998

Browning MD, Dudeck EM, Rapier JL, et al: Significant reductions in synapsin but not synaptophysin specific activity in the brains of some schizophrenics. Biol Psychiatry 34:528–535, 1993

Bruton CJ, Crow TJ, Frith CD, et al: Schizophrenia and the brain: a prospective clinico-neuropathological study. Psychol Med 20:285–304, 1990

Bullmore ET, Brammer M, Harvey I, et al: Cerebral hemispheric asymmetry revisited: effects of handedness, gender and schizophrenia measured by radius of gyration in magnetic resonance images. Psychol Med 25:349–363, 1995

Bullmore ET, O'Connell P, Frangou S, et al: Schizophrenia as a developmental disorder of neural network integrity: the dysplastic net hypothesis, in Neurodevelopment and Adult Psychopathology. Edited by Keshavan MS, Murray RM. New York, Cambridge University Press, 1997, pp 253–266

Cannon M, Jones P, Murray RM, et al: Childhood laterality and later risk of schizophrenia in the 1946 British birth cohort. Schizophr Res 26:117–120, 1997

Casson IF, Clarke CA, Howard CV, et al: Outcomes of pregnancy in insulin dependent diabetic women: results of a five year population cohort study. BMJ 315:275–278, 1997

Castle D, Murray RM: The neurodevelopmental basis of sex differences in schizophrenia. Psychol Med 21:565–575, 1991

Castle DJ, Wessely S, Murray RM: Sex and schizophrenia: effects of diagnostic stringency, and associations with premorbid variables. Br J Psychiatry 162:658–664, 1993

Castle DJ, Wessely S, Van Os J, et al: The effect of gender in age at onset of psychosis, in Psychosis in the Inner City: The Camberwell First Episode Study (Maudsley Monogr No 40) Hove, UK, Psychology Press, 1998, pp 27–36

Christison GW, Casanova MF, Weinberger DR, et al: A quantitative investigation of hippocampal pyramidal cell size, shape and variability of orientation in schizophrenia. Arch Gen Psychiatry 46:1027–1032, 1989

Chua SE, McKenna PJ: Schizophrenia—a brain disease? A critical review of structural cerebral abnormality in the disorder. Br J Psychiatry 166:563–582, 1995

Clouston TS: The Neuroses of Development. Edinburgh, Oliver & Boyd, 1891

Clouston TS: Clinical Lectures on Mental Diseases, 3rd Edition. London, Churchill, 1892

Corrigall RJ, Murray RM: Twin concordance for congenital and adult-onset psychosis: a preliminary study of the validity of a novel classification of schizophrenia. Acta Psychiatr Scand 89:142–145, 1994

Cotter D, Kerwin R, Doshi B, et al: Alterations in hippocampal non-phosphorylated MAP2 protein expression in schizophrenia. Brain Res 765:238–246, 1997

Crawford JR, Besson JAO, Bremner M, et al: Estimation of premorbid intelligence in schizophrenia. Br J Psychiatry 161:69–74, 1992

Crow TJ, Done DJ: Prenatal exposure to influenza does not cause schizophrenia. Br J Psychiatry 161:390–393, 1992

Crow TJ, Ball J, Bloom SR, et al: Schizophrenia as an anomaly of development of cerebral asymmetry: a postmortem study and a proposal concerning the genetic basis of the disease. Arch Gen Psychiatry 46:1145–1150, 1989

Crow TJ, Done DJ, Sacker A: Cerebral lateralization is delayed in children who go on to develop schizophrenia. Schizophr Res 22:181–185, 1996

Davis JO, Bracha HS: Prenatal growth markers in schizophrenia: a monozygotic co-twin control study. Am J Psychiatry 153:1166–1172, 1996

DeLisi LE, Goldin LR, Maxwell E, et al: Clinical features of illness in siblings with schizophrenia and schizoaffective disorder. Arch Gen Psychiatry 44:891–896, 1987

DeLisi LE, Hoff AL, Schwartz AE, et al: Brain morphology in first-episode schizophrenic-like psychotic patients: a quantitative magnetic resonance imaging study. Biol Psychiatry 29:159–175, 1991

DeLisi LE, Sakuma M, Tew W, et al: Schizophrenia as a chronic active brain process: a study of progressive structural change subsequent to the onset of schizophrenia. Psychiatry Res 74:129–140, 1997

Eastwood SL, Burnet PJ, Harrison PJ: Altered synaptophysin expression as a marker of synaptic pathology in schizophrenia. Neuroscience 66:201–206, 1995a

Eastwood SL, McDonald B, Burnet PJ, et al: Decreased expression of mRNAs encoding non-NMDA glutamate receptors GluR1 and GluR2 in medial temporal lobe neurons in schizophrenia. Mol Brain Res 29:211–223, 1995b

Elkis H, Friedman L, Wise A, et al: Meta-analyses of studies of ventricular enlargement and cortical sulcal prominence in mood disorders. Arch Gen Psychiatry 52:735–746, 1995

Falkai P, Bogerts B: Cell loss in the hippocampus in schizophrenics. Eur Arch Psychiatry Neurol Sci 236:154–161, 1986

Fañanas L, Van Os J, Murray RM: Dermatoglyphic a-b ridge count as a possible marker for developmental insult in schizophrenia: replication in two samples. Schizophr Res 20:307–314, 1996

Fearon P, Cotter D, Murray RM: Is the association between obstetric complications and schizophrenia mediated by glutamatergic excitotoxic damage in the foetal/neonatal brain? in Psychopharmacology of Schizophrenia. Edited by Reveley M, Deakin B. London, Arnold (in press)

Feinberg I: Schizophrenia: caused by a fault in programmed synaptic elimination during adolescence. J Psychiatr Res 17:319–334, 1982–1983

Feinberg I: Schizophrenia as an emergent disorder of late brain maturation, in Neurodevelopment and Adult Psychopathology. Edited by Keshavan MS, Murray RM. New York, Cambridge University Press, 1997, pp 237–252

Fish B: Neurobiological antecedents of schizophrenia in childhood. Arch Gen Psychiatry 34:1297–1313, 1977

Foerster A, Lewis S, Owen MJ, et al: Low birth weight and a family history of schizophrenia predict poor premorbid functioning in psychosis. Schizophr Res 5:3–20, 1991a

Foerster A, Lewis S, Owen MJ, et al: Premorbid personality in psychosis: effects of sex and diagnosis. Br J Psychiatry 158:171–176, 1991b

Friston KJ: Functional and effective connectivity in neuroimaging: a synthesis. Hum Brain Map 2:56–78, 1994

Frith CD, Friston KJ, Liddle PF, et al: Willed action and the prefrontal cortex in man: a study with PET. Proc R Soc Lond B Biol Sci 244:241–246, 1991a

Frith CD, Leary J, Cahill C, et al: IV. Performance on psychological tests. Br J Psychiatry 159 (suppl 13):26–29, 1991b

Galaburda AM: Toxicity of plasticity: lessons from a model of developmental learning disorder, in Normal and Abnormal Development of the Cortex. Edited by Galaburda AM, Christen Y. Heidelberg, Germany, Springer, 1997, pp 135–144

Geddes JR, Verdoux H, Takei N, et al: Individual patient data meta-analysis of the association between schizophrenia and abnormalities of pregnancy and labor. Schizophr Bull (in press)

Glantz LA, Lewis DA: Synaptophysin and not RAB3A is specifically reduced in the prefrontal cortex of schizophrenic subjects (abstract). Soc Neurosci Abstr 20:622, 1994

Glantz LA, Lewis DA: Assessment of spine density on layer III pyramidal cells in the prefrontal cortex of schizophrenic subjects (abstract). Soc Neurosci Abstr 21:239, 1995

Green MF, Satz P, Soper HV, et al: Relationship between physical anomalies and age of onset of schizophrenia. Am J Psychiatry 144:666–667, 1987

Green MF, Satz P, Christenson C: Minor physical anomalies in schizophrenia patients and their siblings. Schizophr Bull 20:433–440, 1994

Griffiths TD, Sigmundsson T, Takei N, et al: Minor physical anomalies in familial and sporadic schizophrenia: the Maudsley Family Study. J Neurol Neurosurg Psychiatry 64:56–60, 1998

Guth C, Jones P, Murray RM: Familial psychiatric illness and obstetric complications in early-onset affective disorder. Br J Psychiatry 163:492–498, 1993

Hare E: Temporal factors and trends, including birth seasonality and the viral hypothesis, in Handbook of Schizophrenia, Vol 3. Edited by Nasrallah HA. Amsterdam, Elsevier, 1988, pp 345–377

Harvey I, Ron M, Du Boulay G, et al: Reduction in cortical volume in schizophrenia on magnetic resonance imaging. Psychol Med 23:591–604, 1993

Heckers S, Heinsen YC, Beckman H: Limbic structures and lateral ventricles in schizophrenia: a quantitative postmortem study. Arch Gen Psychiatry 47:1016–1022, 1990

Howard RJ, Graham C, Sham P, et al: A controlled family study of late-onset non-affective psychosis (late paraphrenia). Br J Psychiatry 170:511–514, 1997

Hultman CM, Ohman A, Cnattingius S, et al: Prenatal and neonatal risk factors for schizophrenia. Br J Psychiatry 170:128–133, 1997

Hultman CM, Sparen P, Takei N, et al: Prenatal and perinatal risk factors for schizophrenia, affective psychosis, and reactive psychosis of early onset. Case-control study. BMJ 318:421–426, 1999

Illowski BP, Juliano Dm, Bigelow LB, et al: Stability of CT scan findings in schizophrenia: results of an eight year follow-up study. J Neurol Neurosurg Psychiatry 51:209–213, 1988

Jakob H, Beckmann H: Prenatal developmental disturbances in the limbic allocortex in schizophrenia. J Neural Transm 65:303–326, 1986

Johnstone EC, Crow TC, Frith CD, et al: Cerebral ventricular size and cognitive impairment in chronic schizophrenia. Lancet 2:924–926, 1976

Johnstone EC, Crow TJ, Frith CED, et al: The dementia of dementia praecox. Acta Psychiatr Scand 57:305–324, 1978

Johnstone EC, Owens DGC, Colter N, et al: The spectrum of structural changes in the brain in schizophrenia: age of onset as a predictor of clinical and cognitive impairments and their cerebral correlates. Psychol Med 19:91–103, 1989

Johnstone EC, Bruton CJ, Crow TJ, et al: Clinical correlates of postmortem brain changes in schizophrenia: decreased brain weight and length correlate with indices of early impairment. J Neurol Neurosurg Psychiatry 57:474–479, 1994

Jones P, Rodgers B, Murray RM, et al: Child developmental risk factors for adult schizophrenia in the British 1946 birth cohort. Lancet 344:1398–1402, 1994

Jones P, Rantakallio P, Hartikainen AL, et al: Schizophrenia as a long term outcome of pregnancy and delivery complications: a 28 year follow-up of the 1966 North Finland General Population Birth Cohort. Am J Psychiatry 155:355–364, 1998

Karmiloff-Smith A: Crucial differences between developmental cognitive neuroscience and adult neuropsychology. Developmental Neuropsychology 13:513–524, 1997

Kempley ST, Vyas S, Bower S, et al: Cerebral and renal artery blood flow velocity before and after birth. Early Hum Dev 46:165–174, 1996

Keshavan MS: Neurodevelopment and schizophrenia: quo vadis?, in Neurodevelopment and Adult Psychopathology. Edited by Keshavan MS, Murray RM. New York, Cambridge University Press, 1997, pp 267–277

Kirov G, Jones P, Harvey I, et al: Do obstetric complications cause the earlier age at onset of male compared to female schizophrenics? Schizophr Res 20:117–124, 1996

Kovelman JA, Scheibel AB: A neurohistological correlate of schizophrenia. Biol Psychiatry 19:1601–1621, 1984

Krimer LS, Herman MM, Saunders RC, et al: A qualitative and quantitative analysis of the entorhinal cortex in schizophrenia. Cereb Cortex 7:732–739, 1997

Kunugi H, Takei N, Murray RM, et al: Small head circumference at birth in schizophrenia. Schizophr Res 20:165–170, 1996

Lane A, Colgan K, Moynihan F, et al: Schizophrenia and neurological soft signs: gender differences in clinical correlates and antecedent factors. Psychiatry Res 64:105–114, 1996

Lane A, Kinsella A, Murphy P, et al: The anthropometric assessment of dysmorphic features in schizophrenia as an index of its developmental origins. Psychol Med 27:1155–1164, 1997

Larroche JK: Malformations of the nervous system, in Greenfield's Neuropathology, 4th Edition. Edited by Adams JM, Corsellis JAN, Duchen LW. London, Edward Arnold, 1984, p 385–450

Leboyer M, Filteau MJ, Jay M, et al: No gender effect on age of onset in familial schizophrenia? (letter). Am J Psychiatry 149:1409, 1992

Leviton A, Gilles F: Ventriculomegaly, delayed myelination, white matter hypoplasia, and "periventricular" leukomalacia: how are they related? Pediatr Neurol 15:127–136, 1996

Lewis SW: Computerised topography in schizophrenia 15 years on. Br J Psychiatry 157 (suppl 9):16–24, 1990

Lewis SW: Psychopathology and brain dysfunction: structural imaging studies, in Neurodevelopment and Adult Psychopathology. Edited by Keshavan MS, Murray RM. New York, Cambridge University Press, 1997, pp 178–186

Lewis SW, Murray RM: Obstetric complications, neurodevelopmental deviance and risk of schizophrenia. J Psychiatr Res 21:413–421, 1987

Lewis SW, Murray RM, Owen MJ: Obstetric complications in schizophrenia: methodology and mechanisms, in Schizophrenia: Scientific Progress. Edited by Schultz SC, Tamminga CA. New York, Oxford University Press, 1989, pp 56–59

Lipska BK, Weinberger DR: Delayed effects of neonatal hippocampal damage on haloperidol induced catalepsy and apomorphine-induced stereotypic behaviours in the rat. Brain Res Dev Brain Res 75:213–222, 1993

Lipska BK, Jaskiw GE, Weinberger DR: Postpubertal emergence of hyperresponsiveness to stress and to amphetamine after neonatal excitotoxic hippocampal damage: a potential animal model of schizophrenia. Neuropsychopharmacology 9:67–75, 1993

Lohr JB, Flynn K: Minor physical anomalies in schizophrenia and mood disorders. Schizophr Bull 19:551–556, 1993

Machon RA, Mednick SA, Schulsinger F: The interaction of seasonality, place of birth, genetic risk and subsequent schizophrenia in a high risk sample. Br J Psychiatry 143:383–388, 1983 [Published erratum appears in Br J Psychiatry 151:124, 1987]

McGrath J, Murray RM: Risk factors for schizophrenia: from conception to birth, in Schizophrenia. Edited by Hirsch S, Weinberger DR. Oxford, UK, Blackwell Scientific, 1995, pp 187–205

McGrath JJ, Van Os J, Hoyos C, et al: Minor physical anomalies in the functional psychoses: associations with clinical and putative aetiological variables. Schizophr Res 18:9–20, 1995

McGuire PK, Shah GMS, Murray RM: Increased blood flow in Broca's area during auditory hallucinations in schizophrenia. Lancet 342:703–706, 1993

McGuire PK, Silbersweig DA, Wright I, et al: Abnormal monitoring of inner speech: a physiological basis for auditory hallucinations. Lancet 346:596–600, 1995

McNeil TF: Obstetric factors and perinatal injuries, in Handbook of Schizophrenia, Vol 3. Edited by Tsuang MT, Simpson JC. Amsterdam, Elsevier, 1988, pp 319–344

McNeil TF: Perinatal risk factors and schizophrenia. Selective review and methodological concerns. Epidemiol Rev 17:107–112, 1995

McNeil TF, Kaij L: Obstetric factors in the development of schizophrenia: complications in the births of preschizophrenics and in reproductions by schizophrenic parents, in The Nature of Schizophrenia: New Approaches to Research and Treatment. Edited by Wynne LC, Cromwell RL, Matthysse S. New York, Wiley, 1978, pp 401–429

McNeil TF, Cantor-Graae E, Norstrom LG, et al: Head circumference in 'preschizophrenic' and normal controls. Br J Psychiatry 153:191–197, 1993

Mednick S, Machon RA, Huttunen MO: Adult schizophrenia following prenatal exposure to an influenza epidemic. Arch Gen Psychiatry 45:189–192, 1988

Mellor CS: Dermatoglyphic evidence of fluctuating asymmetry in schizophrenia. Br J Psychiatry 160:467–472, 1992

Murray RM, Lewis SW: Is schizophrenia a neurodevelopmental disorder? BMJ 295:681–682, 1987

Murray RM, Lewis SW, Reveley AM: Towards an aetiological classification of schizophrenia. Lancet 1:1023–1026, 1985

Murray RM, Lewis SW, Owen MJ, et al: The neurodevelopmental origins of dementia praecox, in Schizophrenia: The Major Issues. Edited by Bebbington P, McGuffin P. London, Heinemann, 1988, pp 90–106

Murray RM, O'Callaghan E, Castle DJ, et al: A neurodevelopmental approach to the classification of schizophrenia. Schizophr Bull 18:319–332, 1992

Nasrallah HA, Olson SC, McCalley-Whitters M, et al: Cerebral ventricular enlargement in schizophrenia: a preliminary follow-up study. Arch Gen Psychiatry 43:157–159, 1986

O'Callaghan E, Larkin C, Kinsella A, et al: Familial, obstetric and other clinical correlates of minor physical anomalies in schizophrenia. Am J Psychiatry 148:479–483, 1991a

O'Callaghan E, Sham P, Takei N, et al: Schizophrenia after prenatal exposure to 1957 A2 influenza epidemic. Lancet 337:1248–1250, 1991b

O'Callaghan E, Buckley P, Redmond O, et al: Abnormalities of cerebral structure in schizophrenia on magnetic resonance imaging: interpretation in relation to the neurodevelopmental hypothesis. J R Soc Med 85:227–231, 1992a

O'Callaghan E, Gibson T, Colohan HA, et al: Risk of schizophrenia in adults born after obstetric complications and their association with early onset of illness: a controlled study. BMJ 305:1256–1259, 1992b

O'Callaghan E, Cotter D, Colgan K, et al: Confinement of winter birth excess in schizophrenia to the urban born and its gender specificity. Br J Psychiatry 166:51–54, 1995

Olney JW, Farber NB: Glutamate receptor dysfunction and schizophrenia. Arch Gen Psychiatry 52:998–1007, 1995

Ong WY, Garey LJ: Ultrastructural features of biopsied temporopolar cortex (area 38) in a case of schizophrenia. Schizophr Res 10:15–27, 1993

Owens DGC, Johnstone EC, Bydder GM, et al: Unsuspected organic disease in chronic schizophrenia demonstrated by computerised tomography. J Neurol Neurosurg Psychiatry 43:1065–1070, 1980

Pakkenberg B: Postmortem study of chronic schizophrenic brains. Br J Psychiatry 151:744–752, 1987

Paneth N, Pinto MJ, Gardiner J, et al: Incidence and timing of germinal matrix/intraventricular hemorrhage in low birth weight infants. Am J Epidemiol 137:1167–1176, 1993

Penrice J, Cady EB, Lorek A, et al: Proton magnetic resonance spectroscopy of the brain in normal preterm and term infants, and early changes after perinatal hypoxia-ischemia. Pediatr Res 40:6–14, 1996

Parnas J, Schulsinger F, Teasdale TW, et al: Perinatal complications and clinical outcome within the schizophrenia spectrum. Br J Psychiatry 140:416–420, 1982

Perrone-Bizzozero NA, Sower AC, Bird ED, et al: Levels of the growth associated protein GAP-43 are selectively increased in association cortices in schizophrenia. Proc Natl Acad Sci U S A 93:14182–14187, 1996

Randall PL: Schizophrenia, abnormal connection, and brain evolution. Med Hypotheses 10:247–280, 1983

Rapoport JL, Giedd J, Kumra S, et al: Childhood-onset schizophrenia: progressive ventricular change during adolescence. Arch Gen Psychiatry 54:897–903, 1997

Reveley AM, Reveley MA, Murray RM: Cerebral ventricular enlargement in non-genetic schizophrenia: a controlled twin study. Br J Psychiatry 144:89–93, 1984

Rifkin L, Lewis S, Jones PB, et al: Low birth weight and schizophrenia. Br J Psychiatry 165:357–362, 1994

Roberts GW, Colter N, Lofthouse R, et al: Is there gliosis in schizophrenia? Investigation of the temporal lobe. Biol Psychiatry 22:1459–1468, 1987

Russell AJ, Munro JC, Jones PB, et al: Schizophrenia and the myth of intellectual decline. Am J Psychiatry 154:635–639, 1997

Russell AJ, Munro JC, Jones PB, et al: Is the National Adult Reading Test an accurate measure of premorbid IQ in schizophrenia. Br J Clin Psychol (in press)

Schulsinger F, Parnas J, Petersen ET, et al: Cerebral ventricular size in the offspring of schizophrenic mothers: a preliminary study. Arch Gen Psychiatry 41:602–606, 1984

Sham PC, O'Callaghan E, Takei N, et al: Schizophrenic births following influenza epidemics between 1939 and 1960. Br J Psychiatry 160:461–466, 1992

Sharma T, Lancaster E, Lee D, et al: Brain changes in schizophrenia. Volumetric MRI study of families multiply affected with schizophrenia—the Maudsley Family Study V. Br J Psychiatry 173:132–138, 1998

Sharma T, Lancaster E, Sigmundsson T, et al: Lack of normal pattern of cerebral asymmetry in familial schizophrenic patients and their relatives—the Maudsley Family Study XI. Schizophr Res (in press)

Stefanis M, Frangou S, Yakeley J, et al: Hippocampal volume reduction in schizophrenia is secondary to pregnancy and birth complications. Biol Psychiatry (in press)

Stevens JR, Casanova M, Bigelow L: Gliosis and schizophrenia. Biol Psychiatry 24:727–729, 1988

Stewart A, Kirkbride V: Very preterm infants at fourteen years: relationship with neonatal ultrasound brain scans and neurodevelopmental status at one year. Acta Paediatr Suppl 416:44–47, 1996

Stewart AL, Rifkin L, Amess PN, et al: Brain structure and neurocognitive and behavioural function in adolescents who were born very preterm. Lancet 353:1653–1657, 1999

Susser E, Lin SP: Schizophrenia after prenatal exposure to the Dutch Hunger Winter of 1944–1945. Arch Gen Psychiatry 49:983–988, 1992

Susser E, Neugebauer R, Hoek HW, et al: Schizophrenia after prenatal famine: further evidence. Arch Gen Psychiatry 53:25–31, 1996

Takei N, Sham PC, O'Callaghan E, et al: Schizophrenia: increased risk associated with winter and city birth—a case-control study in 12 regions within England and Wales. J Epidemiol Community Health 49:106–107, 1995

Torrey EF, Rawlings R, Waldman IN: Schizophrenic births and viral diseases in two states. Schizophr Res 1:73–77, 1988

Torrey EF, Miller J, Rawlings R, et al: Seasonality of birth in schizophrenia and bipolar disorder: a review of the literature. Schizophr Res 28:1–38, 1997

Turner SW, Toone BK, Brett-Jones JR: Computerised tomographic scan changes in early schizophrenia. Psychol Med 16:219–225, 1986

Van Os J, Fahy TA, Jones P, et al: Psychopathological syndromes in the functional psychoses: associations with course and outcome. Psychol Med 26:161–176, 1996

Van Os J, Marcelis M, Sham P, et al: Psychopathological syndromes and familial morbid risk of psychosis. Br J Psychiatry 169:241–246, 1997a

Van Os J, Woodruff P, Fañanas L, et al: Temporal origin of cerebral structural abnormalities in schizophrenia: associations with second trimester dermatoglyphic ridge counts (abstract). Schizophr Res 24:158, 1997b

Verdoux H, Geddes JR, Takei N, et al: Obstetric complications and age at onset in schizophrenia: an international collaborative meta-analysis of individual patient data. Am J Psychiatry 154:1220–1227, 1997a

Verdoux H, Takei N, Cassou de Saint-Mathurin R, et al: Seasonality of birth in schizophrenia: the effect of regional population density. Schizophr Res 23:175–180, 1997b

Walker E: Neurodevelopmental aspects of schizophrenia. Schizophr Res 9:151–152, 1993

Walker EF, Lewine RRJ, Neumann C: Childhood behavioral characteristics and adult brain morphology in schizophrenia. Schizophr Res 22:93–101, 1996

Walsh C, Asherson P, Sham P, et al: Age of onset of schizophrenia in multiply affected families is early and shows no sex difference, in Schizophrenia: Breaking Down the Barriers. Edited by Holliday SG, Ancill RJ, MacEwan GW. New York, Wiley, 1996, pp 81–97

Weinberger DR: Implications of normal brain development for the pathogenesis of schizophrenia. Arch Gen Psychiatry 44:660–669, 1987

Weinberger DR, Lipska BK: Cortical maldevelopment, antipsychotic drugs and schizophrenia: a search for common ground. Schizophr Res 16:87–110, 1995

Weinberger DR, Cannon-Spoor E, Potkin SG, et al: Poor premorbid adjustment and CT scan abnormalities in chronic schizophrenia. Am J Psychiatry 137:1410–1413, 1980

Wolyniec PS, Pulver AE, McGrath JA, et al: Schizophrenia: gender and familial risk. J Psychiatr Res 1:17–28, 1992

Woodruff PWR, Murray RM: The aetiology of brain abnormalities in schizophrenia, in Schizophrenia: Exploring the Spectrum of Psychosis. Edited by Ancill R. Chichester, UK, Wiley, 1994, pp 95–144

Woodruff PWR, Wright IC, Bullmore ET, et al: Auditory hallucinations and the temporal cortical response to speech in schizophrenia: a functional magnetic resonance imaging study. Am J Psychiatry 154:1676–1682, 1997a

Woodruff PWR, Wright IC, Shuriquie N, et al: Structural brain abnormalities in male schizophrenics reflect fronto-temporal dissociation. Psychol Med 27:1257–1266, 1997b

Wright IC, Ellison ZR, Sharma T, et al: Mapping of grey matter changes in schizophrenia. Schizophr Res 35:1–14, 1999

Wright P, Takei N, Rifkin L, et al: Maternal influenza, obstetric complications and schizophrenia. Am J Psychiatry 152:1714–1720, 1995

Wright P, Sham PC, Gilvarry CM, et al: Autoimmune diseases in the pedigrees of schizophrenic and control subjects. Schizophr Res 20:261–267, 1996

Depression and Anxiety

CHAPTER 10

Childhood Depression: Is It the Same Disorder?

Richard Harrington, F.R.C.Psych.

Until recently, it was widely believed that depressive disorders were very rare in preadolescent children. Young children were thought to be incapable of experiencing many of the phenomena that are characteristic of depressive disorders in adults. Over the past 20 years, however, there has been a substantial change in the ways in which mood disturbance among the young is conceptualized. The use of structured personal interviews with children as young as 8 years has shown that depressive syndromes resembling adult depressive disorders can and do occur among prepubertal children (Angold et al. 1998). Indeed, the prevailing psychiatric classifications give the impression that depressive disorder in young people is a unitary, well-defined syndrome with core symptoms that are the same across the age span. Thus, in DSM-IV (American Psychiatric Association 1994), the essential criteria for major depression for prepubertal children, adolescents, and adults are similar.

Nevertheless, professional opinion has been divided about whether depressive disorder in preadolescent children really is the same as

This research was supported by the MacArthur Foundation Research Network on Psychopathology and Development. Parts of this chapter are based on a chapter in a volume (No. 11, 1995) of the Association of Child Psychology and Psychiatry Occasional Paper Series, and the author is grateful for permission to reproduce them here.

depressive disorder in adults. This controversy has been fuelled by the finding that the majority of children who meet the criteria for a depressive diagnosis also meet the criteria for a nondepressive disorder as well. The question therefore arises as to whether these children are better regarded as being depressed or as having another kind of mental disorder altogether.

This chapter begins with a brief discussion of some of the issues surrounding the diagnosis of depressive disorder in young people. The evidence for its links with depression in adults is then reviewed. It will be argued that although depressive disorder in adolescence appears to have strong links with depression in adults, the same cannot be said for depression in preadolescent children. The boundaries of preadolescent depression are blurred, and there is as yet little evidence to support its distinctiveness within the broader class of a nondifferentiated global concept of childhood emotional disorder.

Defining Depressive Disorders in Preadolescent Children

Thirty years ago there was considerable skepticism about the notion that depressive disorders could occur in children. However, two developments led to an increasing rate of diagnosis of depressive disorder in young people. The first was the construction, in both the United Kingdom and the United States, of adequate standardized measures focusing specifically on depressive features in childhood (Puig-Antich and Chambers 1978; Rutter et al. 1970). Findings with these measures showed that symptoms of misery in children were frequently reported by teachers, parents, and the children themselves. Moreover, depression was found to be a good discriminator of overall psychopathology. For example, 60% of 10-year-old girls in the Isle of Wight Study (Rutter et al. 1970) with psychopathology, but only 11% of those without disorder, were reported to be miserable on the parental account.

The second development was the use of operationalized diagnostic criteria to define a depressive syndrome in children. Early attempts to operationalize such a syndrome used modified versions of adult criteria for depressive disorder (Pearce 1978; Weinberg et al. 1973). By the late

1970s the full criteria for adult depression were applied to children (American Psychiatric Association 1980). Current research on preadolescent depression tends to assume that if the child meets the appropriate criteria for major depression in DSM-IV, then an adultlike depressive syndrome is present.

However, this is not necessarily the case for several reasons. First, the assessment of depression at all ages depends to an important extent on the person's verbal account of his or her subjective state. Young children do not find it easy to describe how they are feeling and often confuse emotions such as anger and sadness (Kovacs 1986). They have particular difficulty describing certain of the key cognitive symptoms of depression, such as hopelessness and self-denigration. There is evidence of developmental changes in many of the cognitive abilities that may underlie these depressive cognitions. For instance, during middle childhood (ages 7 through 9 years), the self is conceived in outward, physical terms. If asked to describe themselves, children of this age will tend to frame their descriptions in terms of external characteristics or of what they do. It is only by adolescence that young people regularly describe themselves in terms of psychological characteristics (Harter 1983).

Second, most research on major depression in young people has been based on the nonhierarchical system of the third and fourth editions of the *Diagnostic and Statistical Manual of Mental Disorders* (American Psychiatric Association 1980, 1987, 1994). In such nonhierarchical systems, young people may meet the criteria for multiple diagnoses. There is no attempt to determine which problem dominates the clinical picture, and there is no separate category for conditions characterized by two or more problems. Rather, it is assumed that comorbidity between depression and other mental conditions represents the co-occurrence of separate disorders. The problem is that depression in young children frequently occurs in conjunction with other mental disorders. Anderson et al. (1987), for instance, found that of 14 children, aged 11 years, with depressive disorders, 11 had at least one other mental condition. Indeed, 8 of the 14 children had depression, an anxiety disorder, an attention-deficit disorder, and a conduct disorder! This is more than would be expected by chance. Clearly, the frequent co-occurrence of supposedly separate disorders raises the question of whether any of them is a valid diagnostic entity.

The third reason for concern about the validity of depressive disorder in children is that there is only low agreement between children and parents in their reports of depressive symptoms in young people (Harrington and Shariff 1992). When interviewed in a standardized fashion, children tend to report higher levels of misery than noted by their parents (Harrington 1993). It is not clear whether this disparity arises because parents are failing to appreciate serious mood disturbances in their children or, rather, because children are overreacting to, or misperceiving, normal variations in mood. It should also be noted that this discrepancy between subject and informant accounts of depressed mood occurs in adults (Thompson et al. 1982). Nevertheless, it again raises questions about the validity of an adultlike depressive disorder in young children and about the extent of the links between child and adult depression.

Child and Adult Depression

The main research strategies that provide information on similarities and dissimilarities between child and adult depression involve 1) phenomenology, 2) epidemiology, 3) outcome, 4) family-genetic factors, 5) biological markers and neurobiology, 6) drug response, and 7) response to psychological treatments.

Phenomenology

Studies comparing the phenomenology of child and adult depressive disorder have generally found considerable similarities (Kolvin et al. 1991; Mitchell et al. 1988; Nurcombe et al. 1989; Ryan et al. 1987). However, such studies suffer from the potential tautology that entry to the study is determined by meeting the criteria for adult depression. A more stringent test is to use multivariate statistical techniques to derive diagnostic dimensions and categories from ratings of symptoms. In a review of early studies of questionnaire measures of childhood symptoms, Quay (1979) found none in which a clear depressive factor distinct from anxiety emerged among the younger age groups. Recent questionnaire studies, too, have found that depression and anxiety cannot be separated in children, and it has therefore been suggested that the two symptom constellations should be combined in the construct of "negative affectivity" (Compas et al. 1993).

It should be noted, however, that pencil-and-paper questionnaires are a crude way of measuring depression. Studies that have obtained interview data directly from children have tended to find meaningful depression factors. For example, in an epidemiological study that involved interviews with nearly 800 11-year-olds, Williams et al. (1989) reported that depression and anxiety emerged as separate factors in girls. However, studies that have examined developmental trends tend to find that depression does not emerge as a separate factor until early adolescence (Thorley 1987).

Epidemiology

Age and sex trends provide another way of examining connections between child and adult depressive disorders. Depressive disorders show marked variations in rate with age. Both clinic (Kolvin et al. 1991; Zeitlin 1986) and general population studies (Angold et al. 1998; Fleming et al. 1989; Rutter et al. 1970, 1976) have found that severe depressive conditions are relatively infrequent in early and middle childhood and probably reach a peak in late adolescence or early life (Burke et al. 1990; Lewinsohn et al. 1993). These age trends seem to be associated with a change in sex ratio of depressive disorders. In a study of psychiatric clinic patients, Pearce (1974, 1978) found that whereas an operationally defined depressed syndrome was more common in boys before puberty, it was more common in girls after puberty. Several studies in the general population have found that depressive disorders in younger children are equally common in the two sexes or more common in boys, whereas depression in adolescence shows the female preponderance that is found in adults (Angold et al. 1998; Cohen et al. 1993; Fleming et al. 1989). The same finding has been reported in studies of the children of depressed parents (Weissman et al. 1997).

The data on age trends and sex differences are not as consistent as one would like. Some investigators have reported that the size of the sex difference varies according to the threshold used to define disorder (Bailly et al. 1992; Fleming et al. 1989). Moreover, measures may not be comparable across the age span. Nevertheless, depressive disorders do stand out from other conditions in the pattern of age trends and sex differences that emerges during early adolescence. It seems there are important differences between child and adult depression with respect to their epidemiology.

Outcome

The course of a disorder has long been recognized as an important validating feature. There is much evidence that depressive conditions in adult life tend to recur (Angst 1997). There is also evidence that early-onset depressive disorders are associated with an increased risk of depression later in life (Harrington et al. 1990; Kovacs et al. 1984). However, several studies have found that childhood-onset depressive disorders are associated with a lower risk of subsequent depression than adolescent-onset varieties of the disorder. Thus, in our adult follow-up of patients with childhood onset of depression, we divided the probands according to whether the onset of depression was pre- or postpubertal (with the latter including those who were pubescent). Prepubertal and postpubertal depressed case patients differed in their outcomes. Continuity to major depression was significantly lower in prepubertal probands than in postpubertal case patients (Harrington et al. 1990). Adjustment in adulthood was also much worse in the case patients with a later onset, with very poor outcomes (such as suicide or long-term admission to psychiatric inpatient units) virtually confined to the postpubertal group. Similarly, Rao et al. (1993) found that suicide in adult life occurred mainly in adolescent-onset cases of depressive disorder. Goodyer et al. (1997a, 1997b) reported that older age at onset was one of a number of factors that predicted an increased risk of recurrence. It can be concluded that the longitudinal findings support the epidemiological research in suggesting that there are important differences between preadolescent and later-onset forms of depression. Earlier age at onset seems to be associated with a lower risk of subsequent depression.

Family-Genetic Factors

It will be appreciated that the course of a disorder may be affected by many extraneous factors, such as treatment. It is necessary, therefore, to study the relationship between prepubertal and adult depression by means of other indicators of similarity or dissimilarity. One such indicator is family history of depression. Family studies of depressed adults have consistently showed that adult depression is familial. Familial aggregation of depression in adults seems to be due partly to genetic influences (Kendler et al. 1993). Interest in the genetics of child and adolescent depression has been heightened by the finding that in cases of adult depression, earlier age at onset is associated with an increased familial loading for depression (Strober 1992). It has therefore been suggested that preadolescent onset of depression might represent the most heritable form of the disorder (Todd et al. 1993).

Thus far, no genetically informative studies (e.g., those with twin or adoption designs) have had sufficient numbers of individuals to determine whether preadolescent cases with depressive disorder differ from adolescent-onset forms with respect to genetic predisposition. There is, however, some evidence of familial differences between prepubertal and adolescent-onset forms of depression. Thus, in a family-interview study of the depressed pre- and postpubertal case patients described earlier, we found that criminality, intrafamilial discord, and parental criticism toward the child were all significantly more common in the families of prepubertally depressed case patients as compared with postpubertally depressed case patients (Harrington et al. 1997). Also, the relatives of prepubertally depressed case patients were more likely to have a depressive disorder that was comorbid with criminality. These differences were found even when the effects of potential confounding variables, such as conduct disorder, year of birth, type of depression, and gender, were controlled in proportional hazards analyses. Contrary to what might have been expected from studies of age at onset and familial loading in adult samples, we did not find that rates of depression were any higher in the relatives of prepubertally depressed probands than in postpubertally depressed case patients. If anything, the reverse was true: bipolar disorders tended to be more common in the families of case patients with depression of postpubertal onset than in those of patients with depression of prepubertal onset (Harrington et al. 1997).

On the basis of these findings, we hypothesized that prepubertal-onset depression might not, as previously suggested, be highly genetic, but might in fact have a greater environmental component than adolescent-onset depression (Harrington et al. 1997). Some support for this hypothesis comes from recent genetic studies of depressive symptoms. In a twin study, Thapar and McGuffin (1994) found that whereas adolescent depression had a strong genetic component, preadolescent depression was mainly associated with nonshared environmental factors. Similar findings were reported by Eley et al. (1998) in an analysis of the genetic contribution to depressive symptoms in the Colorado Adoption Study. Of course, it may not be possible to generalize these findings to depressive disorders. It must also be added that some family studies of depressed preadolescent children have found very high rates of affective disorders (Neuman et al. 1997). Nevertheless, the evidence thus far supports the idea that prepubertal onset of depression shows important familial, and possibly genetic, differences from adolescent- and adult-onset forms of depression. Specifically, prepubertal-onset cases may be associated with a very high risk of environmental adversity, particularly problems within the family.

Biological Markers and Neurobiology

A large literature has documented a wide range of biological investigations in depressed young people (Yaylayan et al. 1992). The aim has been both to identify a marker that has diagnostic specificity for depression and to understand the physiological processes that may underlie the disorder.

Three types of investigation have provided information on possible developmental differences in the neurobiology of depression. The first is the study of cortisol secretion, measured by investigations such as the dexamethasone suppression test (DST). Several studies have shown that depressed young patients are less likely than nondepressed patients to show suppression of cortisol secretion when the exogenous corticosteroid dexamethasone is administered (Casat and Powell 1988). The specificity of the DST for depressive disorder is slightly greater for adolescents or adults than it is for children (Casat and Powell 1988; Ferguson and Bawden 1988).

The second type of developmentally informative investigation is the study of sleep. Polysomnographic studies of depressed adults have tended to demonstrate abnormalities of sleep, including shortened rapid eye movement (REM) latency (time from the start of sleep to the first period of REM sleep) and reduced slow wave sleep (Benca et al. 1992). Many polysomnographic studies with depressed adolescents have shown sleep abnormalities, mainly of REM sleep (Appelboom-Fondu et al. 1988; Cashman et al. 1986; Emslie et al. 1987; Kutcher et al. 1992; Lahmeyer et al. 1983; Riemann and Schmidt 1993). These generally positive results of polysomnographic studies with depressed adolescents contrast with the mainly negative results of such studies with children, in which, with one or two exceptions (e.g., Emslie et al. 1990), comparisons with depressed patients and control subjects have shown few polysomnographic differences (Dahl et al. 1991; Puig-Antich et al. 1982; Young et al. 1982).

The third type of developmentally informative investigation is the study of growth hormone. A variety of pharmacological challenge agents that stimulate release of growth hormone have been studied in depressed adults. The idea has been to investigate the activity of certain neuronal pathways, particularly the monoamine pathways, because these have been implicated in the etiology of depression. Studies of adults with major depression have tended to show blunted growth hormone response to provocative stimuli (Checkley 1992). Blunted growth hormone response to provocative stimuli has also been demonstrated in prepubertal children both during a major depressive episode (Jensen and Garfinkel 1990; Puig-Antich et al. 1984a; Ryan et al. 1994) and after recovery (Puig-Antich et al. 1984b). Interestingly, however, the results with adolescents have been negative. Though some studies have reported high levels of growth hormone in adolescents with major depression (Kutcher et al. 1991), growth hormone provocation studies with depressed adolescents (Dahl et al. 1992; Jensen and Garfinkel 1990; Kutcher et al. 1991; Waterman et al. 1991) have not found the blunting of growth hormone response that has been reported in prepubertal children.

It seems, then, that sleep abnormalities, and possibly DST response, are less apparent in prepubertal depressed children than in depressed adolescents, whereas growth hormone abnormalities may be more prominent. It is difficult to reconcile these contradictory findings, but in interpreting them a number of methodological points should be noted. First, these types of biological investigations may be influenced by factors other than depression. For example, weight loss can lead to a positive DST (Mullen et al. 1986). Antidepressants can cause blunting of growth hormone response in provocation tests, even if they are stopped months before the test (Cowen and Wood 1991). Second, much biological research in this age group has relied on psychiatrically healthy control groups, raising the question of whether the positive results are specific to depression. All in all, however, the results of biological investigations suggest that prepubertally depressed children show fewer biological abnormalities than depressed adolescents. Depressed adolescents resemble depressed adults in their sleep patterns and in their response to the DST.

Drug Response

One of the main pillars on which the disease concept of depressive disorder in adults has rested is the positive response to antidepressants. Many controlled trials have shown that antidepressants such as tricyclics are significantly better than placebo in the treatment of moderately severe depressive disorders (Paykel 1989). Controlled trials with depressed children and adolescents have, however, failed to find significant benefits of tricyclic antidepressant medication (Hazell et al. 1995). For example, Puig-Antich et al. (1987) found that the proportion of prepubertal children with major depression who responded to imipramine (56%) was not significantly different from that of children who responded to placebo (68%). Negative findings were also reported by Geller et al. (1992) in another study of prepubertal major depression. Placebo-controlled trials of tricyclic antidepressants in adolescents with major depression also found no significant benefits of active drug over placebo (Geller et al. 1990; Kramer and Feiguine 1983; Kutcher et al. 1994; Kye et al. 1996).

There are several possible reasons for the apparently negative findings of studies of tricyclics in children and adolescents (Ryan 1990). First, it is difficult to do randomized drug trials in this age group. Consent must in practice be obtained from two people, and many parents are reluctant to allow their children into a study in which one of the treatments is medication. It may be especially difficult to obtain consent in studies involving tricyclics, for which regular monitoring of cardiac function is required. Second, some tricyclic studies have been based on very severe cases of depression. Indeed, the pooled response rate across the tricyclic trials in both children and adolescents is only around 33% (Hazell et al. 1995), which is much less than the approximately 60% reported in studies with adults. Third, it is likely that juvenile depressive disorders are heterogeneous. Drug effects may be apparent only in certain subgroups. Tricyclic trials have generally used populations that are too small to permit meaningful subgroup analysis. It could be that there is a small effect of medication that would have been detected in larger trials. Fourth, there may be developmental variations in the metabolism of tricyclics, such as in their rate of elimination from the body (Geller 1991), that make it hard to achieve the optimal dosage. Finally, it has been suggested that young people differ from adults both in the relative balance of the cerebral neurotransmitters on which tricyclic antidepressants are thought to act (Strober et al. 1990) and in the hormonal milieu of the brain (Ryan et al. 1986).

A recent report suggests that the selective serotonin reuptake inhibitor fluoxetine may be of benefit in children and adolescents with major depression (Emslie et al. 1997). It is too early to say whether this finding is robust—a previous trial with fluoxetine produced a negative result (Simeon et al. 1990). Nevertheless, it clearly raises the possibility that young people may be more responsive to antidepressants than previously thought, since the study of Emslie and colleagues did not find that children responded differently from adolescents.

In summary, trials of antidepressant medication have thus far not revealed a differential treatment response between preadolescent children and adolescents.

Response to Psychological Treatments

A variety of different psychological treatments have been used to help depressed children, of which the best studied has been cognitive-behavior therapy (CBT). There is evidence that CBT is an effective treatment for clinically depressed adolescents (Brent et al. 1997; Wood et al. 1996). Trials of CBT have generally not included young children and so are of limited value in establishing the degree of similarity between prepubertal and postpubertal depression. In line with the outcome studies, however, it does seem that younger children are more likely to have their symptoms remit than are adolescents (Jayson et al. 1998).

Child and Adolescent Depression

In interpreting the results of the studies reviewed in this chapter, it is important to recognize that there is no external criterion that can act as a "gold standard" against which the degree of similarity between child and adolescent depression can be tested. Each of the tests described in this chapter is fallible. For example, the course of a disorder may be altered by many different factors, including treatment. Just because child and adolescent depression have different outcomes does not necessarily mean that they are different disorders. Similarly, when a young person fails to respond to antidepressants it does not mean that he is not depressed. Any one of a large number of factors could have affected response to treatment.

It should also be borne in mind that the diagnoses that the external criteria are supposed to compare may not be equally reliable. There is evidence that it is harder to diagnose depression reliably in younger children than in adolescents (Edelbrock et al. 1985). Moreover, there may be developmental differences in the methods used to make diagnoses. Studies of depressed prepubertal children have tended to place greater weight on information from the parents than on the interview with the child. For instance, early versions of the Schedule for Affective Disorders and Schizophrenia for School-Aged Children (Kiddie-SADS) (one of the most commonly used instruments in research on depression in young people) began with the parental interview and used the child interview to confirm or refute what the parent said (Puig-Antich and Chambers 1978). By contrast, it has been common practice for the final best-estimate diagnosis of depression in adolescents to be based mainly on the interview with the adolescent. Dissimilarities between child and adolescent depression could, then, be attributed to age differences in diagnostic reliability or in the sources of information that were used to make this diagnosis, or both.

Nevertheless, the distinction between child and adolescent depression is now supported by evidence from a wide variety of different sources. First, marked changes in the epidemiology of depressive disorders occur during adolescence, with the development of a female preponderance and an increase in rates. Second, there is now evidence of developmental differences in outcomes, with adolescent-onset forms of the disorder associated with a higher rate of depression in adult life and a greater risk of completed suicide than preadolescent depression. Third, early- and later-onset depressions seem to differ in terms of family history. In the Maudsley studies, prepubertal onset of depression was associated with an increased familial loading of criminality and family discord compared with adolescent-onset depression (Harrington et al. 1997). It seemed that prepubertal depression was associated with a range of disorders in relatives, including depression, whereas adolescent-onset depression was associated with a more specific loading of depressive disorders only. Findings consistent with the Maudsley studies were reported by Puig-Antich et al. (1989), who demonstrated that prepubertal depression was associated with familial comorbidity of depression, antisocial personality, and alcoholism. The available data suggest, then, that although adolescent depression appears to be strongly linked to major depression in adulthood, there is much less support for the concept of an adultlike depressive syndrome in preadolescents.

If prepubertal depression is not the same as adult depressive disorder, then what have many of us been studying over the past 20 years? There is no doubt that there is something wrong with the dysphoric prepubertal children who have been described in many studies and whom we occasionally see in our clinics. Most of these children are very impaired (Puig-Antich et al. 1985a, 1985b), and some make serious suicide attempts. If not depression, then how should their problems best be conceptualized?

There are two main possibilities. The most parsimonious explanation is that the depression is simply part and parcel of another psychopathological syndrome altogether. Epidemiological studies have shown that in children, misery is associated with a wide range of psychopathology, including conduct disorder and reading retardation, as well as emotional disturbance. For instance, in the Isle of Wight studies of 10-year-olds, depressive features such as depressed mood and lack of smiling were among the best discriminators of overall psychopathology (Rutter et al. 1970). Further support for the idea that depression is best seen as part of another psychopathological syndrome comes from studies of children who have both depression and conduct disorder. We found that the outcomes of children with depression and conduct disorder were identical to those of children with conduct disorder (Harrington et al. 1991); the former evidenced a low rate of depression in adulthood and a high rate of antisocial outcomes, such as criminality. By contrast, young people with "pure" depression had a significantly increased risk of depression in adult life.

The second possibility is that depression in prepubertal children is a valid diagnostic entity, but one distinct from most forms of maturity-onset depression. There is, for example, a literature going back over many years (reviewed by Trad [1986]) about the depressive reactions of infants and young children to extreme stress or deprivation. Such children are said to become withdrawn and anorexic and fail to thrive. Our finding (Harrington et al. 1997) that prepubertal depression was associated with an extremely high rate of intrafamilial relationship problems is consistent with this idea. Alternatively, it could be that prepubertal depression is related to what Winokur (1979) called "depressive spectrum disease." This form of depression is associated with alcoholism and criminality in relatives.

Conclusion

There appear to be important differences between prepubertal- and maturity-onset depressive disorders. Prepubertal-onset disorders are more likely to be associated with adverse family circumstances and with relationship problems within the family. Adolescent-onset disorders show much stronger temporal continuities with adult depressive conditions and share with adult depression a female preponderance. Prepubertal depression is not yet established as a valid diagnostic entity that is distinct from other forms of psychopathology in young children.

References

American Psychiatric Association: Diagnostic and Statistical Manual of Mental Disorders, 3rd Edition. Washington, DC, American Psychiatric Association, 1980

American Psychiatric Association: Diagnostic and Statistical Manual of Mental Disorders, 3rd Edition, Revised. Washington, DC, American Psychiatric Association, 1987

American Psychiatric Association: Diagnostic and Statistical Manual of Mental Disorders, 4th Edition. Washington, DC, American Psychiatric Association, 1994

Anderson JC, Williams S, McGee R, et al: DSM-III disorders in preadolescent children: prevalence in a large sample from the general population. Arch Gen Psychiatry 44:69–76, 1987

Angold A, Costello EJ, Worthman CM: Puberty and depression: the roles of age, pubertal status and pubertal timing. Psychol Med 28:51–61, 1998

Angst J: A regular review of the long term follow up of depression. BMJ 315:1143–1146, 1997

Appelboom-Fondu J, Kerkhofs M, Mendlewicz J: Depression in adolescents and young adults—polysomnographic and neuroendocrine aspects. J Affect Disord 14:35–40, 1988

Bailly D, Beuscart R, Collinet C, et al: Sex differences in the manifestations of depression in young people. A study of French high school students, Part I: prevalence and clinical data. Eur Child Adolesc Psychiatry 1:135–145, 1992

Benca RM, Obermeyer WH, Thisted RA, et al: Sleep and psychiatric disorders: a meta-analysis. Arch Gen Psychiatry 49:651–668, 1992

Brent D, Holder D, Kolko D, et al: A clinical psychotherapy trial for adolescent depression comparing cognitive, family, and supportive treatments. Arch Gen Psychiatry 54:877–885, 1997

Burke KC, Burke JD, Regier DA, et al: Age at onset of selected mental disorders in five community populations. Arch Gen Psychiatry 47:511–518, 1990

Casat CD, Powell K: The dexamethasone suppression test in children and adolescents with major depressive disorder: a review. J Clin Psychiatry 49:390–393, 1988

Cashman MA, Coble P, McCann BS, et al: Sleep markers for major depressive disorder in adolescent patients (abstract). Sleep Res 15:91, 1986

Checkley S: Neuroendocrinology, in Handbook of Affective Disorders, 2nd Edition. Edited by Paykel ES. Edinburgh, Churchill Livingstone, 1992, pp 255–266

Cohen P, Cohen J, Kasen S, et al: An epidemiological study of disorders in late childhood and adolescence, I: age- and gender-specific prevalence. J Child Psychol Psychiatry 34:851–867, 1993

Compas BE, Ey S, Grant KE: Taxonomy, assessment, and diagnosis of depression during adolescence. Psychol Bull 114:323–344, 1993

Cowen PJ, Wood AJ: Biological markers of depression. Psychol Med 21:831–836, 1991

Dahl RE, Ryan ND, Birmaher B, et al: Electroencephalographic sleep measures in prepubertal depression. Psychiatry Res 38:201–214, 1991

Dahl RE, Ryan ND, Williamson DE, et al: Regulation of sleep and growth hormone in adolescent depression. J Am Acad Child Adolesc Psychiatry 31:615–621, 1992

Edelbrock C, Costello AJ, Dulcan MK, et al: Age differences in the reliability of the psychiatric interview with the child. Child Dev 56:265–275, 1985

Eley TC, Deater-Deckard K, Fombonne E, et al: An adoption study of depressive symptoms in middle childhood. J Child Psychol Psychiatry 39:337–345, 1998

Emslie GJ, Roffwarg HP, Rush AJ, et al: Sleep EEG findings in depressed children and adolescents. Am J Psychiatry 144:668–670, 1987

Emslie GJ, Rush AJ, Weinberg WA, et al: Children with major depression show reduced rapid eye movement latencies. Arch Gen Psychiatry 47:119–124, 1990

Emslie GJ, Rush AJ, Weinberg WA, et al: A double-blind, randomized, placebo-controlled trial of fluoxetine in children and adolescents with depression. Arch Gen Psychiatry 54:1031–1037, 1997

Ferguson HB, Bawden HN: Psychobiological measures, in Assessment and Diagnosis in Child Psychopathology. Edited by Rutter M, Tuma AH, Lann IS. New York, Guilford, 1988, pp 232–263

Fleming JE, Offord DR, Boyle MH: Prevalence of childhood and adolescent depression in the community: Ontario Child Health Study. Br J Psychiatry 155:647–654, 1989

Geller B: Psychopharmacology of children and adolescents: pharmacokinetics and relationships of plasma/serum levels to response. Psychopharmacol Bull 27:401–409, 1991

Geller B, Cooper TB, Graham DL, et al: Double-blind placebo-controlled study of nortriptyline in depressed adolescents using a "fixed plasma level" design. Psychopharmacol Bull 26:85–90, 1990

Geller B, Cooper TB, Graham DL, et al: Pharmacokinetically designed double-blind placebo-controlled study of nortriptyline in 6- to 12-year-olds with major depressive disorder. J Am Acad Child Adolesc Psychiatry 31:34–44, 1992

Goodyer IM, Herbert J, Secher SM, et al: Short-term outcome of major depression, I: comorbidity and severity at presentation as predictors of persistent disorder. J Am Acad Child Adolesc Psychiatry 36:179–187, 1997a

Goodyer IM, Herbert J, Tamplin A, et al: Short-term outcome of major depression, II: life events, family dysfunction, and friendship difficulties as predictors of persistent disorder. J Am Acad Child Adolesc Psychiatry 36:474–480, 1997b

Harrington RC: Depressive Disorder in Childhood and Adolescence. Chichester, UK, Wiley, 1993

Harrington RC, Shariff A: Choosing an instrument to assess depression in young people. Newsletter of the Association for Child Psychology and Psychiatry 14:279–282, 1992

Harrington RC, Fudge H, Rutter M, et al: Adult outcomes of childhood and adolescent depression, I: psychiatric status. Arch Gen Psychiatry 47:465–473, 1990

Harrington RC, Fudge H, Rutter M, et al: Adult outcomes of childhood and adolescent depression, II: risk for antisocial disorders. J Am Acad Child Adolesc Psychiatry 30:434–439, 1991

Harrington RC, Rutter M, Weissman M, et al: Psychiatric disorders in the relatives of depressed probands, I: comparison of prepubertal, adolescent and early adult onset forms. J Affect Disord 42:9–22, 1997

Harter S: Developmental perspectives on the self-system, in Handbook of Child Psychology, Vol 4: Social and Personality Development. Edited by Mussen P, Hetherington M. New York, Wiley, 1983, pp 275–385

Hazell P, O'Connell D, Heathcote D, et al: Efficacy of tricyclic drugs in treating child and adolescent depression: a meta-analysis. BMJ 310:897–901, 1995

Jayson D, Wood AJ, Kroll L, et al: Which depressed patients respond to cognitive-behavioral treatment? J Am Acad Child Adolesc Psychiatry 37:35–39, 1998

Jensen JB, Garfinkel BD: Growth hormone dysregulation in children with major depressive disorder. J Am Acad Child Adolesc Psychiatry 29:295–301, 1990

Kendler KS, Neale MC, Kessler RC, et al: A longitudinal twin study of 1-year prevalence of major depression in women. Arch Gen Psychiatry 50:843–852, 1993

Kolvin I, Barrett ML, Bhate SR, et al: The Newcastle Child Depression Project: diagnosis and classification of depression. Br J Psychiatry 159 (suppl 11):9–21, 1991

Kovacs M: A developmental perspective on methods and measures in the assessment of depressive disorders: the clinical interview, in Depression in Young People: Developmental and Clinical Perspectives. Edited by Rutter M, Izard CE, Read RB. New York, Guilford, 1986, pp 435–465

Kovacs M, Feinberg TL, Crouse-Novak M, et al: Depressive disorders in childhood, II: a longitudinal study of the risk for a subsequent major depression. Arch Gen Psychiatry 41:643–649, 1984

Kramer AD, Feiguine RJ: Clinical effects of amitriptyline in adolescent depression: a pilot study. J Am Acad Child Adolesc Psychiatry 20:636–644, 1983

Kutcher S, Malkin D, Silverberg J, et al: Nocturnal cortisol, thyroid stimulating hormone, and growth hormone secretory profiles in depressed adolescents. J Am Acad Child Adolesc Psychiatry 30:407–414, 1991

Kutcher S, Williamson P, Marton P, et al: REM latency in endogenously depressed adolescents. Br J Psychiatry 161:399–402, 1992

Kutcher S, Boulos C, Ward B, et al: Response to desipramine treatment in adolescent depression: a fixed-dose, placebo-controlled trial. J Am Acad Child Adolesc Psychiatry 33:686–694, 1994

Kye CH, Waterman GS, Ryan ND, et al: A randomized, controlled trial of amitriptyline in the acute treatment of adolescent major depression. J Am Acad Child Adolesc Psychiatry 35:1139–1144, 1996

Lahmeyer HW, Poznanski EO, Bellur SN: EEG sleep in depressed adolescents. Am J Psychiatry 140:1150–1153, 1983

Lewinsohn PM, Hops H, Roberts RE, et al: Adolescent psychopathology, I: prevalence and incidence of depression and other DSM-III-R disorders in high school students. J Abnorm Psychol 102:133–144, 1993

Mitchell J, McCauley E, Burke PM, et al: Phenomenology of depression in children and adolescents. J Am Acad Child Adolesc Psychiatry 27:12–20, 1988

Mullen PE, Linsell CR, Parker D: Influence of sleep disruption and calorie restriction on biological markers for depression. Lancet 2:1051–1055, 1986

Neuman RJ, Geller B, Rice JP, et al: Increased prevalence and earlier onset of mood disorders among relatives of prepubertal versus adult probands. J Am Acad Child Adolesc Psychiatry 36:466–473, 1997

Nurcombe B, Seifer R, Scioli A, et al: Is major depressive disorder in adolescence a distinct diagnostic entity? J Am Acad Child Adolesc Psychiatry 28:333–342, 1989

Paykel ES: Treatment of depression: the relevance of research for clinical practice. Br J Psychiatry 155:754–763, 1989

Pearce JB: Childhood depression. Unpublished MPhil thesis, University of London, London, England, 1974

Pearce JB: The recognition of depressive disorder in children. J R Soc Med 71:494–500, 1978

Puig-Antich J, Chambers W: The Schedule for Affective Disorders and Schizophrenia for School-Aged Children. New York, New York State Psychiatric Institute, 1978

Puig-Antich J, Goetz R, Hanlon C, et al: Sleep architecture and REM sleep measures in prepubertal children with major depression during an episode. A controlled study. Arch Gen Psychiatry 39:932–939, 1982

Puig-Antich J, Goetz R, Davies M, et al: Growth hormone secretion in prepubertal major depressive children, II: sleep-related plasma concentration during a depressive episode. Arch Gen Psychiatry 41:463–466, 1984a

Puig-Antich J, Novacenko H, Tabrizi MA, et al: Growth hormone secretion in prepubertal major depressive children, III: response to insulin induced hypoglycemia in a drug-free, fully recovered clinical state. Arch Gen Psychiatry 41:471–475, 1984b

Puig-Antich J, Lukens E, Davies M, et al: Psychosocial functioning in prepubertal major depressive disorders, I: interpersonal relationships during the depressive episode. Arch Gen Psychiatry 42:500–507, 1985a

Puig-Antich J, Lukens E, Davies M, et al: Psychosocial functioning in prepubertal major depressive disorders, II: interpersonal relationships after sustained recovery from affective episode. Arch Gen Psychiatry 42:511–517, 1985b

Puig-Antich J, Perel JM, Lupatkin W, et al: Imipramine in prepubertal major depressive disorders. Arch Gen Psychiatry 44:81–89, 1987

Puig-Antich J, Goetz D, Davies M, et al: A controlled family history study of prepubertal major depressive disorder. Arch Gen Psychiatry 46:406–418, 1989

Quay HC: Classification, in Psychopathological Disorders of Childhood. Edited by Quay HC, Werry JS. New York, Wiley, 1979, pp 1–42

Rao U, Weissman MM, Martin JA, et al: Childhood depression and risk of suicide: preliminary report of a longitudinal study. J Am Acad Child Adolesc Psychiatry 32:21–27, 1993

Riemann D, Schmidt MH: REM sleep distribution in adolescents with major depression and schizophrenia (abstract). Sleep Res 22:554, 1993

Rutter M, Tizard J, Whitmore K (eds): Education, Health and Behaviour. London, Longmans, 1970

Rutter M, Graham P, Chadwick OF, et al: Adolescent turmoil: fact or fiction? J Child Psychol Psychiatry 17:35–56, 1976

Ryan ND: Pharmacotherapy of adolescent major depression: beyond TCAs. Psychopharmacol Bull 26:75–79, 1990

Ryan ND, Puig-Antich J, Cooper T, et al: Imipramine in adolescent major depression: plasma level and clinical response. Acta Psychiatr Scand 73:275–288, 1986

Ryan ND, Puig-Antich J, Ambrosini P, et al: The clinical picture of major depression in children and adolescents. Arch Gen Psychiatry 44:854–861, 1987

Ryan ND, Dahl RE, Birmaher B, et al: Stimulatory tests of growth hormone secretion in prepubertal major depression: depressed versus normal children. J Am Acad Child Adolesc Psychiatry 33:824–833, 1994

Simeon JG, Dinicola VF, Ferguson HB, et al: Adolescent depression: a placebo-controlled fluoxetine treatment study and follow-up. Prog Neuropsycho-pharmacol Biol Psychiatry 14:791–795, 1990

Strober M: Relevance of early age-of-onset in genetic studies of bipolar affective disorder. J Am Acad Child Adolesc Psychiatry 31:606–610, 1992

Strober M, Freeman R, Rigali J: The pharmacotherapy of depressive illness in adolescence, I: an open label trial of imipramine. Psychopharmacol Bull 26:80–84, 1990

Thapar A, McGuffin P: A twin study of depressive symptoms in childhood. Br J Psychiatry 165:259–265, 1994

Thompson WD, Orvaschel H, Prusoff BA, et al: An evaluation of the family history method for ascertaining psychiatric disorders. Arch Gen Psychiatry 39:53–58, 1982

Thorley G: Factor study of a psychiatric child rating scale: based on ratings made by clinicians on child and adolescent clinic attenders. Br J Psychiatry 150:49–59, 1987

Todd RD, Neuman R, Geller B, et al: Genetic studies of affective disorders: should we be starting with childhood onset probands? J Am Acad Child Adolesc Psychiatry 32:1164–1171, 1993

Trad PV: Infant Depression: Paradigms and Paradoxes. New York, Springer-Verlag, 1986

Waterman GS, Ryan ND, Puig-Antich J, et al: Hormonal responses to dextro-amphetamine in depressed and normal adolescents. J Am Acad Child Adolesc Psychiatry 30:415–422, 1991

Weinberg WA, Rutman J, Sullivan L, et al: Depression in children referred to an educational diagnostic center: diagnosis and treatment. J Pediatr 83:1065–1072, 1973

Weissman MM, Warner V, Wickramaratne P, et al: Offspring of depressed parents: 10 years later. Arch Gen Psychiatry 54:932–940, 1997

Williams S, McGee R, Anderson J, et al: The structure and correlates of self-reported symptoms in 11-year-old children. J Abnorm Child Psychol 17:55–71, 1989

Winokur G: A family history (genetic) study of pure depressive disease, in Genetic Aspects of Affective Illness. Edited by Mendlewicz J, Shopsin B. New York, Spectrum, 1979, pp 27–33

Wood AJ, Harrington RC, Moore A: Controlled trial of a brief cognitive-behavioural intervention in adolescent patients with depressive disorders. J Child Psychol Psychiatry 37:737–746, 1996

Yaylayan S, Weller EB, Weller RA: Neurobiology of depression, in Clinical Guide to Depression in Children and Adolescents. Edited by Shafii M, Shafii SL. Washington, DC, American Psychiatric Press, 1992, pp 65–88

Young W, Knowles JB, MacLean AW, et al: The sleep of childhood depressives: comparison with age-matched controls. Biol Psychiatry 17:1163–1168, 1982

Zeitlin H: The Natural History of Psychiatric Disorder in Children. Oxford, UK, Oxford University Press, 1986

11

Offspring at Risk: Early-Onset Major Depression and Anxiety Disorders Over a Decade

Myrna M. Weissman, Ph.D.
Virginia Warner, M.P.H.
Priya Wickramaratne, Ph.D.
Donna Moreau, M.D.
Mark Olfson, M.D.

The topic of this book — understanding the childhood onset of adult psychiatric disorders, the sequence in which psychiatric disorders develop and the form they take in childhood, and how they evolve over the life span — has important public health and preventive implications. Identification of the timing of onset of any disorder could guide interventions either before symptoms begin, by focusing on risk factors, or

This work was supported in part by grant MH-36197 (to M.W.) and 5P30MH43878 (M.W.) and by Research Scientist Development Award K20-MH01042 (M.O.) from the National Institutes of Health. Portions of this chapter are reprinted with permission from Weissman MM, Warner V, Wickramaratne P, et al.: "Offspring of Depressed Parents: 10 Years Later." *Archives of General Psychiatry* 54:932–940, 1997.

at the first signs of illness in high-risk individuals. Prevention could be a realistic goal.

Until recently, there were many obstacles to understanding childhood onset of adult depression. Among these were the lack of concepts and of tools for assessment and the lack of an empirical base. Before the 1970s the conventional wisdom was that depression was primarily a disorder of the middle-aged or elderly and that children rarely get depressed. The question of whether childhood depression existed prompted the National Institute of Mental Health in 1975 to hold its first conference on childhood depression. Two groups with opposing views were identified. At one pole were clinicians who described children with symptoms of depression, some of whom were receiving tricyclic antidepressants. At the other end were scientists who argued that childhood depression is not a distinct clinical syndrome, but rather a condition of childhood development "evanescent in nature and dissipating with time" (Lefkowitz and Burton 1978, p. 716). Consistent with the belief that children did not get depressed was the absence of assessment tools. Lefkowitz and Burton (1978) pointed out that the absence of a body of significant research on objective measurement and epidemiological characteristics reflected the lack of interest and skepticism about the existence of the syndrome in children.

In the 1970s the situation began to change dramatically. The late Joaquim Puig-Antich, M.D., modified the leading diagnostic assessment for adults, the Schedule for Affective Disorders and Schizophrenia (SADS; Endicott and Spitzer 1978), for children (the Kiddie-SADS; Puig-Antich and Chambers 1978). He began a systematic study of the symptom patterns, social functioning, treatment, sleep patterns, and neuroendocrine patterns of children and adolescents with depression and anxiety disorders coming for treatment to Babies Hospital at Columbia University (Puig Antich et al. 1989).

In the late 1980s, the Epidemiologic Catchment Area Study, a community survey of psychiatric disorders and the associated ages at onset in more than 18,000 adults, was launched (Robins and Regier 1991). This study was followed by in the 1990s the National Comorbidity Survey, a community survey of psychiatric disorders in about 9,000 persons (Kessler et al. 1994).

During this decade, a number of studies of the families of patients with depression and anxiety disorders were initiated. The epidemiological studies clearly showed that major depressive disorder (MDD) is associated with an early age at onset. The age-specific rates of first onset of MDD from the 1980 survey of adults and similar data from the subsequent survey in the 1990s are presented in Figures 11–1 and 11–2, respectively. These surveys, as well as the international surveys that followed, made it clear that the peak age at first onset of major depression is in the teens and young adulthood; that prepubertal onset, although uncommon, occurs; and that the rates of MDD are consistently higher in women than in men, even in quite diverse countries (Weissman et al. 1996). Moreover, the results from family-genetic studies showed that early onset of major depression (onset before age 30 years) is the most familial, further suggesting the importance of childhood and adolescent onset of MDD (Weissman et al. 1984).

Longitudinal Study of Offspring at High Risk of Developing Depression

It was against this background that we began a longitudinal study of offspring at high and low risk of developing depression by virtue of their parent's depression. Since it was clear that depression often affected women in their childbearing and childrearing years, we felt that studying the effect on the offspring could have public health implications. Given the increased familial risk of depression in the first-degree relatives of probands with MDD, we expected that the offspring would be at high risk and that if we studied them early enough we would begin to understand the onset, sequence, and course of their disorder.

We have been following up on a cohort of offspring either with one or both parents having MDD (high risk) or with neither parent having MDD (low risk). Follow-up has been carried out over a decade, with the offspring having been assessed three times during this period. The full details of the methods used in this study can be found elsewhere (Weissman et al. 1987, 1997).

At the initial interview, we found that the offspring of depressed parents, ranging in age from 6 to 23 years, compared with those of nondepressed parents, had a significantly increased risk of MDD and anxiety

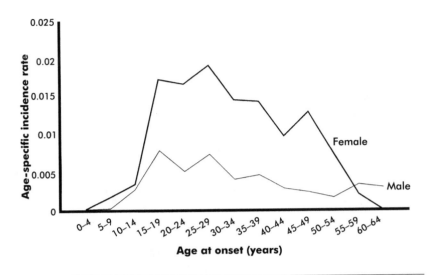

FIGURE 11-1.   *Age-specific incidence rates of depression in the United States, 1980.*
Source. Data from the Epidemiologic Catchment Area Study (N = 18,571) (Robins and Regier 1991).

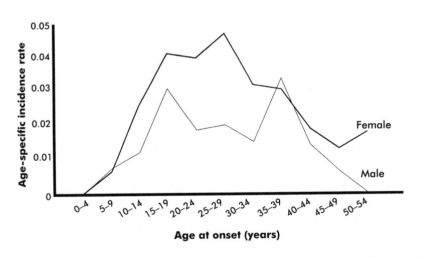

FIGURE 11-2.   *Age-specific incidence rates of major depression in the United States,*
1990.
Source. Data from the National Comorbidity Survey (N = 8,096) (Kessler et al. 1994).

disorders and markedly poorer overall functioning. Two years later, the differences between the groups of offspring were more pronounced, with the offspring of depressed parents continuing to have an increased incidence of depression, high recurrences rates, and slower recovery. There were striking differences in age at onset between each group of offspring. All of the cases of prepubertal-onset depression occurred in the offspring of depressed parents who themselves had early onset of MDD (before age 20 years). No sex differences in the rates of prepubertal-onset MDD were found. After puberty, the female offspring showed a marked increase in onset of MDD that peaked between the ages of 15 and 20 years. For the male offspring, there was a gradual rise in MDD onset after puberty. The results also suggest that the depressed offspring of nondepressed parents had a different course of illness than the depressed offspring of depressed parents and that longer follow-up would be required to capture clinically significant differences between the two groups.

The goal of the original study was to determine whether the lifetime rates of psychopathology, and specifically MDD, in the offspring of depressed probands were greater than those in the offspring of nondepressed parents. Comparisons were made in the overall lifetime rates of disorder (from birth to the time of interview) between the two groups. Because subjects were between the ages of 6 and 23 years, there was a wide variation in their stage of development at the first interview. As a consequence, many of the offspring at the time of first interview had not yet passed through the critical period of risk for the onset of depression, and the estimates of age-specific risks were unstable. With the availability of the 10-year follow-up, more precise estimates could eventually be made of age-specific and cumulative lifetime rates.

During the 10-year follow-up, we found that the offspring of depressed parents, compared with those of nondepressed parents, had higher rates of of MDD and phobias (about threefold higher for both), panic disorder, and alcohol dependence (nearly fivefold higher) (Table 11–1). There was no significant interaction between parental depression status and parental and offspring gender for the risk of MDD, anxiety disorders, or alcohol dependence in offspring (data not shown).

The peak time for the incidence period for MDD for both sexes was between ages 15 and 20 years (Figure 11–3). At all ages, the incidence

TABLE 11–1. *Cumulative rates of DSM-III-R psychiatric disorders (with impairment criteria applied) in offspring, by parental diagnosis*

| Diagnosis in offspring | Parental diagnosis | | Relative risk[c] (95% confidence interval) |
	One or both with MDD,[a] n (%)	Neither with MDD,[b] n (%)	
Any mood disorder	87 (85.3)	20 (37.9)	2.39 (1.46, 3.89)
MDD	64 (56.4)	13 (25.1)	2.50 (1.38, 4.54)
Bipolar disorder	3 (2.3)	0 (0.0)	—[d]
Dysthymia	7 (6.1)	3 (5.7)	0.922 (0.238, 3.58)
Any anxiety disorder	51 (41.7)	8 (15.1)	2.96 (1.41, 6.24)
Phobias	27 (21.0)	4 (7.6)	2.94 (1.03, 8.41)
Panic disorder	14 (13.4)	0 (0.0)	—[e]
OCD	1 (1.9)	1 (0.78)	—[f]
GAD	0 (0.0)	0 (0.0)	—[g]
ADHD	5 (3.9)	2 (3.8)	0.882 (0.166, 4.67)
Any substance abuse	40 (32.0)	14 (27.8)	1.32 (0.715, 2.42)
Alcohol abuse	18 (14.5)	8 (16.0)	0.934 (0.406, 2.15)
Alcohol dependence	21 (21.6)	2 (7.4)	4.93 (1.16, 21.06)
Drug abuse	7 (5.5)	7 (13.6)	0.414 (0.145, 1.18)
Drug dependence	16 (14.5)	1 (1.9)	6.98 (0.925, 52.74)
Schizophrenia	2 (1.8)	0 (0.0)	—[h]
Childhood disorders			
Separation anxiety	16 (12.4)	6 (11.3)	1.08 (0.424, 2.78)
Conduct disorder	44 (34.1)	11 (20.8)	1.88 (0.969, 3.64)[i]

TABLE 11–1. Cumulative rates of DSM-III-R psychiatric disorders (with impairment criteria applied) in offspring, by parental diagnosis (continued)

Diagnosis in offspring	Parental diagnosis		Relative risk[c] (95% confidence interval)
	One or both with MDD,[a] n (%)	Neither with MDD,[b] n (%)	
Childhood disorders (continued)			
Overanxious disorder	17 (13.6)	1 (1.9)	7.22 (0.959, 54.28)
Any of the above diagnoses	99 (78.4)	25 (47.2)	2.18 (1.40, 3.38)

Note. If the offspring reported, in the Schedule for Affective Disorders and Schizophrenia (SADS) or Kiddie-SADS, during an episode of disorder that they sought help, took medication, were hospitalized, or had impaired functioning at work, school, or home, they were considered impaired. Data on impairment were not collected for conduct disorder. ADHD = attention-deficit/hyperactivity disorder; GAD = generalized anxiety disorder; MDD = major depressive disorder. OCD = obsessive-compulsive disorder. [a]Data for 129 offspring. [b]Data for 53 offspring. [c]Adjusted for age and sex of offspring. [d]Two-tailed Fisher exact test = 1.25, df = 1, P = 0.56. [e]Two-tailed Fisher exact test = 6.23, df = 1, P = 0.004. [f]Two-tailed Fisher exact test = 0.427, df = 1, P = 1.00. [g]Not estimable because there were no cases. [h]Two-tailed Fisher exact test = 0.831, df = 1, P = 1.00. [i]Data on impairment were not collected for conduct disorder.
Source. Reprinted with permission from Weissman MM, Wickramaratne PJ, Moreau D, et al.: "Offspring of Depressed Parents: Ten Years Later." *Archives of General Psychiatry* 54:932–940, 1997. Copyright 1997, American Medical Association.

by sex was higher in the offspring of depressed parents than in those of nondepressed parents. The incidence rates declined after age 20 years except for the rates in male offspring, which appeared to decline slightly after age 25. Prepubertal onset is uncommon in general and in our sample occurred primarily in the high-risk offspring. The incidence rates were higher in female than in male adolescents. After age 20 years, the incidence rates were similar in both sexes.

A different pattern was found for any anxiety disorder, including panic disorder, generalized anxiety disorder, agoraphobia, social phobia, simple phobia, separation anxiety, obsessive-compulsive disorder, and overanxious disorder (Figure 11–4). The peak incidence of anxiety in

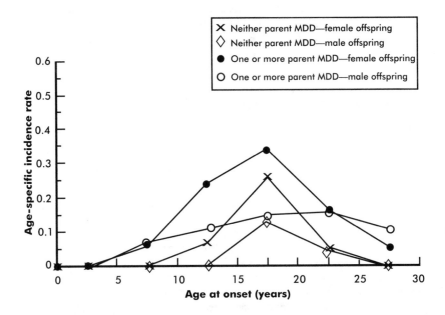

FIGURE 11–3.   *Age-specific incidence rates of major depressive disorder (MDD) by parental MDD and sex of offspring* (N = 182, *lifetime rates*).
Source. Reprinted with permission from Weissman MM, Wickramaratne PJ, Moreau D, et al.: "Offspring of Depressed Parents: Ten Years Later." *Archives of General Psychiatry* 54:932–940, 1997. Copyright 1997, American Medical Association.

the offspring for both sexes occurred much earlier than that of MDD (age range: 5–10 years), especially in the offspring of depressed parents. Among anxiety disorders, phobias and separation anxiety disorder had, on average, the earliest onset (mean ages at onset: 5.2 and 6.6 years, respectively). Overall, the incidence rates for anxiety disorders appear to decline after age 10 years and converge by sex of offspring and parental diagnosis. The incidence rate for alcohol dependence in both sexes of depressed probands increased at ages 15–20 years (Figure 11–5).

The illness severity at the time of the third interview (i.e., at 10-year follow-up) in the offspring who were depressed at the time of the first or second interviews was greater in the offspring of depressed parents than in those of nondepressed parents (Table 11–2). The depressed offspring of depressed parents were less likely to go for treatment when they felt they needed it and less likely to receive treatment when they were depressed. More than 30% of the depressed offspring of depressed

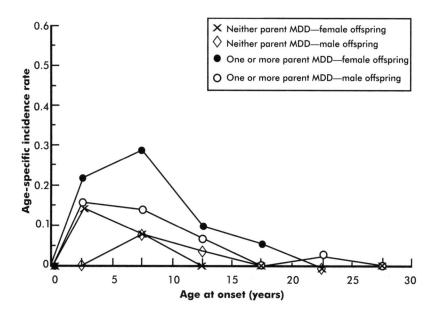

FIGURE 11–4. *Age-specific incidence rates of any anxiety disorder by parental major depressive disorder (MDD) and sex of offspring (N = 182 lifetime).*
Source. Reprinted with permission from Weissman MM, Wickramaratne PJ, Moreau D, et al.: "Offspring of Depressed Parents: Ten Years Later." *Archives of General Psychiatry* 54:932–940, 1997. Copyright 1997, American Medical Association.

parents never received any treatment; in addition, they had more impairment overall, in work and marriage, than the depressed offspring of nondepressed parents and reported more days on which they felt depressed.

Conclusion

As in previous investigations, we found that 1) parental depression increases the risk of depression in the offspring; 2) the course of depression in children, as in adults, is protracted, 3) the morbidity rate is high, and 4) the overall symptom picture in offspring does not vary by the age at onset of the symptoms and does not differ by proband group. The overall rates and burden of illness are greater in the offspring of depressed parents than in those of nondepressed parents. The former continue to

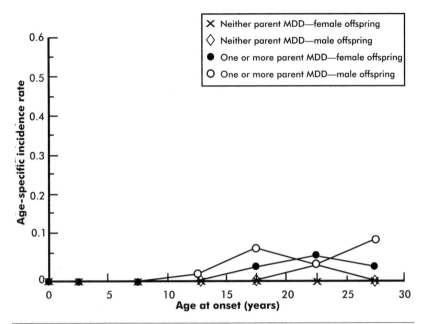

FIGURE 11–5. *Age-specific incidence rates of alcohol dependence by parental major depressive disorder (MDD) and sex of offspring (N = 182 lifetime).*
Source. Reprinted with permission from Weissman MM, Wickramaratne PJ, Moreau D, et al.: "Offspring of Depressed Parents: Ten Years Later." *Archives of General Psychiatry* 54:932–940, 1997. Copyright 1997, American Medical Association.

have markedly higher rates of MDD (threefold higher) and anxiety disorders. As they mature, they also have higher rates of alcohol dependence (fivefold higher) and poorer functioning in work, family, and marriage. The cumulative rate of MDD in the offspring of nondepressed parents (25.1/100) for ages 6–36 years is higher than that in the community sample for ages 15–34 years (17.1/100), and this difference may be explained by our closer surveillance of the sample (i.e., three interviews), as well as by the younger ages of the offspring when interviewing began.

The observed recurrent nature of depression is consistent with findings from longitudinal studies of depressed adults and children. The increased risk of MDD in the offspring of depressed parents is consistent with that found in numerous studies in which the offspring were minors. The familial nature of depression was consistent with that demonstrated in studies in which the probands were depressed children or adults. Although the absolute rates vary with the design and criteria used, the

TABLE 11–2. *Severity of outcome at 10-year follow-up in offspring with any depression at time of first or second interviews, by parental diagnosis*

	Parental diagnosis				
	One or more MDD[a]	Neither MDD[b]			
			Odds ratio[c] (95% CI)		
Did not go for treatment when felt such was needed, n (%)					
	23 (33.3)	1 (4.2)	12.85 (1.61, 102.54)		
GAS ≤71, n (%)					
	32 (40.0)	4 (15.4)	4.34 (1.33, 14.14)		
			Statistic[d]	df	P
Social Adjustment Scale, mean (SD)					
Work	1.84 (1.07)	1.30 (0.324)	−3.66	88.5	0.0004
Social and leisure	1.97 (0.567)	1.89 (0.450)	−0.689	49	0.49
Extended family	1.68 (0.509)	1.46 (0.314)	−2.54	64.6	0.01
Marital	1.88 (0.630)	1.47 (0.358)	−3.05	46.1	0.003
Parental	1.44 (0.402)	1.22 (0.405)	−1.44	23.2	0.16
Family	1.78 (0.601)	1.61 (0.502)	−1.37	44.3	0.18
Overall	1.80 (0.455)	1.59 (0.332)	−2.56	55.2	0.01
No. of days depressed during follow-up, mean (SD)					
	118 (401)	11 (49)	−2.33	86	0.02
			Statistic[e]	df	P
Ever out of work in last 5 years because of psychopathology, n (%)					
	11 (13.7)	1 (3.8)	1.92	1	0.29[f]
Number of MDD episodes during follow-up, n (%)					
0	53 (66.2)	23 (88.4)			
1	23 (28.7)	2 (7.6)			
2+	4 (5.0)	1 (3.8)	5.10	2	0.08
Suicide gestures or attempts, n (%)					
	13 (16.2)	3 (11.5)	0.340	1	0.75[f]

TABLE 11–2.   *Severity of outcome at 10-year follow-up in offspring with any depression at time of first or second interviews, by parental diagnosis* (continued)

| | Parental diagnosis | | | | |
	One or more MDD[a]	Neither MDD[b]	Statistic[e]	*df*	*P*
Treatments over 10 years,[g] *n* (%)					
Outpatient treatment	33 (67.4)	6 (100.0)	2.76	1	0.16[f]
Hospitaliza-tion	4 (8.2)	3 (50.0)	8.42	1	0.02[f]
Any treat-ment	33 (67.4)	6 (100.0)	2.76	1	0.16[f]

Note. Numbers of offspring from which data on parental diagnosis are derived vary, as specified in table notes, because of missing data. CI = confidence interval; GAS = Global Assessment Scale. MDD = major depressive disorder.
[a]Data for 80 offspring, except in category of treatment over 10 years, in which data for 49 offspring are represented.
[b]Data for 26 offspring, except in category of treatment over 10 years, in which data for 6 offspring are represented.
[c]Adjusted for age and sex of offspring. [d]T statistic is used for continuous variables.
[e]Chi-square statistic is used for dichotomous variables. [f]Two-tailed Fisher exact test.
[g]Treatment for MDD for offspring with any depression at time of third interview (10-year follow-up).
Source. Reprinted with permission from Weissman MM, Wickramaratne PJ, Moreau D, et al.: "Offspring of Depressed Parents: Ten Years Later." *Archives of General Psychiatry* 54:932–940, 1997. Copyright 1997, American Medical Association.

magnitude of the effect of familial depression (i.e., a two- to threefold increased risk) is consistent across high-risk and family studies.

More shifts to bipolar disorders occurred among the offspring of depressed parents than in the offspring of nondepressed parents, but the overall rate of bipolar disorder (2.3% in the offspring of depressed parents) was lower than that reported by other investigators. Of note, some of the offspring have not fully passed through the age at risk for the onset of bipolar disorder.

Prepubertal onset of MDD is uncommon, and it did not occur in the offspring of the nondepressed parents. The peak first onset of MDD in middle and late adolescence is consistent with the findings from epide-miological studies of depressive disorders in adolescents and adults. This peak is consistent in female offspring regardless of proband diagnosis, and this suggests a consistent vulnerability period for focus on detection and intervention. Why the rates should increase so abruptly in young females in middle and late adolescence and early adulthood is still unclear and is an area for further research. Parental affective disorders further increase the risk of first onset in adolescents. However, affective disorders in parents may serve as an identifier of a constellation of risk factors. High rates of comorbid anxiety disorders in depressed parents may be a factor. Alternatively, early expression of anxiety disorders could constitute an underlying vulnerability to psychopathology related to shared genetic or environmental factors.

The current findings support initiatives aimed at early detection and possible treatment intervention in the parents of depressed offspring and the offspring of depressed parents. Physicians who specialize in pediat-rics and adolescent medicine, as well as internists, family physicians, and child psychiatrists, are particularly well positioned to inquire about the mental health history of their patients' parents.

Alternatively, psychiatrists who treat adult patients should inquire about the clinical status of the offspring. Successful treatment of parental depression may provide primary prevention by reducing the symptoms of depression that may impair parenting. Secondary prevention may be achieved through the early detection and treatment of high-risk offspring who exhibit early or minor forms of anxiety, depressive, or substance abuse disorders. Finally, the aggressive treatment of established MDD (i.e., tertiary prevention) may reduce the high level of social impairment characteristically found in the depressed offspring of depressed parents.

Only a small proportion of young people with mental disorders receive adequate mental health treatment. In the current study, a large number of the offspring who perceived a need for mental health care accessed no treatment whatsoever. One possible explanation is that the offspring of depressed parents develop negative attitudes toward mental health treatment because they associate it with their parents' chronic course of illness. Alternatively, the depressed parent may deny that his or her offspring have the same disorder. A better understanding of how parental factors influence the seeking of health care for offspring may help public health planners extend treatment to this vulnerable and underserved population. There are now strong financial incentives to limit treatment costs. Our data suggest that outcomes research should assess the impact of parental depression on the offspring over time.

References

Endicott J, Spitzer RL: A diagnostic interview: the Schedule for Affective Disorders and Schizophrenia. Arch Gen Psychiatry 35:837–844, 1978

Kessler RC, McGonagle KA, Zhao S, et al: Lifetime and 12-month prevalence of DSM-III-R psychiatric disorders in the United States: results from the National Comorbidity Survey. Arch Gen Psychiatry 51:8–19, 1994

Lefkowitz MM, Burton N: Childhood depression: a critique of the concept. Psychol Bull 85:716–726, 1978

Puig-Antich J, Chambers W: The Schedule for Affective Disorders and Schizophrenia for School-Aged Children. New York, New York State Psychiatric Institute, 1978

Puig-Antich J, Goetz D, Davies M, et al: A controlled family history study of prepubertal major depressive disorder. Arch Gen Psychiatry 46:406–418, 1989

Robins LN, Regier DA (eds): Psychiatric Disorders in America: The Epidemiologic Catchment Area Study. New York, Free Press, 1991

Weissman MM, Wickramaratne PJ, Merikangas KR, et al: Onset of major depression in early adulthood: increased familial loading and specificity. Arch Gen Psychiatry 41:1136–1143, 1984

Weissman MM, Gammon GO, John K, et al: Children of depressed parents: increased psychopathology and early onset of major depression. Arch Gen Psychiatry 44:847–853, 1987

Weissman MM, Bland RC, Canino GJ, et al: Cross-National Epidemiology of Major Depression and Bipolar Disorder. JAMA 276:293–299, 1996

Weissman MM, Wickramaratne PJ, Moreau D, et al: Offspring of depressed parents: ten years later. Arch Gen Psychiatry 54:932–940, 1997

CHAPTER 12

When Is Onset?
Investigations Into Early
Developmental Stages of
Anxiety and Depressive
Disorders

Hans-Ulrich Wittchen, Ph.D., Dipl.Psych.
Roselind Lieb, Ph.D., Dipl.Psych.
Peter Schuster, Dipl.Psych.
Albertine J. Oldehinkel, Ph.D.

Over the past two decades, general population studies have used standardized diagnostic instruments such as the Diagnostic Interview Schedule (DIS; Robins et al. 1981) or the Composite International Diagnostic Interview (CIDI; World Health Organization 1990) to study the epidemiology of anxiety and depressive disorders (see, e.g., Angst and Dobler-Mikola 1985; Burke et al. 1991; Eaton et al. 1994; Kessler et al. 1994, 1996; Magee et al. 1996; Robins and Regier 1991; Wittchen 1994; Wittchen and von Zerssen 1987; Wittchen et al. 1994, 1998b, 1998c). These studies have found that anxiety and depressive disorders, as defined by DSM-III (American Psychiatric Association 1980), DSM-III-R (American Psychiatric Association 1987), or DSM-IV (American

Psychiatric Association 1994), occur frequently, with lifetime prevalences of up to 20%, even in adolescents and young adults. They often co-occur (i.e., are comorbid) and have different distributions of age at onset. Specific phobias, for example, manifest themselves for the first time predominantly in childhood or adolescence, whereas agoraphobia and panic disorder most frequently start in early adulthood. Depressive disorders and generalized anxiety disorder are associated with a higher age at onset, with increasing cumulative incidence throughout adulthood.

When the considerable degree of "within anxiety disorder comorbidity" (e.g., between specific phobias, agoraphobia, and panic disorder) is taken into account, epidemiological studies further suggest that in cases of comorbidity, anxiety precedes the onset of depressive disorders and primary and pure depressive disorders clearly occur less frequently than secondary comorbid depression. More detailed retrospective analyses also suggest that temporal primary anxiety disorders substantially increase the risk for secondary depression (Kessler et al. 1996; Wittchen 1996; Wittchen and Vossen 1995).

These findings have recently received considerable renewed research interest, especially from developmental perspectives. Focusing on the nature of associations between disorders, studies have examined, for example, the links between primary separation anxiety and secondary agoraphobia (Gittelman and Klein 1985), the role of primary anxiety disorders in the subsequent development of depressive disorders (Wittchen et al. 1991), and the course and outcome of depressive disorders (Kessler et al. 1996, 1998; Reed and Wittchen 1998; Wittchen and Essau 1989). By and large, these findings from large-scale adult epidemiological studies are consistent with those from prospective and retrospective child and adolescent studies, which used different categorical and dimensional diagnostic schedules and more refined assessment strategies, including multiple informants. For example, three groups of investigators (Lewinsohn et al. 1993, 1994, 1995; Garrison et al. 1989; McGee et al. 1992) all found similarly high prevalences and patterns of age at onset.

However, a number of serious concerns have been raised regarding the validity of age-at-onset findings and retrospective lifetime estimation of childhood disorders:

1. General skepticism has been expressed about the adequacy of dealing with childhood and adolescent anxiety and depressive disorders as "encapsulated entities" (Achenbach 1985; Anthony 1985).

2. Doubts have been expressed about the suitability of standardized diagnostic interviews such as the DIS or the CIDI, originally developed for adults. In particular, the standardized use of symptom and diagnostic questions for all ages, the use of strict categorical thresholds in determining diagnostic prevalence, and the restricted diagnostic coverage (exclusion of childhood disorders) need to be mentioned. In childhood disorders, one might expect different phenomenological presentations of key syndromes and different cognitive abilities in the comprehension of complex symptom questions.

3. Because many of the above-mentioned findings were not based on prospective longitudinal designs, concerns were also expressed about the reliability and accuracy of retrospective evaluations of lifetime disorders and the determination of age-at-onset characteristics of childhood syndromes and diagnoses.

4. It has not yet been determined to what degree and with what limitations categorical diagnostic procedures used in adult diagnostic instruments such as the CIDI or the DIS are adequate strategies to appropriately evaluate onset and onset characteristics in childhood. Recall bias in dating onset has been suggested as one major concern, especially when adults are asked about the first onset of their condition, which might have been decades earlier in adolescence or early childhood. Consistent with this skepticism, retrospective age cohort–specific analyses of age at onset have suggested that such bias might indeed be considerable (Burke et al. 1990, 1991; Magee et al. 1996).

Other, more general methodological concerns refer to the way age at onset is determined by most diagnostic instruments, including the DIS and CIDI. For example, simply asking the subject within the complex series of diagnostic questions "When was the first time you . . ." (the standard form of onset question in both the DIS and CIDI) might not offer enough stimulation to the subject to start a careful memory search (Kessler et al. 1998). Furthermore, among diagnostic instruments, and even within the same instrument, there is often considerable variation in the way onset of a disorder is assessed. For some diagnoses (e.g., major depression and manic syndromes), the CIDI, for example, requires all diagnostic criteria specified by DSM-IV to be met. For other disorders (e.g., panic disorder and phobias), however, it requires only the presence and first occurrence of key syndromes (e.g., a panic attack) or specific symptoms (e.g., an unreasonably strong fear in certain cued situations). Such inconsistency in the assessment of age at onset might not be trivial. To take a more straightforward example: Is onset of influenza measured as the point in time when someone starts sneezing or as the time the full picture, including fever, is manifest? The variability in assessment of age at onset might therefore affect not only findings of disorder-specific onset characteristics but also causal inferences regarding the determination of primary and secondary disorders and temporal patterns of comorbidity.

In this chapter, we investigate how different methods of assessing age at onset of DSM-IV anxiety and depressive disorders in a representative population sample of adolescents affect disorder-specific age-at-onset characteristics and temporal characteristics of comorbidity. The data come from a prospective longitudinal community study, the Early Developmental Stages of Psychopathology (EDSP) study, which originally involved 1,395 community respondents from 14–17 years of age at baseline. All respondents were personally interviewed with the Munich-CIDI (M-CIDI; Wittchen and Pfister 1997), and a more refined assessment method for age at onset was used. Further separate personal interviews were conducted with the respondent's parents to collect symptom, diagnostic, and developmental information about the respondent's parents, as well as their children, in order to compare parent and offspring information. Limiting the subsequent analyses to 14- to 17-year-olds had the advantage of limiting the influence of potential recall bias in assessment of those anxiety disorders expected to become apparent early in life.

After describing the study design and methods of the EDSP, we present prevalence and incidence findings. We then address, more specifically, the following issues:

1. The age at which and the consistency over time with which adolescent community respondents report the first onset of specific anxiety and depressive disorders when the CIDI standard onset questions are used ("When was the first time you had . . .?)

2. The effect of using onset information based on key features of a disorder (standard onset) compared with onset information based on the full diagnostic picture (peak onset)

3. Differences in age at onset between respondents who are able to remember clearly the first time they had the syndrome and those who are not able to recall the onset clearly

4. The frequency with which the respondents' parents report information about the child's early development concerning biological, psychological, and developmental vulnerabilities and risks (These findings from the family-history component of the EDSP will also be examined with regard to specificity to anxiety and depressive disorders.)

We end the chapter by discussing the implications of various ways of determining symptom-, syndrome- and disorder-based onsets, emphasizing primary and secondary disorders and temporal comorbidity patterns.

Methods

The EDSP study is a research program funded by the German Ministry of Research and Technology and is designed to collect data on the prevalence, risk factors, comorbidity, and course of mental disorders. In this study, the specific emphasis is on substance use disorders in two major age groups: 14- to 17-year-olds and 18- to 24-year-olds at baseline.

Design

The EDSP is a prospective longitudinal study with a family-history component consisting of a baseline survey and two follow-up surveys approximately 15 and 30 months after the baseline (Figure 12–1). Separate personal interviews with the respondents' parents were carried out both to obtain information about the respondents' somatic, psychological, and social childhood development and childhood disorders and to assess symptoms, syndromes, and diagnoses of mental disorders in the parents. In this chapter, we report only on findings from the baseline survey and the first follow-up of the 14- to 17-year-olds, and we also include some of the family-history findings (for a full description of the study, see Wittchen et al. 1998b, 1998c).

At baseline, *lifetime and 12-month prevalence* rates were obtained for symptoms, key syndromes, and the full diagnostic picture. This information allowed us to evaluate syndromes present during the past 12 months and those present only prior to the 12 months preceding the baseline assessment. At follow-up, both the 12-month psychopathology and diagnoses and the interval psychopathology were evaluated to calculate the *incidence* (i.e., new cases of a disorder [individual was not previously affected at baseline or prior to baseline]) and the overall *cumulative lifetime incidence* (i.e., baseline lifetime or 12-month cases plus new cases).

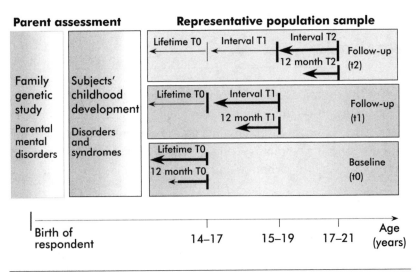

FIGURE 12–1.　*Early Developmental Stages of Psychopathology (EDSP) study: design and diagnostic information (see text for details).*

Samples

Community Respondents

The total sample was drawn from the 1994 Bavarian government registry of residents in metropolitan Munich, with all registrants expected to be 14–24 years of age during the first half of 1995 eligible for selection. For the purposes of this chapter, as noted earlier, only 14- to 17-year-olds are considered. Because the study was designed as a longitudinal panel with special interest in the development of psychopathological syndromes and disorders, and because of the low birth rates in the youngest birth cohort, 14- to 15-year-olds were sampled at twice the probability at which 16- to 21-year-olds were sampled, and 22- to 24-year-olds were sampled at half this probability.

Sample size (raw and weighted number of respondents) and response rates for the sample of 14- to 17-year-olds are summarized in Table 12–1. Of the 1877 individuals aged 14–17 years in the sample at baseline, 1,395 were located and interviewed. Sampled individuals who were not located were disproportionately older and uncontactable because either they had moved outside the metropolitan Munich area sometime between the time of their registration and the beginning of the study in 1995 or they could not be associated with the listed address during the fieldwork period. The response rate at baseline was 74.3%. Refusal to participate (12.2%) was by far the most frequent reason for nonresponse, followed by reported lack of time (3.8%). Other reasons for nonresponse were failure to contact anyone in the identified household (2.1%) and failure to contact the sampled individual in an identified household (3.0%). To account for the differential sampling probabilities and the nonresponse, we adjusted the data for age, sex, and geographic location to match the distribution of the sampling frame.

Of the 14- to 17-year-old subjects in the baseline sample, most (89%) were still attending school, 9.6% were currently in training for a job, and less than 1% were either already in the workforce, unemployed, or had dropped out of school (Tables 12–2 and 12–3). The majority of students (54.7%) were attending college-preparatory–level high school (*Gymnasium*); 19.7% of the students were attending intermediate-level high school (*Realschule*), and 10.2% were in short-course high school (*Hauptschule*). Almost all respondents (97.8%) were living with their

TABLE 12–1. *Sample size and response rates at baseline (t0) and follow-up (t1), by gender, in a sample of respondents from the Early Developmental Stages of Psychopathology (EDSP) study aged 14–17 years at baseline*

Sample	Total	Males	Females
Community sample			
Baseline sample (aged 14–17 years), n	1,877	963	914
Baseline (t0) completed interviews			
n	1,395	714	681
Response rate, % weighted	74.3	74.1	74.5
Follow-up (t1) completed interviews			
n	1,228	637	591
Response rate, % weighted	88.0	89.2	86.8
Parents sample			
Parent interviews			
n	1,053	541	512
Response rate, % weighted	95.7	84.9	86.6

parents at the time of the baseline interview. The majority of respondents (61.4%) were classified as belonging to the middle class, with only 4.7% belonging to the lower class. Subjective financial status was described by the majority as good (56.9%) or very good (13.2%), with only 3.8% describing a bad or a very bad situation.

At follow-up, 1,228 respondents were successfully reinterviewed (response rate of 88.0%). Considerably more subjects at follow-up, compared with baseline, either were in job training (21.0% at follow-up vs. 9.6% at baseline), were employed (3.8% vs. 0.8%), or had entered university (1.0% vs. 0%). The proportion of subjects living with their parents was slightly lower at follow-up compared with baseline (95.3% vs. 97.8%). No remarkable changes had occurred concerning social class and financial situation.

Community Respondents' Parents

A separate family study was conducted with the parents of respondents aged 14–17 years at baseline. Because we intended to assess detailed

TABLE 12–2. *Distribution of sociodemographic variables at baseline in a sample of respondents from the EDSP study aged 14–17 years*[a]

	Total ($n = 1,395, n_w = 921$)			Men ($n = 714, n_w = 464$)			Women ($n = 681, n_w = 456$)		
	n	n_w	$\%_w$	n	n_w	$\%_w$	n	n_w	$\%_w$
Employment									
School	1,290	819	89.0	653	405	87.2	637	415	90.0
University	...	...	...	...	...	...	...	...	...
Job training	91	88	9.6	52	51	11.0	39	37	8.1
Employed	7	7	0.8	4	5	1.0	3	3	0.7
Unemployed	2	1	0.1	1	1	0.1	1	1	0.1
Other	5	4	0.5	4	3	0.7	1	1	0.2
School type (current)									
Hauptschule	166	94	10.2	106	60	12.9	60	34	7.4
Realschule	297	181	19.7	144	87	18.8	153	94	20.6
Gymnasium	769	504	54.7	376	238	51.2	393	266	58.3
Fachoberschule	9	8	0.9	4	4	0.8	5	4	0.9
Other	49	33	3.6	23	16	3.5	26	17	3.7
No school	105	101	11.0	61	59	12.8	44	42	9.2
Living arrangement									
With parents	1,372	901	97.8	704	456	98.2	668	445	97.5
Alone	15	14	1.5	8	8	1.6	7	6	1.4
With partner	...	...	...	...	...	...	...	...	...
With other	8	6	0.7	2	1	0.2	6	5	1.1
Social class									
Lowest	4	3	0.3	3	2	0.3	1	1	0.2
Lower middle	61	41	4.4	40	27	5.8	21	14	3.1
Middle	867	565	61.4	416	267	57.5	451	298	65.3
Upper middle	378	259	28.1	209	140	30.1	169	119	26.0
Upper	52	34	3.7	29	19	4.0	23	15	3.4
None of the above	33	19	2.1	17	10	2.2	16	9	2.0

TABLE 12–2. *Distribution of sociodemographic variables at baseline in a sample of respondents from the EDSP study aged 14–17 years[a] (continued)*

	Total ($n = 1{,}395, n_w = 921$)			Men ($n = 714, n_w = 464$)			Women ($n = 681, n_w = 456$)		
	n	n_w	$\%_w$	n	n_w	$\%_w$	n	n_w	$\%_w$
Financial situation									
Very bad, bad	49	35	3.8	25	18	3.9	24	17	3.6
Not good or bad	362	241	26.2	197	129	27.8	165	112	24.6
Good	802	524	56.9	397	256	55.1	405	268	58.7
Very good	182	121	13.2	95	61	13.2	87	60	13.2

Note. n = unweighted number of respondents; n_w = weighted number of respondents; $\%_w$ = weighted percentage.
[a]None of the respondents were married.

information about natal complications, as well as psychological and somatic symptoms in infancy and early childhood, for each respondent by parent interview, we interviewed predominantly the mothers of the respondents. Only if the mother was not available (dead or not locatable) was the father interviewed. A total of 1,053 (1,026 mothers, 27 fathers) direct parent interviews were conducted in the family study investigation (response rate of 86%). Nonresponse among parents was predominantly due to refusal to participate (12.9%), with lack of time (0.5%) and failure to contact parents (0.7%) accounting for only a very small proportion of the nonresponse.

Symptom and Diagnostic Assessments

Symptom and diagnostic assessments at baseline and first follow-up were based mainly on the computer-assisted personal interview (CAPI) lifetime (T0) and 12-month (T1) change version of the M-CIDI (Wittchen and Pfister 1997; Wittchen et al. 1995a). In the parent investigation, symptom and diagnostic information was assessed by a modified family-genetic version of the M-CIDI (Lachner and Wittchen 1997). (For a detailed discussion of the M-CIDI and how it differs from the World Health Organization's CIDI, see Wittchen et al. 1998c and Lachner et al. 1998.) Briefly, the M-CIDI is a modified version of the World Health

TABLE 12–3. *Distribution of sociodemographic variables at follow-up in a sample of respondents from the EDSP study aged 14–17 years at baseline (see Table 12–2)*

	Total (n and n_w = 1,228)			Men (n = 636, n_w = 619)			Women (n = 592, n_w = 609)		
	n	n_w	$\%_w$	n	n_w	$\%_w$	n	n_w	$\%_w$
Employment									
School	938	882	70.8	477	432	69.8	461	450	73.9
University	8	13	1.0	...	...	...	8	13	2.1
Job training	228	258	21.0	132	147	23.8	96	111	18.2
Employed	33	47	3.8	17	24	3.9	16	23	3.8
Unemployed	5	6	0.5	2	3	0.4	3	3	0.5
Other	16	22	1.8	8	13	2.1	8	9	1.5
School type (current)									
Hauptschule	25	20	1.6	13	10	1.6	12	10	1.6
Realschule	194	159	13.0	108	89	14.3	86	70	11.6
Gymnasium	635	623	50.8	313	292	47.2	322	331	54.4
Fachoberschule	41	40	3.2	18	18	2.9	23	22	3.6
Other	43	40	3.2	25	23	3.8	18	16	2.7
No school	290	346	28.2	159	187	30.2	131	159	26.2
Living arrangement									
With parents	1,186	1,169	95.3	621	598	96.6	565	571	93.9
Alone	17	23	1.9	6	8	1.3	11	15	2.5
With partner	10	17	1.4	3	6	0.9	7	11	1.8
With other	15	19	1.5	6	7	1.2	9	12	1.9
Social class									
Lowest	4	4	0.4	3	3	0.5	1	1	0.2
Lower middle	65	69	5.6	40	43	7.0	25	26	4.2
Middle	693	690	56.2	339	333	53.8	354	357	58.6
Upper middle	438	437	35.6	238	224	36.2	200	213	35.0
Upper	19	19	1.6	14	13	2.1	5	6	1.0
None of the above	9	8	0.7	2	2	0.4	7	6	1.0

TABLE 12–3.   *Distribution of sociodemographic variables at follow-up in a sample of respondents from the EDSP study aged 14–17 years at baseline (see Table 12–2) (continued)*

	Total (n and n_w = 1,228)			Men (n = 636, n_w = 619)			Women (n = 592, n_w = 609)		
	n	n_w	$\%_w$	n	n_w	$\%_w$	n	n_w	$\%_w$
Financial situation									
Very bad, bad	52	56	4.6	32	33	5.3	20	24	3.9
Not good or bad	314	322	26.3	157	159	25.8	157	163	26.8
Good	695	681	55.6	360	342	55.3	335	340	55.9
Very good	165	166	13.6	86	84	13.7	79	82	13.4
Marital status									
Married	1	2	0.1	...	...	...	1	2	0.3
Not married	1,227	1,226	99.9	637	619	100.0	590	607	99.7

Note. n = unweighted number of respondents; n_w = weighted number of respondents; $\%_w$ = weighted percentage.

Organization's CIDI, version 1.2, that is supplemented by questions to cover criteria from DSM-IV and ICD-10 (World Health Organization 1992) (Wittchen and Pfister 1997; Wittchen et al. 1995a).

The M-CIDI allows for the assessment of symptoms, syndromes, and diagnoses of 48 mental disorders (not counting various subtypes of main disorders), providing information about onset, duration, and clinical and psychosocial severity. The diagnostic findings reported in this chapter are based on the M-CIDI/DSM-IV algorithms (Pfister and Wittchen 1995), but without use of the DSM-IV hierarchy rules, unless otherwise stated in the text. The M-CIDI includes numerous features that have been developed and tested in several methodological studies with the CIDI or modifications thereof (Wittchen et al. 1995a, 1995b):

- Use of symptom lists and memory aids that are assembled in a separate response booklet to improve lifetime recall, ease memory search, and shorten length of the interviews in the somatization and anxiety section

- Visual presentation of symptom and criteria lists to help the proband answer questions designed to assess onset and recency of reported symptoms
- Implementation of dimensional ratings in various sections for the assessment of impairment associated with core syndromes
- Specific rating of key syndromes for their first, worst, and most recent occurrence (see below), with additional questions to allow derivation of pure cross-sectional measures
- Inclusion of additional specific modules and self-rating questionnaires to assess chosen psychological constructs of special research interest in the M-CIDI as well as a separate response booklet for an accurate assessment of symptoms, syndromes, and diagnoses (An overview of the different psychological constructs, together with their assessment instruments, is provided in Table 12–4.)
- Implementation of separate current and lifetime ratings for the degree of impairment in various social roles (e.g., work, school, leisure time, partner) for each diagnostic section
- Addition of more open-ended questions describing the person's problems, allowing the clinical editor to judge the appropriateness of the CIDI ratings
- Inclusion of syndrome-based coding in some sections rather than the symptom-specific probe questions of the original CIDI
- Deletion of many of the CIDI skip rules in several diagnostic sections to allow for the study of subthreshold conditions (i.e., mixed anxiety-depression disorders and brief recurrent syndromes) and to improve the ability to measure more subtle changes in diagnostic status (because considerably less diagnostic stability is expected in adolescents than in adults)

Furthermore, the M-CIDI attempts a more detailed assessment of age at onset (Table 12–5) by separating onset questions for symptoms, syndromes, and diagnosis, as well as responses of those subjects who can clearly and exactly remember the first onset. Moreover, because the M-CIDI has separate summary questions to assess *diagnostic* age at onset—age at which the full set of diagnostic criteria were first met ("peak onset")—in addition to the CIDI questions, which base age at onset on first presence of key features only ("standard onset"), the effect of these

TABLE 12–4. *Measures used in the EDSP study to assess major psychological constructs*

Domain	Measure	Reference
Baseline interview		
Health behavior	Fragebogen zur Erfassung des Gesundheitsverhaltens	Dlugosch and Krieger 1994
Psychiatric symptom distress	Symptom Checklist–90— Revised	Derogatis 1986
Behavioral inhibition	Retrospective Self-Report of Inhibition	Resnick et al. 1992
Premenstrual symptoms	Premenstrual Symptom Scale	Wittchen 1995
Daily hassles	Daily Hassles Scale	Perkonigg and Wittchen 1995b
Life events	Münchner Ereignis Liste	Wittchen 1987
Self-esteem	Vergleich von Kompetenzen Skala	Lachner and Wittchen 1997
Problem-solving competence	Problemlösekompetenz Skala	Perkonigg and Wittchen 1995a
Self-esteem	Aussagen Liste zum Selbst-wertgefühl für Kinder und Jugendliche	Schauder 1991
Familial psycho-pathology	M-CIDI module for family history information	Wittchen et al. 1995a
First follow-up interview		
Recalled parental rearing behavior	Fragebogen zum erinnerten Erziehungsverhalten	Schumacher et al., in press
Resilience	Resilience Scale[a]	Wagnild and Young 1993
Daily hassles	Daily Hassles Scale	Perkonigg and Wittchen 1995b
Premenstrual symptoms	Premenstrual Symptom Scale	Wittchen 1995
Mood (survey)	Stimmungs Skala[a]	Bohner et al. 1991
Affect lability	Affect Lability Scales[a]	Harvey et al. 1989

TABLE 12–4. *Measures used in the EDSP study to assess major psychological constructs* (continued)

Domain	Measure	Reference
First follow-up interview (*continued*)		
Life events	Münchner Ereignis Liste	Maier-Diewald et al. 1983
Depression (attribution)	Reason for Depression Questionnaire[a]	Addis et al. 1995
Alcohol outcome expectancies	Effects of Drinking Alcohol Scale	Leigh and Stacy 1993
Family study		
Familial relationships	Subjektives Familienbild	Mattejat 1993
Family functioning	Family Assessment Device	Epstein et al. 1983
Parental educational style	Skala elterlicher Erziehungsmaßnahmen	Lachner and Wittchen 1997
Early development history	Child Behavior Checklist[b]	Achenbach 1992
Natal complications	Mannheimer Eltern Interview[b]	Esser et al. 1989
Somatic and psychopathological symptoms in infancy and early childhood	Mannheimer Eltern Interview[b]	Esser et al. 1989
ADHD	M-CIDI (module for ADHD)	Lachner and Wittchen 1997
Conduct disorder	M-CIDI (module for conduct disorder)	Lachner and Wittchen 1997
Oppositional defiant disorder	M-CIDI (module for oppositional defiant disorder)	Lachner and Wittchen 1997
Familial psychopathology	M-CIDI (module for family history information)	Lachner and Wittchen 1997
Help-seeking behavior in infancy and childhood	M-CIDI (specific questions on help-seeking behavior)	Lachner and Wittchen 1997

Note. M-CIDI = Munich Composite International Diagnostic Interview; ADHD = attention-deficit/hyperactivity disorder.
[a]Modified version.
[b]Selected questions.

two alternative assessment modes for age at onset can be explored. Throughout this chapter, we use the term *standard onset* to the onset as determined in the standard way with the CIDI and *peak onset* to refer to the onset of the full disorder.

The mean duration for completing the CAPI M-CIDI, including questionnaires, was 77 minutes. The decision to use the CAPI M-CIDI was made after pilot testing showed that CAPI interviews reduced the length of interview administration and helped avoid interviewer coding, skip rule, and probe question errors.

Family Study Information and Variables

For the present analyses, we focus on the following groups of variables:

1. Ten prenatal (e.g., infections of mother), 8 perinatal, and 10 post-natal (e.g., low birthweight) conditions and complications grouped together into one natal risk index with three levels of natal risk: no natal risk, moderate natal risk, and severe natal risk (Table 12–6)
2. Eighteen clinically significant sensory (e.g., poor hearing or sight), physical (e.g., epilepsy, asthma, allergies), or mental (e.g., enuresis, sleep disturbance) syndromes, conditions, or disabilities, along with information about the age at onset and recency of each
3. Type of specific childhood disorders (oppositional defiant disorder, conduct disorder, various forms of attention-deficit and hyperactivity disorders) and age at onset for each
4. Timing of and reason for professional help seeking for childhood mental problems as well as resulting diagnoses
5. Measures of marked affect lability in childhood as assessed by an affect lability scale for childhood problems

Reliability and Validity of the M-CIDI

The psychometric properties of the M-CIDI have been investigated in various locations and samples (Lachner et al. 1998; Wittchen and Pfister 1997; Wittchen et al. 1998a). Test-retest reliability findings for 14- to 24-year-olds ($n = 60$) (Wittchen et al. 1998a) examined by two independent interviewers were as follows: The average time interval between interviews (independent readministration by different interviewers) was

TABLE 12–5. *Assessment of age at onset in the anxiety and depression section of the CIDI, the M-CIDI, and the family study of the EDSP study*

Onset question type	Examples and remarks
Standard CIDI onset	
For symptoms	**Specific phobia:** "When was the first time you experienced such an unreasonably strong fear of heights?" [When more than a year ago: "How old were you then?"]
For syndromes and diagnoses	**Panic disorder:** "When was the first time you had such an unexpected, sudden spell or attack of feeling anxious or very uneasy and had at least four of the symptoms you mentioned, such as . . . [mention up to four symptoms previously endorsed]"
Extended M-CIDI questions	For each standard age-at-onset question (examples refer to panic attack):
Exactly recall	"Can you remember *exactly and clearly* the very first time you had such a spell or attack?" [If no: "At about what age?"]
First signs	"Can you remember exactly and clearly the very first time you had *any of things* from the list in front of you [respondent's list with all signs and symptoms]?"
Peak	"Can you remember exactly and clearly the very first time all the things from the list in front of you *occurred together*, that is, in about the same month?" [If no: "At about what age do you think you had . . . ?"]
Memory aids (visual response list)	All symptom and criteria questions are supported by visual response lists. Items endorsed were marked to help the respondent to remember to recognize all the relevant symptoms in complex age-at-onset summary questions when giving the answer.
Parental assessment (age at onset and recency for key syndromes of offspring)	"Please look at the list M4: Did your child ever suffer from any of the problems, symptoms, or illnesses after birth? Please mark all that apply and tell me at about what age they occurred for the first and the last time."

Note. CIDI = Composite International Diagnostic Interview; M-CIDI = Munich Composite International Diagnostic Interview.

TABLE 12–6. *Natal complications covered in the natal risk index*

No natal risk

Moderate natal risk (at least one of the following complications):

Strong nausea	Fetal malpresentation or cesarean section as birth complication
Diabetes mellitus	Pulmonary edema
Severe iron deficiency	Severe jaundice
Serious infection	Birth trauma
Shingles	Pseudocroup
Premature contractions or cerclage in pregnancy	Low birthweight
Excessive blood loss	Blood group incompatibility
Umbilical cord complications	Omphalitis
Forceps or vacuum extraction	Obstructive bronchial asthma
Precipitate delivery	Pneumonia or pylorospasm in the newborn

Severe natal risk (at least one of the following complications):

German measles	Premature placental separation or difficult delivery as birth complication
Abortion attempt	Severe cardiac difficulties
Placental insufficiency	Anoxia
Sepsis	Congenital infections
Shingles	Very weak muscle tone
Anemia	Convulsions
Excessively high or low blood pressure	Respiratory paralysis
Excessive bleeding/placental anomalies or hydramnios in pregnancy	Extreme preterm delivery
Poisoned amniotic fluid	Congenital immunodeficiency or reduced neonatal reflexes in the newborn

Note. In defining these three levels of risk, all reported natal complications were rated by cooperating clinicians.

38.5 days. Reliability for lifetime DSM-IV diagnosis was high for most disorders (kappa values above 0.65); the exceptions were bipolar disorder (0.64), any somatoform disorder (0.62), any eating disorder (0.56), and generalized anxiety disorder (0.45).

The procedural validity of the M-CIDI (Reed et al. 1998) was established in three ways: 1) by comparing the M-CIDI output to the output from the Structured Clinical Interview for DSM-IV, 2) by comparing the diagnostic output to the output from the Munich Diagnostic Checklist (Hiller et al. 1994), and 3) by comparing clinical consensus diagnoses with the M-CIDI output. Kappa values in a sample of 68 inpatients and outpatients, with the clinician diagnostic checklist taken as the gold standard, were as follows: single-episode and recurrent major depression, 0.96 and 0.95, respectively; bipolar disorder, 0.88; dysthymia, 0.54; social phobia, 0.80; other specific phobias, 0.64; panic disorder, 0.63; substance use disorder, 0.86; somatoform disorders, 0.50; posttraumatic stress disorder, 0.85; and obsessive-compulsive disorder, 0.90.

Interviewers, Interviewer Training, and Fieldwork

The survey staff for the baseline and follow-up investigations consisted of 39 clinically experienced interviewers (psychologists and health survey researchers). All interviewers had undergone several screening stages and were finally chosen from the initial group of 67 applicants. They received 2 weeks of training that included the CIDI standard training components. This training period was followed by at least 10 practice interviews that were closely monitored by our staff. Immediately prior to the beginning of each wave, one day of prefield training was held to stress important points and techniques and to increase the motivation of the interviewers. To assist interviewers in establishing contact or dealing with technical issues and to answer any questions from probands, a telephone hotline was installed.

To attain the maximum level of participation, several special efforts were made during the study:

1. Addresses of at least four contacts were given to another interviewer of the opposite sex, and overall at least 10 attempts at contact (with

a maximum of 15) were made at different times of the day and week, including weekends.

2. Interviewers who were especially successful at contacting were trained for recontacting difficult-to-contact probands.
3. Motivational letters with a telephone card enclosed and the request to call back were sent to 100 unreachable probands.
4. Up to DM 60 (U.S.$40) was offered to motivate the last, indecisive probands.

After the probands were contacted by letter and phone, a time and location for the interview was established. Most interviews took place at the time of first contact in the probands' homes. At the beginning of the interview, the written data protection explanation was given to the probands as well as a gift as an incentive for participation. The standard gift was two telephone cards, each worth DM 12 (U.S.$8).

The interviewers were closely monitored throughout the field period by clinical editors. The interviewers were required to contact the editors at the beginning of the study after having completed three to five interviews and, throughout the field period, when submitting completed interviews. This procedure gave the interviewers an opportunity to receive help with technical and content aspects of the interview. It also ensured that within a week of submission of the interview data to the clinical editor, interviews were checked according to a standard procedure for both formal consistency and appropriate recording techniques. During these weekly editing sessions, detailed feedback was given to every interviewer so that errors could be avoided in later interviews. The personal feedback for interviewers was maintained throughout the study to ensure a high quality of administration and to motivate the interviewers. The editors also gave the interviewers instructions for the reassessment of missing values or questionnaires. The correct administration of interviews was checked by random follow-up phone calls to probands.

The parental interviews were also conducted by highly trained interviewers (14 clinical interviewers, 13 nonclinician interviewers) shortly after the first follow-up investigation. As in the surveys with the probands (the procedure for which was just described), the interviewers were closely monitored by our clinical editors to guarantee the quality of the parent interviews.

Analysis

In this chapter, we report findings only for the following diagnoses, which occurred at sufficiently high frequencies: specific phobias, separation anxiety disorder, agoraphobia, social phobia, panic disorder, and depressive disorder (major depression and dysthymia). All data reported, unless otherwise stated, were weighted to adjust for the complex sampling weighting scheme (14- to 15-year-olds were oversampled) as well as for nonresponse. Prevalence and incidence estimates were computed with SAS (SAS Institute, Inc., Cary, NC) and SUDAAN (Research Triangle Institute, Research Triangle Park, NC). The SAS LIFETEST procedure was used to compute life-table estimates for age-at-onset analyses. Although hazard rates allow a much more detailed picture of age-at-onset characteristics, cumulative incidence curves are presented throughout this chapter to facilitate the recognition of differences between curves.

Results

Prevalence and Incidence at Baseline and Follow-Up

Table 12–7 presents the weighted lifetime and 12-month prevalence and incidence of specific DSM-IV anxiety and depressive disorders at baseline in the population aged 14–17 years and at first follow-up. Information about other mental disorders assessed is also presented. At baseline, overall, 21.3% of the population reported having had at least one of the anxiety disorders. Specific phobias were reported most frequently (17.1%), followed by separation anxiety disorder (4.5%), social phobia (3.7%), and agoraphobia (2.8%). Depressive disorders were less common (8.0% [major depression, 6.7%; dysthymia, 1.7%]). Comparison of the ratio between lifetime prevalence and 12-month prevalence among anxiety disorders (21.3% lifetime vs. 14.5% at 12 months) and among depressive disorders (8.0% lifetime vs. 4.8% at 12 months) suggests a slightly higher persistence of diagnostic status for anxiety disorders. It is noteworthy that even in this young age group, about one-third

TABLE 12–7. *Prevalence and incidence of anxiety and depressive disorders at baseline and follow-up in a sample of respondents from the EDSP study aged 14–17 years at baseline (N = 1228)*

	Baseline (t0) findings				Follow-up (t1) findings					
	Lifetime		12-month		Incidence		12-month		Cumulative lifetime[a]	
DSM-IV diagnosis	n	$\%_w$	n	$\%_w$	n	$\%_w$	n	$\%_w$	n	$\%_w$
Any depression	92	8.0	59	4.8	72	6.7	99	8.5	164	14.2
Major depression	72	6.7	39	3.4	66	6.0	80	6.8	138	12.2
Dysthymia	24	1.7	23	1.6	20	1.8	24	2.1	44	3.5
Any anxiety disorder	268	21.3	181	14.5	75	8.0	126	10.4	343	27.7
Panic attack[b]	39	3.2	23	1.9	31	2.7	30	2.5	70	5.8
Panic disorder	9	0.7	4	0.3	8	0.6	10	0.8	17	1.3
Agoraphobia	30	2.8	22	2.4	11	0.8	15	1.2	41	3.6
Social phobia	48	3.7	37	2.9	22	2.1	25	2.3	70	5.8
GAD	3	0.3	2	0.2	1	0.1	1	0.1	4	0.4
Separation anxiety disorder	55	4.5	…	…	…	…	…	…	55	4.5
Any specific phobia	217	17.1	139	10.9	59	5.7	94	7.7	276	21.8
Animal	66	5.4	46	3.8	19	1.7	28	2.5	85	7.0
Natural	40	2.9	27	1.8	6	0.5	8	0.6	46	3.4
Blood/injury	55	4.5	32	2.6	18	1.4	25	1.9	73	5.8
Situational	28	2.6	22	2.0	14	1.3	15	1.4	42	4.0
Other	11	0.9	8	0.7	2	0.1	2	0.1	13	1.1
NOS	78	6.0	38	2.9	24	2.1	28	2.2	102	8.0
Any other anxiety disorder	9	0.9	4	0.4	6	0.4	7	0.5	15	1.3
OCD	6	0.6	3	0.3	3	0.2	3	0.2	9	0.8
PTSD	4	0.5	2	0.3	3	0.2	4	0.3	7	0.7

TABLE 12–7. Prevalence and incidence of anxiety and depressive disorders at baseline and follow-up in a sample of respondents from the EDSP study aged 14–17 years at baseline (N = 1228) (continued)

	Baseline (t0) findings				Follow-up (t1) findings				
	Lifetime		12-month		Incidence		12-month		Cumulative lifetime[a]	
DSM-IV diagnosis	n	$\%_w$	n	$\%_w$	n	$\%_w$	n	$\%_w$	n	$\%_w$
Any substance use disorder[c]	164	16.1	155	15.2	172	15.1	252	20.2	336	28.7
Nicotine	119	11.5	112	10.8	100	8.3	152	12.5	219	18.9
Alcohol	66	7.2	56	6.2	115	9.6	128	10.4	181	16.1
Drugs	25	2.2	22	1.9	28	2.5	37	3.1	53	4.6
Any somatoform disorder[d]	25	2.7	18	1.8	57	4.8	59	5.1	82	7.3
Any eating disorder	12	1.1	11	1.0	9	1.0	5	0.5	21	2.1
Any other disorder	10	1.4	15	1.3	18	1.5	17	1.4	34	2.8
Any of the above	456	39.0	342	29.8	204	25.6	433	35.2	660	54.6
One	321	26.8	264	22.7	...	...	326	26.0	387	31.2
Two	95	8.4	57	5.0	...	...	87	7.5	192	16.1
Three	32	3.0	19	1.8	...	...	16	1.4	56	5.0
Four or more	8	0.8	2	0.1	...	...	4	0.3	25	2.3

Note. Raw *n* and weighted prevalences ($\%_w$) are reported in prevalence columns. GAD = generalized anxiety disorder; NOS = not otherwise specified; OCD = obsessive-compulsive disorder; PTSD = posttraumatic stress disorder.
[a]t0 + t1.
[b]Not a DSM-IV disorder per se, but criteria included in DSM-IV because such attacks occur in the context of several anxiety disorders.
[c]Twelve-month diagnoses for substance disorders require that all necessary diagnostic criteria be fulfilled in the past 12 months. Cases in which there is partial remission are not counted.
[d]Includes persistent pain, hypochondriasis, and somatization.

had two or more of the lifetime disorders listed in the table (when only any specific phobia was used and subtypes of specific phobias were not taken into account).

At follow-up, 19 months later, a considerable number of new cases (25.6%)—those in which the criteria for diagnosis had not been met previously—were observed. When the rates at baseline were taken into account, incidence rates were highest for depressive disorders (6.7%), panic disorder (0.6%), and social phobia (2.1%), with the resulting overall cumulative lifetime incidences of 14.2% for depressive disorders, 1.3% for panic disorder, and 5.8% for social phobia. Incidence rates were considerably lower for specific phobias (5.7%) relative to baseline prevalence (17.1%).

The overall comorbidity was also considerably increased at follow-up, with the diagnostic criteria for at least two disorders being fulfilled in almost one-half of all cases (when comorbidity between subtypes of specific phobia is not considered). Markedly different patterns of comorbidity emerged for anxiety and depressive disorders (Figure 12–2). At baseline, 59.0% of all anxiety disorders were pure disorders, with this proportion dropping to 39.3% at follow-up. The proportion of pure depressive disorders, already considerably lower (31.1%) than that of pure anxiety disorders at baseline, dropped further, to only 16.5% at follow-up. In 68.9% cases of depression at follow-up, there was comorbidity with at least one anxiety disorder, and there were particularly strong increases in the multimorbidity pattern (with depression, anxiety, and others increasing from 16.5% to 30.9%).

Onset of Anxiety and Depressive Disorders

The data in Table 12–7 suggest that depressive disorders are of later onset than most types of anxiety disorders, particularly phobic disorders. In order to examine diagnosis-specific patterns of age at onset and their stability over the follow-up period, we examined the cumulative age-at-onset curves for the baseline and follow-up findings separately. Computing separate baseline and follow-up cumulative incidence curves not only gives a detailed description of age-at-onset characteristics of each disorder but also provides a measure of consistency of respon-

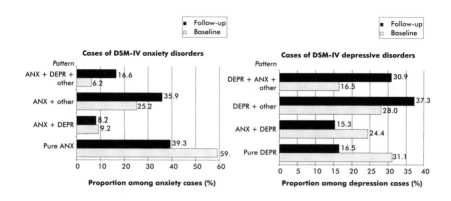

FIGURE 12–2. *Patterns of lifetime comorbidity at baseline and follow-up in a sample of respondents from the EDSP study aged 14–17 years at baseline.* ANX = anxiety disorder; DEPR = depressive disorder.

dents' answers regarding age at onset. *Consistency* here refers to the notion that, ideally, age at onset reported for incident cases at follow-up should not predate the age at onset given at baseline.

Figure 12–3 depicts the cumulative incidence of depressive disorders by age at onset as assessed from responses to the standard CIDI question *"When was the first time you had a period of two weeks or more when you felt (depressed/lost interest/other equivalents) and also had some of the other problems you mentioned (such as . . . [a list of all depressive symptoms endorsed is given])?"* The risk for first onset of depressive disorder steadily rose beginning at about age 12 years, with a marked and steady increase in the cumulative incidence among the baseline sample up to age 17. By the follow-up at age 19, the incidence had increased further. There was considerable stability in respondents' answers between baseline and follow-up, as indicated by the nearly complete overlap of the two curves in Figure 12–3 before age 14 years. In almost no incident case at follow-up did the respondent indicate having had onset of the disorder prior to the baseline examination.

Evaluation of the cumulative incidence of anxiety disorders by age at onset as assessed from responses to the standard CIDI question reveals a different picture (Figure 12–4). In more than two-thirds of cases of anxiety disorder, the respondent reported an early onset, specifically,

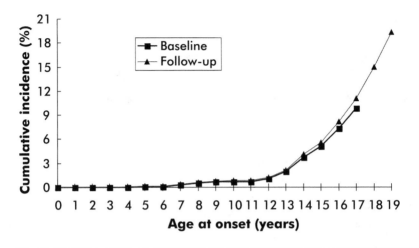

FIGURE 12–3.   *Cumulative incidence of depressive disorders, by age at onset, in a sample of respondents from the EDSP study aged 14–17 years at baseline.*

before age 14 years. Only relatively few incident cases were observed after the age of 14 and during follow-up for specific and social phobias. The only exceptions were the two less prevalent disorders of panic disorder and agoraphobia (Figure 12–5). Whereas for depressive disorders there was considerable stability in respondents' answers across time, for anxiety disorders there was some discrepancy between the information on age at onset gathered at baseline and follow-up. This discrepancy suggests that in many incident cases the respondent reporting a threshold anxiety at follow-up indicated an onset of the condition well before the baseline examination.

Ideally, such a discrepancy should not be found, since such early onset should already have been reported at baseline. As seen in Figure 12–5, this discrepancy is most pronounced in panic disorder and specific phobias and less marked in agoraphobia and social phobia. The effect is also evident for all subtypes of DSM-IV specific phobias (not shown separately in Figure 12–5), with no clear differences between phobias with predominantly very early onset (prior to age 10 years), such as animal and blood injury phobias, and those specific phobias with later

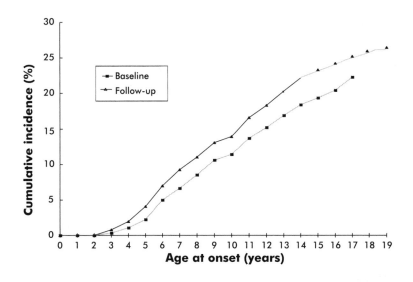

FIGURE 12–4. *Cumulative incidence of any anxiety disorder, by age at onset, in a sample of respondents from the EDSP study aged 14–17 years at baseline.*

onset, such as natural/environmental, situational, and other types (Figure 12–6).

Among several possible explanations for these inconsistencies in reporting age at onset, forgetting that one had the disorder at baseline was found to be an an unlikely hypothesis. A systematic review of the baseline symptom reports revealed that almost all subjects had already reported the respective fears and associated symptoms of anxiety. However, these symptoms failed to meet the full diagnostic threshold for a diagnosis. Thus, it is likely that a considerable proportion of subjects with subthreshold cases at baseline who developed the full disorder at follow-up based their age-at-onset report on the presence of the first or earlier significant signs and not the full diagnostic picture. The likelihood of this hypothesis is increased by the fact that the CIDI standard age-at-onset questions for anxiety disorders, unlike those for depressive disorders, do not clearly refer to the onset of the full diagnostic picture, but rather to selected key features, such as the occurrence of the first unexpected spontaneous panic attack in panic disorder or the occurrence of any unreasonably strong fear in social and specific phobias.

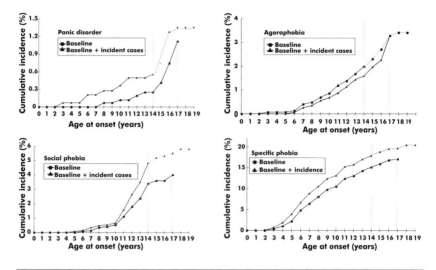

FIGURE 12–5.   *Cumulative incidence of specific anxiety disorders, by age at onset, in a sample of respondents from the EDSP study aged 14–17 years at baseline.*

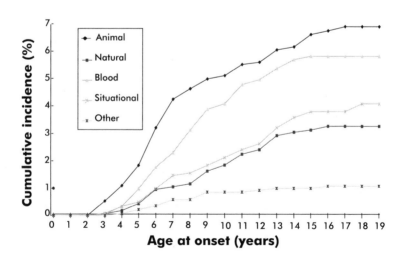

Age at onset (years)

FIGURE 12–6.   *Cumulative incidence of DSM-IV subtypes of specific phobias, by age at onset, in a sample of respondents from the EDSP study aged 14–17 years at baseline.*

Standard Versus Peak Age at Onset

To examine the issue of the effects of type of onset reported, we compared the cumulative lifetime age-at-onset curves for the syndrome-based standard CIDI questions and the diagnosis-based peak questions of the M-CIDI for panic disorder, social phobia, and agoraphobia (Figure 12–7). The respective diagnostic peak CIDI questions ensure, as in the assessment of onset in depression, that the respondent takes into account all relevant diagnostic features before answering the onset question.

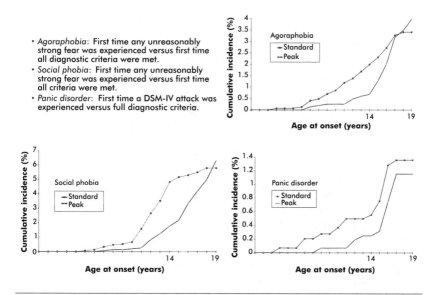

* *Agoraphobia*: First time any unreasonably strong fear was experienced versus first time all diagnostic criteria were met.
* *Social phobia*: First time any unreasonably strong fear was experienced versus first time all criteria were met.
* *Panic disorder*: First time a DSM-IV attack was experienced versus full diagnostic criteria.

FIGURE 12–7. *Effects of age-at-onset definitions (standard vs. peak) on cumulative lifetime incidence of specific anxiety disorders in a sample of respondents from the EDSP study aged 14–17 years at baseline.*

The "peak" definition results in a considerably lower proportion of early-onset cases, especially among prepubertal respondents with panic disorder, with steeper increases in risks after age 14 years. For phobic disorder this effect is clearly visible only after age 9 (agoraphobia) and 12 (social phobia). Overall, the peak onset definition, compared with the standard onset definition, results in a significantly higher average age at onset for panic disorder (mean age peak: 14.0 vs. 11.7 years; $P <$ 0.05), agoraphobia (14.4 vs. 12.0 years; $P < 0.001$) and phobias (14.2 vs.

11.7 years; $P < 0.001$). It is also noteworthy that in 52% of panic, 34 % of agoraphobia, and 37% of social phobia cases the standard and the peak age at onset were identical.

Thus, it can be concluded that age at onset based on the key features of the disorder only (i.e., standard CIDI procedure) results in slightly lower mean ages at onset than does the ("peak") diagnostic age-at-onset strategy.

Recall of First Onset of Anxiety Disorder

Kessler et al. (1998) recently demonstrated, for respondents aged 15–55 years in the National Comorbidity Survey, that accurate remembrance of the first occurrence has a substantial effect on respondents' reports of age at onset. We were interested in whether this finding could be replicated for more-recent-onset cases among individuals aged 14–17 years. Depending on diagnosis, 23%–32% of respondents with anxiety disorders overall, but only 4% of those with depressive disorder, indicated not being able to clearly remember the first time they had their disorder (standard onset). We suspect that these respondents, especially those with childhood-onset disorders such as specific phobias, tended to shift their age at onset into the past and tended to answer more frequently than those clearly remembering from the beginning that they had had their disorder. Although we compared the cumulative age-at-onset curves, as well as onset codes, for all diagnoses, no remarkable or statistically significant differences were found. Age at onset for panic was 11.8 years among those clearly remembering the onset vs. 11.7 years among those not clearly remembering; for agoraphobia, 11.8 years vs. 12.1 years; for social phobia, 11.8 vs. 11.0; and for specific phobias, 8.1 vs. 7.4.

Primary Anxiety and Secondary Depressive Disorders

Having shown in the previous analyses in this chapter that estimations of age at onset are significantly affected by the assessment mode, we now turn to the question of whether the assessment mode also results in different patterns of temporality in subjects with comorbidity. Figure 12–8 shows the frequency with which any of the disorders examined occurs either as the only or, if comorbid, the primary condition (defined

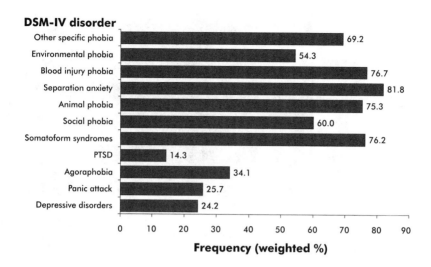

FIGURE 12–8. *Frequency at which some of the DSM-IV disorders examined in the EDSP study occurred either as the only or, if comorbid, the primary condition among respondents aged 14–17 years at baseline.* A primary condition was defined as having occurred at least 1 year before the onset of the second disorder on the basis of the standard CIDI age-at-onset question. PTSD = posttraumatic stress disorder.

as having occurred at least 1 year before the onset of the second disorder on the basis of the standard CIDI age-at-onset question). Because we assumed that there was some syndrome overlap for the age groups studied, we also included other forms of mental disorders (e.g., somatoform disorders, substance-related disorders, other anxiety and stress-related disorders, eating disorders) for this examination. It appears from these analyses that depressive disorders, panic attacks, agoraphobia, and posttraumatic stress disorder rarely occur as the only condition or the temporally primary condition. The most frequent early disorders were separation anxiety (81.8%), subtypes of specific phobias (except for the environmental types), and somotoform disorders and syndromes (76.2%).

Figure 12–9 shows the temporal relationship of comorbid disorders when the, diagnostically speaking, stricter, peak-onset definition (i.e., when all diagnostic criteria are fulfilled) is used consistently across disorders. Whenever anxiety disorders were involved in the comorbidity pattern, the anxiety disorders were almost always the primary condition.

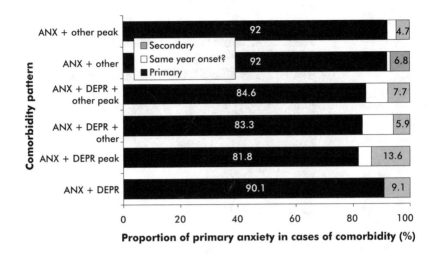

FIGURE 12–9.   *Comorbidity patterns of DSM-IV disorders, defined by stricter, peak-onset criteria, in a sample of respondents from the EDSP study aged 14–17 years at baseline.* The DSM-IV disorders included for consideration in this figure are those shown in Figure 12–8. ANX = anxiety disorder; DEPR = depressive disorder.

The only conditions preceding anxiety disorders in significant proportions were somatoform conditions. Depressive disorders were almost always secondary conditions. It is also noteworthy that a depressive disorder and an anxiety disorder, as reported by respondents, very rarely had their onset within the same year. Thus, the sequential comorbidity pattern was not affected by the assessment mode of onset used. Strictly defined DSM-IV depressive disorders rarely occurred early or as the only or primary condition.

Parental Information: Vulnerability and Early Developmental Risk Factors

Shifting emphasis from the respondents' reports to the parents' information given about the child's development, we examined the frequency with which the parents reported conspicuous signs of disorder considerably earlier than the adolescent in the interview. On the assumption that a considerable proportion of early childhood conditions might not be reliably remembered by the respondents, we focused on five fairly broad groups of variables from the independent family study, ranging

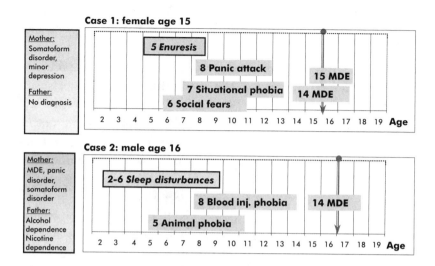

FIGURE 12–10. *Two case examples from family study sample of respondents from the EDSP study.* Blood inj. = blood injury; MDE = major depressive episode.

from birth complications through childhood syndromes to specific childhood disorders.

We mapped the parents' and the respondents' information graphically on a life chart (Figure 12–10) to look for, in particular, any indications that depressive syndromes were frequently reported by the parents considerably earlier than by the respondents. The two case records in Figure 12–10 provide some background information about the information used.

Each case contains a summary of the parents' psychopathology followed by a summary of the child's developmental history. This summary separates diagnostic information given by the parents (boxed) and respondents (shaded) and represents onsets of key features and the full disorder as assessed in the M-CIDI.

The frequencies of five groups of variables among adolescents and young adults with anxiety or depressive disorders, or both, were compared with those among subjects without mental disorders (Table 12–8). Overall, only three variables were significantly related to onset of anxiety and depressive disorders: clinically significant signs of affect lability in childhood (odds ratio [OR] = 2.01), early mental health treatment for some psychological reason (OR = 1.51), and any conduct or oppositional defiant disorder (OR = 1.91). Further, these associations seem to be highest in the group with comorbid disorders (anxiety and depressive disorders).

Analysis of the pre-, peri-, and postnatal complications reported by mothers (group 1) revealed that almost two-thirds of the subjects with any affective or anxiety disorder had some indication for at least one such complication. However, these complications were quite unspecific; almost identical frequencies were observed in subjects with no mental disorder. Similarly, no significant or specific associations were found for sensory, physical, and mental disabilities or for the specific psychological and psychophysiological syndromes assessed. In only one category—childhood pain syndromes—did the association come close to reaching statistical significance. Clinically significant signs of affect lability in early childhood were the strongest and most consistent indicator, especially for depressive disorders. For almost 50% of those with pure depression and 41% of those with comorbid depression—compared with only 20% in the reference group—at least one of the five key questions for affect lability was endorsed. Among the other variables, any professional help seeking, mostly reported for nondepressive symptoms, was significantly related to pure and comorbid depression, whereas early-childhood conduct disorder was related only to comorbid depression and anxiety.

To summarize, whereas natal complications and early sensory, physical, and mental disabilities are obviously fairly nonspecific in predicting anxiety and depressive disorders among adolescents, signs of affect lability in early childhood (by parents' report), professional help seeking, and early DSM-IV childhood disorders seem to be more specific childhood expressions of later anxiety and depressive disorders.

In a final explorative analysis, therefore, we examined whether onset characteristics for major depressive disorders, as ascertained by the respondents' M-CIDI algorithms, differed from age at onset as judged by the parents. In particular, we were interested in the degree to which age at onset for depression shifts forward when age-at-onset ratings of parents are used. In light of the low base rates for most of the significantly related variables—the exception being affect lability, which was not completely unexpected—we did not find any significant changes overall.

Discussion

Using longitudinal prospective data from a generalized population sample assessed with a modified version of the CIDI, we examined patterns of age at onset in a group of 14- to 17-year-old community subjects. Limiting the study to subjects aged 14–17 years offered several advantages. First, in terms of the cognitive and social development, this group is fairly homogeneous, with regard to, for example, the cognitive ability of understanding and answering the diagnostic interview questions. Second, in this age group a considerable proportion of anxiety disorders have just manifested themselves or will during the follow-up period, and thus we were able to get more accurate information regarding recent onset than other adult epidemiological surveys. Third, the mobility in this age group is not yet high, with the vast majority of subjects still living with their parents; these circumstances kept attrition low and enabled us more easily to get information from the parents about the child's development and mental health status.

However, several limitations of the study should also be mentioned. Concerning the exploration of onset characteristics, the study was a natural post hoc analysis and not an experiment that systematically examined the effect of age-at-onset assessment strategies, so we were restricted to data collected with the modified version of the M-CIDI. Further, the M-CIDI allows the examination of only two of the many possible variations in the assessment of age at onset of anxiety disorders—namely, the study of the effect of the question "Can you clearly remember the very first time?" and the effects of standard CIDI onset questions about anxiety disorder, which usually refer to key syndromes and features of the disorder—as opposed to questions that ascertain that the respondent has taken into account the full set of diagnostic criteria when giving his or her estimate. In conducting such analyses, we also refrained from examining gender-specific differences, mainly because of the lack of statistical power. It should also be mentioned that age-at-onset comparisons of parents and offspring are necessarily restricted to a fairly broad syndrome level and thus lack the high level of detail available from respondents when the M-CIDI is used.

With these limitations in mind, our findings suggest, consistent with

TABLE 12–8.   *Early indicators of anxiety/depression in a sample of respondents from the EDSP study aged 14–17 years at baseline (parents' information)*

	\multicolumn{4}{c}{Respondent diagnostic status at t_0/t_1}		
	\multicolumn{2}{c}{No threshold Dx^a}	\multicolumn{2}{c}{Any ANX/ DEPR Dx^b}	Univariate,
	n	$\%_w$	n	$\%_w$	OR (95% CI)
Pre-, peri-, and postnatal risk					
No indication	196	39.5	138	37.5	1.00 (. . .)
Mild/probable indication	137	29.2	108	30.8	1.11 (0.79, 1.54)
Severe/definite indication	152	31.3	119	31.7	1.07 (0.77, 1.48)
Sensory disabilities					
Poor sightedness, crosseye, poor hearing	16	2.9	11	3.3	1.15 (0.52, 2.55)
Impaired coordination or awkwardness	16	3.8	7	2.3	0.60 (0.26, 1.39)
Speech defects	15	3.7	14	3.3	0.87 (0.41, 1.83)
Any sensory disabilities	46	10.2	28	7.7	0.73 (0.45, 1.19)
Physical disabilities					
Physical disability, visible	18	3.5	15	4.0	1.16 (0.57, 2.39)
Physical disability, not visible	15	3.5	4	1.3	0.36 (0.13, 1.02)
Any physical disability	33	6.9	17	4.6	0.64 (0.35, 1.18)
Selected symptoms of mental disorders					
Sleep disturbances	28	5.5	30	8.1	1.50 (0.87, 2.59)
Elimination disorder symptoms (enuresis/encopresis)	21	4.5	16	4.0	0.88 (0.44, 1.75)
Tics	9	1.7	2	0.4	0.23 (0.04, 1.35)
Any symptom of mental disorder	53	10.7	46	11.9	1.13 (0.73, 1.73)
Somatic conditions					
Allergy, hay fever	108	21.5	82	23.4	1.11 (0.80, 1.54)
Diabetes	1	0.4	2	0.6	1.38 (0.19, 10.09)
Asthma	16	2.6	18	4.8	1.86 (0.88, 3.90)
Whooping cough	139	30.2	106	31.4	1.05 (0.78, 1.41)
Epilepsy or other convulsive disorders	9	2.0	9	2.1	1.07 (0.40, 2.83)
Pain troubles	15	3.2	20	5.8	1.87 (0.95, 3.67)
Any somatic condition	225	46.2	188	52.8	1.30 (0.99, 1.71)
Marked affect lability in childhood	101	20.2	121	33.8	2.01* (1.47, 2.75)
Early help seeking for					
Depression	16	3.7	12	2.7	0.73 (0.33, 1.62)
Other conditions	77	15.4	79	21.6	1.51* (1.06, 2.15)
Any condition	93	19.1	91	24.4	1.36 (0.98, 1.90)
DSM-IV childhood disorders					
ADHD	17	3.3	11	3.8	1.16 (0.55, 2.42)
Conduct disorder/ODD	14	2.6	17	4.9	1.91* (1.03, 4.00)

Note. ADHD = attention-deficit/hyperactivity disorder; ANX = anxiety disorder; n_w = weighted n; ODD = oppositional defiant disorder; OR = odds ratio.

| Respondent diagnostic status at t_0/t_1 | | | | | | | | |
| Only ANX[c] | | | Only DEPR[d] | | | ANX and DEPR[e] | | |
n	$\%_w$	OR	*n*	$\%_w$	OR	*n*	$\%_w$	OR
83	36.6	1.00	34	46.8	1.00	21	29.9	1.00
65	30.5	1.12	23	31.5	0.90	20	31.0	1.39
77	33.0	1.13	17	21.7	0.58	25	39.1	1.65
3	1.2	0.41	2	2.1	0.72	6	11.2	4.28*
4	2.0	0.53	1	2.1	0.55	2	3.4	0.90
9	3.3	0.88	2	2.0	0.52	3	4.5	1.22
14	5.7	0.53	5	6.2	0.58	9	15.3	1.59
9	3.7	1.05	4	6.6	1.94	2	2.4	0.67
1	0.5	0.13*	2	3.9	1.13	1	1.0	0.26
9	3.7	0.51	5	8.3	1.21	3	3.3	0.46
22	10.1	1.93*	4	3.8	0.67	4	6.5	1.18
10	3.6	0.81	1	0.9	0.20	5	8.5	1.97
2	0.7	0.39	...	...	...	...	...	...
32	13.4	1.30	5	4.7	0.41	9	14.9	1.47
53	24.4	1.17	16	20.6	0.94	13	23.4	1.11
1	0.6	1.53	1	0.9	2.22	...	...	...
9	3.0	1.14	6	8.5	3.42*	3	6.3	2.48
70	34.4	1.21	19	24.7	0.75	17	29.4	0.95
4	1.7	0.87	3	3.1	1.60	2	2.2	1.11
12	5.7	1.81	5	8.3	2.72*	3	3.6	1.12
120	55.0	1.42*	37	48.0	1.07	31	51.3	1.22
61	27.0	1.46*	33	46.8	3.46*	27	40.8	2.71*
8	2.9	0.78	1	1.8	0.47	3	3.3	0.88
40	17.3	1.14	22	27.0	2.02*	17	29.3	2.27*
48	20.2	1.07	23	28.8	1.71	20	32.6	2.04*
4	2.1	0.61	1	1.7	0.51	6	11.6	3.85*
8	3.4	1.30	2	3.5	1.35	7	11.2	4.68*

CI = confidence interval; DEPR = depressive disorder; Dx = diagnosis;
*P < 0.05; [a]$n = 485$, $n_w = 468$; [b]$n = 365$, $n_w = 368$; [c]$n = 225$, $n_w = 219$; [d]$n = 74$, $n_w = 78$; [e]$n = 66$, $n_w = 70$.

the majority of epidemiological surveys (Kessler et al. 1996; Lewinsohn et al. 1993), the following:

1. Threshold depressive disorders are predominantly disorders of late-adolescent or adult onset that show a strong increase at follow-up. Most anxiety disorders, especially specific phobias, and social phobia, however, occur considerably earlier, mostly in childhood, before the age of 12 years.

2. The finding that threshold depressive disorders are predominantly disorders of late-adolescent or adult onset is fairly robust across the different assessment modes for age onset. Determining the age at onset by taking into account the presence of the full diagnostic picture, in general, shifts onset to slightly higher ages. This effect was found to be strongest for social phobia and agoraphobia, with a mean shift in age at onset of approximately 2–3 years. The size of the shift did not affect the temporality pattern in comorbid anxiety disorders; it might, however, have led to significant changes with regard to intra-anxiety comorbidity patterns, which were not examined here.

3. Unlike Kessler et al. (1998), we did not find any significant effect for age at onset with regard to the entry question "Can you exactly remember . . ." Although for some disorders there were indications that those who were not able to clearly remember the very first age at onset chose the answer "I have had it all my life" slightly more often, there was no significant difference in age at onset. This question might function in young respondents (as in older respondents) as a trigger for the respondent to think hard and to stimulate a memory search for a particularly clear recollection before giving an answer (Kessler et al. 1998), but it does not appear to result in significantly different answers in this age group. One practical and technical implication of this exploration concerning different assessment modes for determining onset of anxiety and depressive disorder is that future studies should use ratings of onset for the key feature of a disorder consistently for all diagnoses examined. Unlike the inconsistent standard strategy incorporated in the DIS and CIDI, such a procedure will minimize artificial differences in onset between disorders and can be used more reliably in the evaluation of the earliest signs of a disorder.

Turning to the more theoretical implications of our findings, we also demonstrated that, irrespective of the way information about age at onset is collected, most forms of anxiety disorders (with panic disorder and generalized anxiety being the exceptions) are early and first primary diagnoses, whereas most depressive disorders are later and secondary diagnoses. With our more refined assessment methodology, we confirmed with good overall agreement (Burke et al. 1990, 1991; Kessler et al. 1994; Lewinsohn et al. 1995; Magee et al. 1996; Marks 1970) that specific phobias (particularly animal phobias and blood injury phobias) are usually the earliest disorders, followed by generalized social phobia, panic attacks, agoraphobia, and panic disorder. Separation anxiety disorder, somatoform conditions, and, less impressively in terms of their specificity, conduct disorders were the only conditions preceding primary anxiety disorder in a small but noteworthy proportion of the sample. The considerably later onset of depressive disorders, with only a few respondents having depression of prepubertal first onset, is consistent with the findings of the majority of other such studies (Wittchen 1994). It must be noted, however, that our study revealed slightly earlier age-at-onset patterns of first occurrence than most adult epidemiological studies (Kessler et al. 1998). This difference might be a reflection of our design, which possibly allowed us to get more valid estimates about onset than those obtained in studies that use samples of older subjects.

In light of the more recent etiological interest in studying sequential comorbidity, especially the effects of primary disorders on secondary depressive disorders, our findings reveal considerable robustness of temporality effects. Even in the strictest assessment of age at onset, the vast majority of anxiety disorders preceded the onset of a depressive disorder by some years. Together with the finding that pure and primary depressions are extremely rare, it is remarkable that the independent exploratory analysis of the parents' information about the child's development and their estimations about the earliest age at onset did not reveal a different picture. The one noteworthy exception was the parents' rating of childhood conditions, especially early signs of mood lability, that seem to be precursors of depressive and comorbid conditions later in life. Given, however, that this association was found in only about 20% of all cases with anxiety and depressive disorders, the overall predictive value is not impressive. In future analyses, we will examine the pathogenic implications of the sequential comorbidity patterns in more detail by focusing on early developmental risks and vulnerabilities.

References

Achenbach T: Assessment of anxiety in children, in Anxiety and the Anxiety Disorders. Edited by Tuma A, Maser J. Hillsdale, NJ, Lawrence Erlbaum, 1985, pp 707–734

Achenbach TM: Manual for the Child Behavior Checklist/2–3 and 1992 Profile. Burlington, University of Vermont, 1992

Addis ME, Truax P, Jacobson NS: Why do people think they are depressed? The Reasons for Depression Questionnaire. Psychotherapy 32:476–483, 1995

American Psychiatric Association: Diagnostic and Statistical Manual of Mental Disorders, 3rd Edition. Washington, DC, American Psychiatric Association, 1980

American Psychiatric Association: Diagnostic and Statistical Manual of Mental Disorders, 3rd Edition, Revised. Washington, DC, American Psychiatric Association, 1987

American Psychiatric Association: Diagnostic and Statistical Manual of Mental Disorders, 4th Edition. Washington, DC, American Psychiatric Association, 1994

Angst J, Dobler-Mikola A: The Zurich Study—a prospective epidemiological study of depressive, neurotic and psychosomatic syndromes, IV: recurrent and nonrecurrent brief depression. Eur Arch Psychiatry Neurol Sci 234:408–416, 1985

Anthony EJ: Discussion of chapters by Gittelman and Klein and Achenbach: a clinician's perspective, in Anxiety and the Anxiety Disorders. Edited by Tuma A, Maser J. Hillsdale, NJ, Lawrence Erlbaum, 1985, pp 403–412

Bohner G, Hormuth SE, Schwarz N: Die Stimmungsskala: Vorstellung und Validierung einer deutschen Version des "Mood Survey." Diagnostica 37:135–148, 1991

Burke KC, Burke JD Jr, Regier DA, et al: Age at onset of selected mental disorders in five community populations. Arch Gen Psychiatry 47:511–518, 1990

Burke KC, Burke JD Jr, Rae DS, et al: Comparing age at onset of major depression and other psychiatric disorders by birth cohorts in five US community populations. Arch Gen Psychiatry 48:789–795, 1991

Derogatis LR: SCL-90-R: Self-Report Symptom Inventory. Weinheim, Germany, Beltz, 1986

Dlugosch GE, Krieger W: Fragebogen zur Erfassung des Gesundheitsverhaltens. Frankfurt am Main, Swets, 1994

Eaton WW, Kessler RC, Wittchen H-U, et al: Panic and panic disorders in the United States. Am J Psychiatry 151:413–420, 1994

Epstein NB, Baldwin LM, Bishop DS: The McMaster Family Assessment Device. Journal of Marriage and Family Therapy 9:171–180, 1983

Esser G, Blanz B, Geisel B, et al: Mannheimer Eltern Interview. Weinheim, Germany, Beltz, 1989

Garrison CZ, Schluchter MD, Schoenbach VJ, et al: Epidemiology of depressive symptoms in young adolescents. J Am Acad Child Adolesc Psychiatry 28:343–351, 1989

Gittelman R, Klein DF: Childhood separation anxiety and adult agoraphobia, in Anxiety and the Anxiety Disorders. Edited by Tuma A, Maser J. Hillsdale, NJ, Lawrence Erlbaum, 1985, pp 389–402

Harvey PD, Greenberg BR, Serper MR: The Affective Lability Scales: development, reliability, and validity. J Clin Psychol 45:786–793, 1989

Hiller W, Dichtl G, Hecht H, et al: Testing the comparability of psychiatric diagnoses between ICD-10 and DSM-III-R. Psychopathology 27:19–28, 1994

Kessler RC, McGonagle KA, Zhao S, et al: Lifetime and 12-month prevalence of DSM-III-R psychiatric disorders in the United States: results from the National Comorbidity Survey. Arch Gen Psychiatry 51:8–19, 1994

Kessler RC, Nelson CB, McGonagle KA, et al: Comorbidity of DSM-III-R major depressive disorder in the general population: results from the US National Comorbidity Survey. Br J Psychiatry 168 (suppl 30):8–21, 1996

Kessler RC, Wittchen H-U, Abelson JM, et al: Methodological studies of the Composite International Diagnostic Interview (CIDI) in the U.S. National Comorbidity Survey. International Journal of Methods in Psychiatric Research 7:33–55, 1998

Lachner G, Wittchen H-U: Münchener Composite International Diagnostic Interview, M-CIDI (familiengenetische Version). Elternbefragung, Version 2.0. München, Max-Planck-Institut für Psychiatrie, Eigendruck, 1997

Lachner G, Wittchen H-U: Familiär übertragene Vulnerabilitätsmerkmale für Alkoholmißbrauch und abhängigkeit, in Abhängigkeit und Mißbrauch von Alkohol und Drogen. Edited by Watzl H, Rockstroh B. Göttingen, Germany, Hogrefe, 1997, pp 43–90

Lachner G, Wittchen H-U, Perkonigg A, et al: Structure, content and reliability of the Munich-Composite International Diagnostic Interview (M-CIDI). Substance use sections. Eur Addict Res 4(1–2):28–41, 1998

Leigh BC, Stacy AW: Alcohol Outcome Expectancies: scale construction and predictive utility in higher order confirmatory models. Psychol Assess 5:216–229, 1993

Lewinsohn PM, Hops H, Roberts RE, et al: Adolescent psychopathology, I: prevalence and incidence of depression and other DSM-III-R disorders in high school students. J Abnorm Psychol 102:133–144, 1993

Lewinsohn PM, Roberts RE, Seeley JR, et al: Adolescent psychopathology, II: psychosocial risk factors for depression. J Abnorm Psychol 103:302–315, 1994

Lewinsohn PM, Rohde P, Seeley JR: Adolescent psychopathology, III: the clinical consequences of comorbidity. J Am Acad Child Adolesc Psychiatry 34:510–519, 1995

Magee WJ, Eaton WW, Wittchen H-U, et al: Agoraphobia, simple phobia, and social phobia in the National Comorbidity Survey. Arch Gen Psychiatry 53:159–168, 1996

Marks IM: The classification of phobic disorders. Br J Psychiatry 116:377–386, 1970

Maier-Diewald W, Wittchen H-U, Hecht H, et al: Die Münchener Ereignisliste (MEL)—Anwendungsmanual. München, Max-Planck-Institut für Psychiatrie, Eigendruck, 1983

McGee R, Feehan M, Williams S, et al: DSM-III disorders from age 11 to age 15 years. J Am Acad Child Adolesc Psychiatry 31:50–59, 1992

Mattejat F: Subjektive Familienstrukturen. Untersuchungen zur Wahrnehmung der Familienbeziehungen und zu ihrer Bedeutung für die psychische Gesundheit von Jugendlichen. Göttingen, Hogrefe, 1993

Perkonigg A, Wittchen H-U: Problemlösekompetenz-Skala. Research Version. München, Max-Planck-Institut für Psychiatrie, Eigendruck, 1995a

Perkonigg A, Wittchen H-U: The Daily Hassles Scale. Research Version. München, Max-Planck-Institut für Psychiatrie, Eigendruck, 1995b

Pfister H, Wittchen H-U: M-CIDI Computerprogramm. München, Max-Planck-Institut für Psychiatrie, Klinisches Institut, 1995

Reed V, Wittchen H-U: DSM-IV panic attacks and panic disorder in a community sample of adolescents and young adults: how specific are panic attacks? J Psychiatr Res 32:335–345, 1998

Reed V, Gander F, Pfister H, et al. To what degree does the Composite International Diagnostic Interview (CIDI) correctly identify DSM-IV disorders? Testing validity issues in a clinical sample. International Journal of Methods in Psychiatric Research 7(3)142–155, 1998

Reznick JS, Hegeman JM, Kaufman ER, et al: Retrospective and concurrent self-report of behavioral inhibition and their relation to adult mental health. Development and Psychopathology 4:301–321, 1992

Robins LN, Regier DA (eds): Psychiatric Disorders in America: The Epidemiologic Catchment Area Study. New York, Free Press, 1991

Robins JN, Helzer JE, Crougham R, et al: NIMH Diagnostic Interview Schedule, Version III. Rockville, MD, National Institute of Mental Health, 1981

Schauder Th: The Statement List for the Self-Esteem of Children and Young People. Weinheim, Germany, Beltz, 1991

Schumacher J, Eisemann M, Brähler E: Rückblick auf die Eltern: der Fragebogen zum erinnerten elterlichen Erziehungsverhalten (FEE). Diagnostica (in press)

Wagnild GM, Young HM: Development and psychometric evaluation of the Resilience Scale. Journal of Nursing Management 1:165–178, 1993

Wittchen H-U: Münchener Ereignis Liste (MEL). Research Version. München, Max-Planck-Institut für Psychiatrie, Eigendruck, 1987

Wittchen H-U: Reliability and validity studies of the WHO-Composite International Diagnostic Interview (CIDI): a critical review. J Psychiatr Res 28:57–84, 1994

Wittchen H-U: Premenstrual Symptom Scale. Research Version. München, Max-Planck-Institut für Psychiatrie, Eigendruck, 1995

Wittchen H-U: What is comorbidity? Fact or artefact? (editorial). Br J Psychiatry 168 (suppl 30):7–8, 1996

Wittchen H-U, Essau CA: Comorbidity of anxiety disorders and depression: does it affect course and outcome? Journal of Psychiatry and Psychobiology 4:315–323, 1989

Wittchen H-U, Pfister H (eds): DIA-X-Interviews: Manual für Screening-Verfahren und Interview; Interviewheft Längsschnittuntersuchung (DIA-X-Lifetime); Ergänzungsheft (DIA-X-Lifetime); Interviewheft Querschnittuntersuchung (DIA-X-12 Monate); Ergänzungsheft (DIA-X-12Monate); PC-Programm zur Durchführung des Interviews (Längs- und Querschnittuntersuchung); Auswertungsprogramm. Frankfurt, Germany, Swets & Zeitlinger, 1997

Wittchen H-U, Vossen A: Implikationen von Komorbidität bei Angststörungen. Ein kritischer Überblick. Verhaltenstherapie Praxis Forschung Perspektiven 5(3):120–133, 1995

Wittchen H-U, Zerssen D von (Hrsg): Verläufe behandelter und unbehandelter Depressionen und Angststörungen. Eine klinisch-psychiatrische und epidemiologische Verlaufsuntersuchung. Berlin, Springer, 1987

Wittchen H-U, Essau CA, Krieg JC: Anxiety disorders: similarities and differences of comorbidity in treated and untreated groups. Br J Psychiatry 159 (suppl 12):23–33, 1991

Wittchen H-U, Knäuper B, Kessler RC: Lifetime risk of depression. Br J Psychiatry 165 (suppl 26):16–22, 1994

Wittchen H-U, Beloch E, Garczynski E, et al: Münchener Composite International Diagnostic Interview (M-CIDI, Paper-Pencil 2.2, 2/95). München, Max-Planck-Institut für Psychiatrie, Klinisches Institut (Eigendruck), 1995a

Wittchen H-U, Kessler R, Zhao S, et al: Reliability and clinical validity of UM-CIDI DSM-III-R generalized anxiety disorder. J Psychiatr Res 29:95–110, 1995b

Wittchen H-U, Lachner G, Wunderlich U, et al: Test-retest reliability of the computerized DSM-IV version of the Munich-Composite International Diagnostic Interview (M-CIDI). Soc Psychiatry Psychiatr Epidemiol 33:568–578, 1998a

Wittchen HU, Nelson GB, Lachner G: Prevalence of mental disorders and psychosocial impairments in adolescents and young adults. Psychol Med 28:109–126, 1998b

Wittchen H-U, Perkonigg A, Lachner G, et al: Early developmental stages of psychopathology study (EDSP): objectives and design. Eur Addict Res 4(1–2):18–27, 1998c

World Health Organization: Composite International Diagnostic Interview (CIDI). Geneva, World Health Organization, Division of Mental Health, 1990

World Health Organization: International Classification of Diseases, 10th Revision. Geneva, World Health Organization, 1992

13

Very-Early-Onset Bipolar Disorder: Does It Exist?

Gabrielle A. Carlson, M.D.

Anthony and Scott (1960) first documented the occurrence in children of strictly defined, noncomorbid, uncomplicated manic-depressive illness almost 40 years ago. Since then, a number of reports have been added to this body of literature (for review, see Carlson 1990, 1994). However, as will be seen later in this chapter, the occurrence of uncomplicated, noncomorbid bipolar disorder in young children is quite rare, with the frequency apparently increasing as puberty/adolescence approaches (Carlson 1983). On the other hand, it has become quite clear that a significant number of clinically referred children have conditions that meet at least the symptom criteria for mania. How *frequently* bipolar disorder in children occurs thus becomes the more pertinent and controversial question, and the question of frequency is contingent on how bipolar disorder is defined.

A second question relevant to discussion of very-early-onset bipolar disorder pertains to what continuity exists between youth and adult bipolarity. This question is usually addressed in two ways: 1) Did an adult with bipolar disorder have prodromal symptoms in childhood? (e.g.,

This chapter was prepared with the support of grants from the National Institute of Mental Health (MH-44733 and MH-44801). I gratefully acknowledge the assistance of the Suffolk County Mental Health Project staff, Kevin L. Kelly, Ph.D., and the Stony Brook University Hospital 12-N Inpatient Staff.

Lish et al. 1994), and 2) Will a child whose condition meets the criteria for mania grow up to have adult manic depression?

This focus of this chapter is on the second question. The first part of the chapter is devoted to a discussion of definition. The second part presents data to clarify the relationship between youth and adult bipolar disorder.

Manic Symptoms

Just as depression can be defined as a symptom, a syndrome, and a disorder, so can mania. The hallmark of mania is elated, expansive, irritable, or volatile mood. These kinds of mood disturbance, composing the A criterion from DSM-III, DSM-III-R, and DSM-IV (American Psychiatric Association 1980, 1987, 1994), have become the subject of the screening question in structured interviews used to make diagnoses in clinical and nonclinical samples. Such mood disturbance is synonymous with emotional lability. The manic syndrome consists of symptoms of mania (the B criterion in DSM) without a discrete onset or offset (i.e., episode). To maintain some clarity of definition, it is best to reserve the diagnosis *bipolar disorder* for those cases in which there are episodes of mania that can be distinguished from episodes of depression or phases of euthymia.

It is unclear whether emotional lability or manic symptoms represent a generalized symptom of central nervous system hyperarousal in a medically diseased state (e.g., organic affective personality as described in DSM-III and DSM-III-R), a subclinical manifestation of a psychopathological state (see, e.g., Akiskal 1992), a temperamental trait (see, e.g., Tanguay 1997), or all of these.

Manic Symptoms in Neurological Disorders

There are four psychopathological states in which emotional lability appears as a cardinal feature. The first is in association with neurological disorders. The adult psychiatry literature is replete with case reports of manic symptoms occurring after a stroke or as part of a metabolic disorder. In its full-blown state, this occurrence of symptoms is called *secondary mania* (for review, see Evans et al. 1995). This phenomenon is observed in children as well. Swedo and Pekar, in Chapter 5 of this volume, emphasize the importance of the symptom of emotional lability in the early diagnosis of a poststreptococcal movement disorder (Sydenham's chorea), accompanied by emotional and obsessive-compulsive symptoms. In a follow-up study of children 1 year after a moderate to serious closed head injury, Gerring et al. (1998) found that emotional lability was a very common sequela. It was most serious in children who either developed attention-deficit/hyperactivity disorder (ADHD) *after* the head injury or had their ADHD symptoms exacerbated by the injury. In these cases, three characteristics quadrupled in severity: emotional lability, symptoms of ADHD, and aggressive behavior. Some children, in fact, met the symptom criteria for mania on structured interview (J. P. Gerring, personal communication, October 10, 1997).

Organic personality syndrome (or disorder) has been the time-honored designation for behaviors secondary to some sort of brain disease that occurs in clear consciousness. This syndrome has been characterized by "lability and shallowness of affect and impairment of judgment" (DSM-II; American Psychiatric Association 1968) or, in greater detail, "affective instability, e.g., marked shifts from normal mood to depression, irritability, or anxiety," "recurrent outbursts of aggression or rage that are grossly out of proportion to any precipitating psychosocial stressors," "markedly impaired social judgment, e.g., sexual indiscretions," "marked apathy and indifference," and "suspiciousness or paranoid ideation" (DSM-III-R; American Psychiatric Association 1987, p. 115). Although this syndrome has been eliminated from DSM-IV because of its lack of specificity, and it is apparently necessary to be able to define the central nervous system lesion in order to give someone the diagnosis of "mood disorder secondary to . . .," it is clear that chronic mood and behavior dysregulation can be associated with known and probably unknown central nervous system pathology.

Manic Symptoms in Psychotic-Like Disorders

Emotional lability accompanies other serious psychopathology in children. Just as there has been a long history of disentangling schizophrenia

with affective symptoms from psychotic bipolar disorder in adults, iron-
ically, emotional lability or dysregulation appears to complicate disorders in children that, years ago, had been designated as "childhood
schizophrenia." As is described elsewhere in this volume (see Chapter
8), Dr. Rapoport and colleagues, in their efforts to recruit a population
of children with narrowly defined schizophrenia, found that 30% of their
referred sample had "complex developmental disorders and brief
psychotic symptoms that did not meet DSM-III-R criteria for schizophrenia" (see Kumra et al. 1998; McKenna et al. 1994). Criteria for this
syndrome—individuals with which are referred to as "multidimensionally impaired"—consist of

> nearly daily periods of emotional lability disproportionate to precipi-
> tants; poor ability to distinguish fantasy from reality as evidenced by
> ideas of reference and brief perceptual disturbances during stressful
> periods or while falling asleep; impaired interpersonal skills despite
> desire to initiate social interactions with peers; cognitive deficits indi-
> cated by multiple deficits in information processing; absence of formal
> thought disorder. (Kumra et al. 1998, p. 92)

As was seen in Gerring et al.'s (1998) description of children with
brain injury, a high proportion of multidimensionally impaired children
(84%) meet the criteria for ADHD. The disorder is also characterized
by very early onset and considerable disability.

Manic Symptoms in Pervasive Developmental Disorders

Another research group interested in autism and pervasive developmental disorders found a population of children who did not meet the
narrow criteria for infantile autism. Towbin et al. (1993) described a
condition called "multiple complex developmental disorder." Recognizing that this condition possibly encompasses children previously
described as "schizophrenic," "borderline," or "atypical" or as having
"childhood onset pervasive developmental disorder," the authors
admitted that they did not know what the ultimate course of the condition in this group of children would be.

Multiple complex developmental disorder comprises three categories of symptoms that have an impact on affect/mood, cognitive function, and social interaction, respectively. The major affective symptoms of this condition include "regulation of affective state and anxiety" that is "impaired beyond that seen in children of comparable mental age mani-fested by . . . intense generalized anxiety, diffuse tension or irritability"; "unusual fears and phobias"; "recurrent panic episodes"; "episodes lasting from minutes to days of behavioral disorganization or regression"; "significant and wide emotional variability with or without environ-mental precipitants"; and "high frequency of idiosyncratic anxiety reac-tions such as sustained periods of uncontrollable giggling, giddiness, laughter, or 'silly' affect that is inappropriate in the context of the situ-ation" (Towbin et al. 1993, p. 777).

Symptoms vaguely similar to those of psychosis include "impaired cognitive processing (thinking disorder) manifested by . . . irrationality, sudden intrusions on normal thought process, magical thinking, neol-ogisms or nonsense words repeated over and over, desultory thinking, blatantly illogical bizarre ideas"; "confusion between reality and fantasy life"; "perplexity and easy confusability (trouble with understanding ongoing social processes and keeping one['s] thoughts 'straight')"; and "delusions, including fantasies of personal omnipotence, paranoid preoccupations, overengagement with fantasy figures, grandiose fanta-sies of special powers, and referential ideation" (Towbin et al. 1993, p. 777).

Multiple complex developmental disorder sounds similar to the multidimensional impairment described earlier, though there is closer continuity with the pervasive developmental disorders in the category of "consistent impairments in social behavior and sensitivity"—for example, "social disinterest, detachment, avoidance or withdrawal in the face of evident competence (at times) of social engagement, partic-ularly with adults." Attachments "may appear friendly and cooperative but very superficial, based primarily on receiving material needs." There is an "inability to initiate or maintain peer relationships." Also present are "disturbed attachments displaying high degrees of ambivalence to adults, particularly parents/caregivers, as manifested by clinging, overly controlling, needy behavior, and/or aggressive, oppositional behavior" and "profound limitations in the capacity of empathy or to read or under-stand others['] affects accurately" (Towbin et al. 1993, p. 777).

The point in describing these as yet unvalidated conditions is to emphasize that two completely independent groups, with completely different theoretical and research orientations, have recognized the existence of a group of children with unusual behavior characterized by a significant mood component that does not meet the criteria for bipolar disorder (manic depression) and psychotic symptoms of insufficient intensity or duration to meet the criteria for schizophrenia, but in whom significant comorbidity and disability exist.

Manic Symptoms and ADHD

ADHD has become the biggest focus in the controversy about whether hyperactive, inattentive children with emotional lability really exhibit mania or "just have ADHD." Both Biederman's group (Biederman et al. 1995; Faraone et al. 1997; Wozniak et al. 1995) and Geller's group (Geller et al. 1998) have chosen "uncomplicated ADHD" as a comparison category to point out the discreteness of childhood mania. Again, however, a look back into the history of "the hyperactive child" syndrome reveals that it was initially designated as including a good deal of emotional lability, sleep disturbance, and variation in behavior. Although hyperactivity and short attention span were the first two symptoms detailed in Laufer and Denhoff's (1957, pp. 464–464) original description of the hyperkinetic behavior syndrome in children, variability was the third. Laufer and Denhoff noted that "[b]ehavior is unpredictable, with wide fluctuations in performance." Other symptoms included impulsiveness and inability to delay gratification, irritability ("fits of anger are easily provoked"), and explosiveness ("reactions of these children are often almost volcanic in their intensity"). Other relevant observations made by Laufer and Denhoff were that in infancy "the baby may have been exceedingly irritable and cried readily" and that sleep problems are common, with early waking and "rampaging through the house in hyperactive, noisy and sleep-disturbing play." Not surprisingly, in DSM-I (American Psychiatric Association 1952), before the designation of "hyperkinetic reaction of childhood" was introduced, the diagnoses "passive-aggressive personality," "anxiety reaction," and "emotionally unstable character" were used to describe such children's conditions (Laufer et al. 1957). Our current comorbidities are oppositional defiant disorder, various anxiety disorders, and bipolar disorder. In tracing the elimination of impulsivity, low frustration tolerance, variability, and so forth from the criteria for ADHD, it would appear that it was the lack of reliability and lack of specificity, not the absence of association, that resulted in these symptoms being phased out of our clinical picture of ADHD (D. Cantwell, personal communication, January 1996). The law of unintended consequences may have resulted in a reconfiguring of ADHD such that some children initially described as exhibiting "hyperkinetic" behavior would be reconceptualized now as having a "bipolar" condition, at least in terms of onset from birth, redefinition of variability as "episodes," and irritability, explosiveness, and impulsiveness.

In conclusion, clinicians have been associating emotional lability with ADHD-type behaviors and psychotic illness–like behaviors for many years and labeling them in different ways. This longstanding recognition suggests an intrinsic and enduring association between these sets of behaviors. One suspects the disagreement is less about the identification of the type of child being described and more about the appropriate label (severe ADHD, schizophrenia spectrum, pervasive developmental disorder spectrum, organic brain disorder, childhood mania).

Nonclinical Samples

How often does one observe emotional lability in a nonclinical population? Estimates of rates of emotional lability from several epidemiological studies range from 5% to 10% (Table 13–1). Furthermore, the symptom of frequent mood change, or "elated, expansive or irritable mood," is associated with other more definitive psychopathology, at least as elicited by structured interview. The association of ADHD, oppositional defiant disorder/conduct disorder, substance use disorder, and anxiety and depression with labile mood is observed, then, even in a nonclinical population. Another example of the association between behavior and mood variability is that seen in the Berkeley Guidance Study (Caspi et al. 1990). Children with ill tempers (judged by severity and frequency of temper tantrums) were followed up at age 30 years, and a personality Q-sort was conducted. The researchers found significant correlations between childhood ill temper and items like "tends

TABLE 13–1.   *Prevalence of symptoms of emotional lability in three community studies*

	Carlson and Kashani (1988)	Lewinsohn et al. (1995)	Tohen and Goodwin (1995)
Sample	Adolescents, ages 14–16 years	Adolescents, ages 14–18 years	Adults
Prevalence/ Definition	10%	5.7%	5.4%
	Moods up and down quickly	Distinct period of elevated, irrita-ble, and expan-sive mood	1 week of euphoria or irritability (ECA)
	Proportion of sample (%)		
Rates of disorder in subjects with emotional lability			
Major depres-sion	60	48.5	
Anxiety disorder	50	32.0	
Disruptive be-havior disorder	40	18.6	
Substance use disorder	N/A	23.7	

Note. ECA = Epidemiologic Catchment Area study; N/A = not applicable.

toward under-control of needs and impulses," "tends to perceive many different contexts in sexual terms," "sees what he can get away with," "is self-dramatizing," "is irritable," "is guileful," "has fluctuating moods," "is a talkative individual," "is self-indulgent," "is gregarious," and "initiates humor." It would appear from these data that manic symptoms or symptoms of emotional lability in the general population are not uncommon and, like manic symptoms in clinically referred children, are associated with both externalizing and internalizing symptoms, both in childhood and in adulthood.

Manic Syndrome

The *manic syndrome* is defined as either euphoria or irritability and the presence of four other symptoms of mania. *There is no requirement that these represent a change in behavior.* Moreover, since mania is probably the ultimate externalizing disorder (i.e., others are more troubled by the manifestations than the manic person is), if the manic episode is not observed by others, it is fair to say that it probably is not occurring. Therefore, it is quite appropriate to consider getting information about manic symptoms and the manic syndrome from people who live with or see regularly the person in question. When such information was obtained with the Diagnostic Interview for Children and Adolescents (Herjanic and Reich 1982) for a sample of 14- to 16-year-olds in Columbia, Missouri, 13.3% of the children were found to have what was termed mania without either episode or severity defined (Carlson and Kashani 1988). I am unaware of a similar study in prepubertal children.

In a clinical sample, it is possible for me to address both the outpatient clinic and inpatient service at the State University of New York at Stony Brook. For the past 10 years, we have been using a DSM-based parent- and teacher-rated checklist, the Child Symptom Inventory (Gadow and Sprafkin 1994), as part of our clinical database. To answer the question of how frequently a "manic syndrome" is occurring in our clinic, I examined rates of manic symptoms as screened with this checklist and the frequency with which parents endorsed at least five symptoms of mania in a sample of children aged 6–18 years. Except for "unusually explosive and irritable," which increased with age (reflecting a referral bias as much as anything), the rates for symptoms of the manic syndrome were remarkably stable at about 9% (Table 13–2).

TABLE 13–2.   *Rates of parent-reported manic symptoms (%) in a sample of referred outpatients*

	Age groups (years)			
	6–10	11–12	13–15	16–18
"Unusually cheerful"	10.0	11.5	15.7	12.1
"Unusually irritable"	21.0	24.6	36.7	39.3
≥5 manic symptoms on the CSI	9.0	9.8	9.6	9.1

Note. CSI = Child Symptom Inventory.
Source. G. A. Carlson, unpublished data, 1998.

Independent verification for this finding comes from a more systematic examination carried out in the Long Island Follow-Up Study (LIFUS; J Loney, H. Salisbury, G. A. Carlson, et al., submitted), in which 250 boys, ages 6–10 years, were evaluated with the Diagnostic Interview for Children and Adolescents, Parent and Child Version (Herjanic and Reich 1982). These boys were referred to the study from the clinic; an ADHD parent support group, CHADD (Children and Adults with Attention Deficit/Hyperactivity Disorder); and schools. The community was invited to refer boys with behavior or emotional problems, since the study was interested in examining comorbidity of both. We found that the criteria for a manic syndrome were met in 9.3% of the boys (Carlson et al. 1998b). Finally, using the DSM-III-R version of the Child Symptom Inventory, we found that 52% of parents endorsed five or more symptoms of mania for the 5- to 12-year-old patients hospitalized on the psychiatric inpatient unit between 1988 and 1992 (Carlson and Kelly 1998) (Table 13–3). In both the LIFUS and the inpatient samples, the children had the same range of diagnoses on structured interview as that reported for children with manic symptoms—namely, high rates of ADHD, oppositional defiant disorder, conduct disorder, and mood disorder. In addition, symptom correlations for these disorders were significant, ranging from 0.3 to 0.47.

Although we have not yet examined the long-term implications of the manic syndrome in the LIFUS sample, several significant observations can be made about the inpatient sample (Carlson and Kelly 1998). First, children with parent-reported manic symptoms, compared with those with no such parent-reported symptoms, were also seen by their teachers as having more manic symptoms prior to admission. Furthermore, these observations were corroborated by the inpatient staff on the basis of several factors from the rating scales used to evaluate the children weekly. The children with manic symptoms were significantly more disinhibited, overactive, inattentive, and euphoric than their nonmanic counterpart, and they had higher rates of comorbid conduct disorder and mood disorder and of conduct disorder alone. In the nonmanic group, the rates of depression alone were higher. Bipolar disorder (manic-depressive illness) was equally represented in both groups, though children in the nonmanic group were admitted during a depressed phase of their illness. Most important, children with manic

TABLE 13–3. *Manic symptoms on the Child Symptom Inventory in a psychiatrically hospitalized group of children*

Periods lasting 2 days or more in which child:	Proportion endorsing[a] (%)
Is extremely active (goes nonstop)	58.3
Does reckless or silly things	54.3
Is explosive and irritable	53.5
Switches rapidly from one topic to another	44.1
Talks excessively	53.5
Needs only a few hours of sleep at night	34.6
Believes that he or she has special abilities or can do things that are unrealistic	23.6
Is abnormally cheerful	16.5

[a]Endorsement was for "often" or "very often."
Source. Carlson and Kelly 1998.

symptoms needed an average of 2 weeks longer to achieve the same level of stability as their nonmanic peers.

Given the consistent finding of comorbid symptoms of externalizing disorder that occur with manic symptoms, it seemed relevant to ask whether the increased severity observed in children with manic symptoms or manic syndrome is a function of comorbidity (i.e., whether having more than one disorder is likely to increase the level of dysfunction), or whether there is a unique morbidity conferred by the manic symptoms themselves. To examine this question, in the LIFUS study we compared the 23 children with the manic syndrome with the next child seen in the study and a comparison group matched for symptoms of ADHD, oppositional defiant disorder, and conduct disorder (Carlson et al. 1998a). Scores from the Child Behavior Checklist (Achenbach 1991), which has been used to describe other samples of outpatients with manic symptoms (e.g., Biederman et al. 1995; Faraone et al. 1997; Wozniak et al. 1995), were used as the basis for comparison. We found that most of the significant differences between the groups completely disappeared. One measure for which there was still a significant difference in scores between groups was the depression/anxiety factor (Figure 13–1); this suggests that the "emotionality" factor remains even in the absence of the aggression/ADHD behaviors.

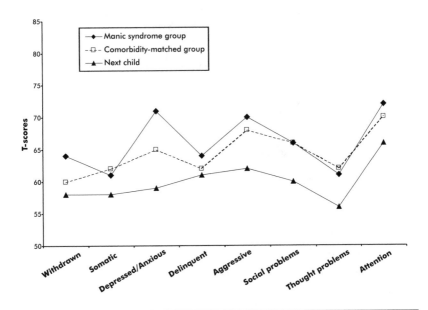

FIGURE 13–1. *Child Behavior Checklist factor scores for children with the manic syndrome compared with those for the next child seen in the study and a comparison group matched for symptoms of attention-deficit/hyperactivity disorder, oppositional defiant disorder, and conduct disorder.* A T-score of 50 is the normative sample mean. Each 10 points is one standard deviation. The manic symptom group is two standard deviations above the normative sample (as developed by Achenbach) in depression, aggression, and attention.

There did not appear to be a real difference in pattern between the LIFUS and inpatient samples, in which the diagnosis of manic syndrome was assigned, and the Massachusetts General Hospital sample, in which the diagnosis of bipolar disorder was given. What is clear is that the more disturbed the sample, the higher the factor scores, with this pattern especially evident with the aggression and social problems factors (Figure 13–2).

Bipolar Disorder

Comorbidity is a very apparent issue among children who are said to meet the criteria for bipolar disorder. In fact, in prepubertal children, uncomplicated, noncomorbid bipolar disorder is extremely rare. That conservative statement is made because some studies do not specifically mention the percentage of children without any comorbidity (Table 13–

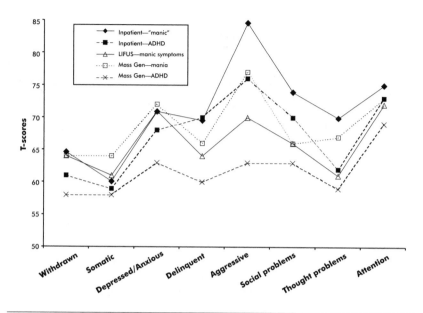

FIGURE 13–2. *Child Behavior Checklist factor scores for five samples of children with mania/manic symptoms and attention-deficit/hyperactivity disorder (ADHD).* See Figure 13–1 for explanation of T-scores. LIFUS = Long Island Follow-Up Study (Carlson et al. 1998a); Mass Gen = Massachusetts General Hospital (Faraone et al. 1997).

4). With adolescence, this picture begins to change, though the extent of such change seems to depend on the sample, the age of the sample, and the focus of the study. For instance, a sample gathered for a drug trial is less likely to have teens with substance abuse because that is an exclusion criterion for treatment. In addition to the presence of comorbidity, heavy loading of bipolar disorder and unipolar depression is the other prominent feature of early-onset bipolar disorder (Strober et al. 1988; Todd et al. 1993). However, what has not been ascertained are the rates of *comorbid* bipolar disorder versus *uncomplicated* bipolar disorder in the first-degree relatives of children with comorbidity.

To summarize, emotional lability is the common denominator of manic symptoms, syndrome, and disorder. This dimension, trait, or behavior appears to engender high rates of other psychopathology and to complicate the disorders or conditions with which it occurs.

TABLE 13–4. *Comorbidity in samples of children and adolescents with bipolar disorder*

	Rate of comorbidity in sample (%)					
Comorbid disorder	Faraone et al. 1997 (N = 68)	Geller et al. 1994 (N = 9)	Kafantaris et al. 1998 (N = 48)	Faraone et al. 1997 (N = 17)	Kovacs and Pollock 1995 (N = 26)	Carlson et al. 1997 (N = 28)
Age group	Children	Children	Teenagers	Teenagers	Teenagers	Teenagers/ young adults[a]
ADHD	93	88.9	20.8	59	NR	39.3[b]
ODD	91	N/A	18.8	71	NR	
Conduct disorder	38	22.2[c]	4.2	35	54.0	32.0
Special education	38	N/A	[NR]	41	N/A	32.1
Anxiety disorder	56	66.6?	33.3	59	N/A	21.4
Depressive disorder	60	22.2	31.3	76	100.0	50.0
Substance abuse/ dependence[d]	0	NR	NR	35	NR	50.0
Psychosis	31	?	48.0	35	NR	100.0
No comorbidity	0	0	31.0	NR	11.5	10.7

Note. ADHD = attention-deficit/hyperactivity disorder; N/A = not applicable; NR = not reported; ODD = oppositional defiant disorder.
[a]Ages 15–20 years.
[b]Combined conduct disorder/ODD.
[c]"Severe."
[d]Includes alcohol abuse or dependence.

Relationship of Childhood and Adult Bipolarity

In children, behavior disorders and mania frequently co-occur. This relationship also occurs in adults. Data from the Epidemiologic Catchment Area (ECA) study (Regier et al. 1984) allow us to examine conduct disorder symptoms and their implications in adults who endorse manic symptoms on the Diagnostic Interview Schedule (Robins et al. 1981). In an analysis of ECA data, only 18- to 29-year-old subjects were examined, to minimize the cohort effect, and the hypothesis was made that substance abuse would likely be continuous with conduct disorder in adolescence. The subjects with mania were divided into two groups on the basis of whether they also had substance/alcohol use or dependence. The rates of conduct disorder were almost four times higher in the manic subjects with substance/alcohol use or dependence than in those with mania alone (Table 13–5). As a continuous variable, five conduct disorder symptoms occurred in the manic subjects with substance/alcohol use or dependence, in contrast to two in the subjects with mania alone (Carlson et al. 1998a). In fact, the number of conduct disorder symptoms in the subjects with bipolar disorder without comorbid substance/alcohol abuse of dependence was no higher than that in the general, nonmanic population (Table 13–6). This suggests that at least in young adults who endorse a lifetime episode of mania, behavior problems are not a common feature unless subsequent substance use disorders develop.

Another data set with which it is possible to explore the relationship between youth psychopathology and adolescent/adult bipolar disorder derives from the Suffolk County Mental Health Project (Bromet et al. 1992). For this study, more than 600 patients hospitalized with a first episode of psychosis were recruited from all of the psychiatric hospitals in Suffolk County, New York. Clinical data from various sources—the treating psychiatrist, hospital chart, school records (when possible), significant other (when possible), and diagnostic instruments—were used at baseline to help a team of psychiatrists make a consensus diagnosis. The diagnostic instruments used were the Structured Interview for Schizotypy (Kendler et al. 1989); the Cannon-Spoor Premorbid

TABLE 13–5. *Rates of conduct disorder among manic subjects from the Epidemiologic Catchment Area study aged 18–29 years with or without substance/alcohol abuse or dependence*

Conduct disorder	Substance abuse/ dependence[a] (n = 25)	No substance abuse/dependence (n = 27)	P
n (%)	13 (52)	4 (14.8)	<0.01
Mean no. (SD) of symptoms	4.9 (2.8)	1.9 (1.8)	<0.0001

Note. SD = standard deviation.
[a]Includes alcohol abuse or dependence.
Source. Data from Carlson et al. 1998a; Regier et al. 1984.

TABLE 13–6. *Relation of adolescent conduct disorder symptoms to bipolar disorder with and without comorbid substance/alcohol abuse or dependence among subjects from the Epidemiologic Catchment Area study aged 18–29 years*

	Rates of adolescent conduct disorder symptoms (%)				
	Trouble at school	Drunk before age 15 years	Lying	Fighting	Stealing
Substance abuse[a]/BP (n = 25)	56.0**	60.0**	60.0**	24.0	68.0*
BP I only (n = 27)	11.1**	11.1**	37.0**	7.4	29.6*
No substance abuse[a] or BP (n = 4,296)	11.0	9.2	15.6**	7.7	20.3

Note. BP = bipolar disorder; BP I = bipolar I disorder.
[a]Includes alcohol abuse or dependence.
*P < 0.01. **P < 0.001.
Source. Carlson et al. 1998a.

Adjustment Scale (Cannon-Spoor et al. 1982), a questionnaire used to elicit childhood developmental and behavior problems; and the Structured Clinical Interview for DSM-III-R (Spitzer et al. 1992). Of the eligible sample, 72% agreed to be in the study. Individuals in the sample were reinterviewed in person at 6 months and 2 years and by telephone at 3, 12, and 18 months. At the time of this writing, 125 subjects who completed their 2-year follow-up, having been initially admitted for a manic episode, have been given a consensus diagnosis of definite bipolar disorder.

To understand the impact of age at onset on the phenomenology and 2-year course of the disorder, we compared two groups of patients: those with a first episode of mania before age 21 years and those with a first episode after age 30 years (G. A. Carlson and E. J. Bromet, unpublished data, 1998). Rates of uncomplicated bipolar disorder were much higher in the patients with a first episode after age 30 (Table 13–7). Similarly, there was a clear female preponderance after age 30. Closer scrutiny reveals very few men with a first episode after age 30 who did not have another psychiatric disorder, usually substance use, of earlier onset that had frequently, but not always, remitted by their first episode of mania. Also evident is that rates of behavior disorders and active substance/alcohol abuse or dependence were significantly higher in the patients between the ages of 15 and 20 years. It may be that this age range constitutes the major onset period in which drugs and alcohol have been used long enough for the criteria for abuse and dependence to be met. In this sample, rates of lifetime substance/alcohol abuse or dependence were similar in both age groups, but men in the older group had largely stopped this behavior with time.

Family history was obtained from the subject and, when possible, his or her significant other. Those taking the history were aware of the diagnosis, but they were not aware of any relevance of age at onset to frequency of particular disorders in relatives. Although rates of illness, reported as the percentage of patients with a first-degree relative with a positive history (bipolar disorder and overall affective disorder) were high in both groups, there was no difference between groups (Table 13–8).

Is there a relationship between age at onset, comorbidity, and outcome? More than two decades ago, I published the results of a follow-up study of manic-depressive patients with early- or late-onset of the disorder (Carlson et al. 1977). In a sample of patients hospitalized on the research unit of the National Institute of Mental Health (NIMH), subjects aged 20 years and younger were compared with subjects with onset of the disorder after age 45 years. Onset was determined retrospectively. In addition, although the patients with early-onset disorder had clearly reported episodes before age 20, virtually none had been treated

TABLE 13–7.   *Adolescent and adult bipolar disorder: sample characteristics and rates of prior psychopathology among subjects from the Suffolk County Mental Health Project*

| | Age at first episode (years) | | |
	Ages 15–20	Ages 30+	Significance
Sample size (*n*)	28	34	
Male, %	64.3	23.5	$\chi^2 = 10.4, P < 0.001$
Manic and depressive episodes, %	50.0	38.8	NS
Prior psychopathology, %			
None	10.7	50.0	$\chi^2 = 10.8, P < 0.001$
Externalizing disorder	39.3	14.7	$\chi^2 = 48.0, P < 0.05$
Special education	32.1	13.3	N/A
Early substance/alcohol use disorders	50.0	20.6	$\chi^2 = 5.9, P < 0.025$
Anxiety/depressive disorders	21.4	26.5	NS

Note. NS = not significant.
Source. G. A. Carlson and E. J. Bromet, unpublished data, 1998.

and absolutely none had been hospitalized. Nevertheless, on a 4-point scale of outcome, 60% of both the early- and late-onset groups were functioning quite well, 20% were clearly symptomatic and impaired but functioning, and 20% were chronically ill. When the same rating scale as in the 1977 NIMH study was used, the outcomes in the subsample from the Suffolk County Mental Health Project described earlier did not differ very much from those in the 1977 NIMH sample (Table 13–8). When a continuous scale was used, however, the average functioning of the patients over age 30 was significantly better than that of the young group.

An attempt is ongoing to replicate the findings with the ECA sample for patients between the ages of 18 and 29 years to determine the specific impact of child/adolescent-onset externalizing disorder, child/adolescent-onset internalizing disorder (i.e., anxiety disorder or a first episode of depression), and lack of comorbidity prior to age 18 years. Reported herein are data for a subsample of bipolar patients (N = 63) from the

TABLE 13–8. *Adolescent and adult bipolar disorder: outcome, substance use, and family history among subjects from the Suffolk County Mental Health Project at 2-year follow-up*

	Age at first episode (years)		
	Ages 15–20	Ages 30+	Significance
Sample size (*n*)	28	34	
Outcome, %			
Excellent/Good	50.0	70.0	
Fair	35.7	26.5	
Poor	14.3	2.9	
Average function (out of 4)	2.75 (1.0)	3.2 (0.9)	$t = 1.7, P < 0.05$ $\chi^2 = 8.1, P < 0.01$
Substance abuse/dependence[a] at 2 years, %	28.6	2.9	
Family history, %			
Affective disorder	54.0	44.0	
Bipolar disorder	33.0	25.0	
Substance use disorders	50.0	44.0	
Mood and substance use disorders	33.3	26.5	

[a]Includes alcohol abuse/dependence.
Source. G. A. Carlson, unpublished data, 1998.

Suffolk County Mental Health Project, including the subjects between ages 21 and 29 years (*n* = 40), who constitute a majority of the bipolar sample. The subsample is taken from the first 300 patients with a first hospitalization for psychosis enrolled on whom 2-year follow-up is complete.

It is apparent (Table 13–9) that the subjects with child/adolescent-onset externalizing disorder account for the male preponderance and the poor outcome. They also account for much of the chronic substance abuse that is occurring, for although lifetime and substance use problems were different between groups at onset, the subjects persisting in their substance abuse habits were mainly those with prior externalizing disorder psychopathology. It is interesting that the patients with comorbidity also had more recurrence of manic, but not depressive, episodes over the 2-year period, though medication treatment was not different between groups. A number of behavior problems, taken from one section of the Structured Interview for Schizotypy, correlated significantly with measures in several functional areas (Table 13–10). In general, a higher number of behavior problems in adolescence was correlated with poorer outcome, recurrence of mania, and continued substance use.

Early-Onset Bipolarity and Comorbidity

Systematically acquired treatment data on early-onset bipolarity and comorbidity are scant and inconclusive. Strober et al. (1988) found that adolescents with mania who had preadolescent ADHD responded less well to lithium carbonate than did adolescents with uncomplicated bipolar disorder. On the other hand, Kafantaris et al. (1998) found that both groups responded equally well or poorly. Many of the subjects in that sample had psychotic disorders, however, and required simultaneous treatment with neuroleptics. Carlson et al. (1992), in a double-blind study of a small sample of prepubertal children with a manic syndrome and ADHD, found that the combination of lithium and methylphenidate worked more effectively to improve inattention and overactivity than either drug alone. Geller et al. (1998) reported on 25 adolescent subtance abusers with bipolar disorder who were randomized to lithium or placebo in a double-blind study. The investigators found that 46% of the subjects treated with lithium showed improvement in their overall function (indicated by a score on the Children's Global Assessment Scale [Shaffer et al. 1983] of 65 or higher) compared with 8% of the subjects receiving placebo. Clearly, the samples in these studies were small and the measures of outcome and improvement were coarse, and only in the study by Carlson et al. (1992) were issues of comorbidity examined separately.

Conclusion

Manic symptoms, whether they are part of a full-fledged disorder or are present only as symptoms or in a syndrome state, seem to represent

TABLE 13–9.   *Outcome of bipolar disorder in a sample of subjects from the Suffolk County Mental Health Project with and without child/adolescent comorbidity*

	No child/ adolescent disorder	Other or no comorbidity with onset before 18 years	Childhood externalizing disorder	P
Sample size, n	18	14	8	
Male, n (%)	10 (55.6)	7 (46.5)	7 (87.5)	
Special education—lifetime, n (%)	3 (16.6)	2 (15.4)	6 (75.0)	0.01
Substance abuse/dependence[a]				
Lifetime, n (%)	6 (33.3)	9 (64.2)[b]	7 (87.5)[c]	NS
At index admission, n (%)	4 (22.2)	6 (42.9)	7 (87.5)	NS
At 24 months, n (%)	0	2 (14.3)	5 (62.5)	0.05
Number of new episodes of mania	0.37	0.57	2.10	0.01
Patients with mania by 24 months, n (%)	1 (5.6)	7 (35.7)	7 (87.5)	0.1
Number of new episodes of depression	0.55	0.43	1.00	NS
Treatment, n (%)				
Taking medication for entire follow-up	10 (55.6)	6 (42.9)	5 (63.3)	NS
Lithium alone	4 (22.2)	5 (35.7)	0	NS
Lithium and neuroleptic	8 (44.4)	5 (35.7)	4 (50)	NS
Neuroleptic alone	3 (16.7)	0	1 (12.5)	NS

TABLE 13–9.   *Outcome of bipolar disorder in a sample of subjects from the Suffolk County Mental Health Project with and without child/adolescent comorbidity* (continued)

	No child/ adolescent disorder	Other or no comorbidity with onset before 18 years	Childhood externalizing disorder	P
Treatment, *n* (%) *(continued)*				
Antidepressant ever	6 (33.3)	0	2 (25.0)	NS
No medication		3[d]	2[e]	
Outcome, no. of subjects				
Excellent	7	4	0	
Good	6	5	0	
Fair	4	4	4	
Poor	1	2	4	
Overall outcome (4 = best)	3.2	2.7	2.0	0.02

[a]Includes alcohol abuse/dependence.
[b]8 drug, 9 alcohol.
[c]7 drug, 6 alcohol.
[d]Two doing well.
[e]Both doing poorly.
Source. G. A. Carlson and E. J. Bromet, unpublished data, 1998.

considerable psychopathology. Since explosive, unpredictable aggressive behavior is an important part of emotional lability/manic symptoms, the exacerbation of any disorder in which aggression already occurs is not surprising. We suspect that much of what is being called "bipolar disorder" with comorbidity represents manic symptoms/emotional lability occurring as part of the psychopathology of the other disorder. In that regard, manic symptoms are like psychotic symptoms: they presage serious psychopathology but are not, in and of themselves, diagnostic of any particular disorder. In fact, if we have learned anything over the past 100 years in trying to distinguish schizophrenia from mania, it should be that cross-sectional symptoms alone are not sufficient. The

TABLE 13–10. *Correlation of various measures of outcome and number of behavior problems in a sample of manic subjects (N = 63) from the Suffolk County Mental Health Project*

	R	P
Overall outcome	−0.57	0.001
Work level (24 months)	−0.52	0.005
Global Assessment of Functioning (6-month best)	−0.50	0.005
Global Assessment of Functioning (24-month best)	−0.46	0.005
New episodes of mania	0.41	0.01
Continued substance abuse/ dependence[a]	0.70	0.0001

[a]Includes alcohol abuse/dependence.

same can be said of attentional symptoms. Although inattention is certainly a prominent part of ADHD, the presence of attentional symptoms is not pathognomonic of this disorder. Nevertheless, their presence certainly increases the likelihood that considerable cognitive impairment will be present. This conclusion, moreover, does not diminish genetic implications, since it may well be that dimensions, rather than disorders, are what is heritable.

That said, there is certainly evidence that manic-depressive illness/ bipolar disorder can begin some years after the onset of an externalizing disorder. The combination is, not surprisingly, no more benign than either disorder alone. Whether the combination represents the co-occurrence of two disorders or a subtype of one or the other has yet to be proven, in part because parental comorbidity has yet to be considered in genetic studies.

References

Achenbach TM: Manual for the Child Behavior Checklist 4–18 and 1991 Profile. Burlington, University of Vermont, Department of Psychiatry, 1991

Akiskal HS: Delineating irritable and hyperthymic variants of the cyclothymic temperament. J Personal Disord 6:326–342, 1992

American Psychiatric Association: Diagnostic and Statistical Manual: Mental Disorders. Washington, DC, American Psychiatric Association, 1952

American Psychiatric Association: Diagnostic and Statistical Manual for Mental Disorders, 2nd Edition. Washington, DC, American Psychiatric Association, 1968

American Psychiatric Association: Diagnostic and Statistical Manual for Mental Disorders, 3rd Edition. Washington, DC, American Psychiatric Association, 1980

American Psychiatric Association: Diagnostic and Statistical Manual for Mental Disorders, 3rd Edition, Revised. Washington, DC, American Psychiatric Association, 1987

American Psychiatric Association: Diagnostic and Statistical Manual for Mental Disorders, 4th Edition. Washington, DC, American Psychiatric Association, 1994

Anthony EJ, Scott P: Manic depressive psychosis in childhood. J Child Psychol Psychiatry 1:53–72, 1960

Biederman J, Wozniak J, Kiely K, et al: CBCL Clinical Scales discriminate prepubertal children with structured-interview-derived diagnosis of mania from those with ADHD. J Am Acad Child Adolesc Psychiatry 34:464–471, 1995

Bromet EJ, Schwartz JE, Fennig S, et al: The epidemiology of psychoses: the Suffolk County Mental Health Project. Schizophr Bull 18:243–255, 1992

Cannon-Spoor H, Potkin SG, Wyatt RJ: Measurement of premorbid adjustment in chronic schizophrenia. Schizophr Bull 8:471–484, 1982

Carlson GA: Bipolar affective disorders in childhood and adolescence, in Affective Disorders in Childhood and Adolescence: An Update. Edited by Cantwell DP, Carlson GA. New York, Spectrum, 1983, pp 61–84

Carlson GA: Annotation: child and adolescent mania—diagnostic considerations. J Child Psychol Psychiatry 31:331–341, 1990

Carlson GA: Adolescent bipolar disorder, in Handbook of Depression in Children and Adolescents. Edited by Reynolds WM, Johnnson HF. New York, Plenum, 1994, pp 41–60

Carlson GA, Kashani JH: Manic symptoms in a non-referred adolescent population. J Affect Disord 15:219–226, 1988

Carlson GA, Kelly KL: Manic symptoms in psychiatrically hospitalized children—what do they mean? J Affect Disord 51:123–136, 1998

Carlson GA, Davenport YB, Jamison KR: A comparison of outcome in adolescent and late-onset bipolar manic-depressive illness. Am J Psychiatry 134:919–922, 1977

Carlson GA, Rapport MD, Pataki CS, et al: The Effects of Methylphenidate and lithium on attention and activity level. J Am Acad Child Adolesc Psychiatry 31:262–270, 1992

Carlson GA, Bromet EJ, Jandorf L: Conduct disorder and mania — what does it mean in adults? J Affect Disord 48:199–205, 1998a

Carlson GA, Loney J, Salisbury H, et al: Young referred boys with DICA-P manic symptoms versus two comparison groups. J Affect Disord 51:113–122, 1998b

Caspi A, Elder GH, Herbener ES: Childhood personality and the prediction of life course patterns, in Straight and Devious Pathways From Childhood and Adulthood. Edited by Robins LN, Rutter M. New York, Cambridge University Press, 1990, pp 13–35

Evans DL, Byerly MJ, Greer RA: Seconday mania: diagnosis and treatment. J Clin Psychaitry 56 (no 3, suppl):31–37, 1995

Faraone SV, Biederman J, Wozniak J, et al: Is comorbidity a marker for juvenile-onset mania? J Am Acad Child Adolesc Psychiatry 36:1046–1055, 1997

Gadow KD, Sprafkin J: Child Symptom Inventories Manual. Stony Brook, New York, Checkmate Plus, 1994

Geller B, Fox LW, Clark KA: Rate and predictors of prepubertal bipolarity during follow-up of 6- to 12-year-old depressed children. J Am Acad Child Adolesc Psychiatry 33:461–468, 1994

Geller B, Cooper TB, Sun K, et al: Double-blind and placebo-controlled study of lithium for adolescent bipolar disorders with secondary substance dependency. J Am Acad Child Adolesc Psychiatry 37:171–178, 1998

Gerring JP, Brady KD, Chen A, et al: Premorbid prevalence of attention-deficit hyperactivity disorder and development of secondary attention-deficit hyperactivity disorder after closed head injury. J Am Acad Child Adolesc Psychiatry 37:647–654, 1998

Herjanic B, Reich W: Development of a structured psychiatric interview for children: agreement between child and parent on individual symptoms. J Abnorm Child Psychol 10:307–324, 1982

Kafantaris V, Coletti DJ, Dicker R, et al: Childhood psychiatric histories of bipolar adolescents: association with family history, psychosis and response to lithium treatment. J Affect Disord 51:153–164, 1998

Kendler KS, Lieberman JA, Walsh D: The Structured Interview for Schizotypy (SIS): a preliminary report. Schizophr Bull 15:559–571, 1989

Kovacs M, Pollock M: Bipolar disorder and conduct disorder in childhood and adolescence. J Am Acad Child Adolesc Psychiatry 34:715–723, 1985

Kumra S, Jacobson LK, Lenane M, et al: "Multidimensionally impaired disorder": is it a variant of very early-onset schizophrenia. J Am Acad Child Adolesc Psychiatry 37:91–99, 1998

Laufer MW, Denhoff E: Hyperkinetic behavior syndrome in children. J Pediatr 50:463–474, 1957

Laufer MW, Denhoff E, Solomons G: Hyperkinetic impulse disorder in children's behavior problems. Psychosom Med 19:38–49, 1957

Lewinsohn PM, Klein DN, Seeley JR: Bipolar disorder in community sample of older adolescents: prevalence, phenomenology, comorbidity and course. J Am Acad Child Adolesc Psychiatry 34:454–463, 1995

Lish JD, Dime MS, Whybrow PC, et al: The National Depressive and Manic-Depressive Association (DMDA) survey of bipolar members. J Affect Disord 31:281–294, 1994

McKenna K, Gordon CT, Lenane M, et al: Looking for childhood-onset schizophrenia: the first 71 cases screened. J Am Acad Child Adolesc Psychiatry 33:636–644, 1994

Regier DA, Myers JK, Kramer M, et al: The NIMH Epidemiologic Catchment Area Program: historical context, major objectives, and study population characteristics. Arch Gen Psychiatry 41:934–941, 1984

Robins LN, Helzer JE, Croughan J, et al: National Institute of Mental Health Diagnostic Interview Schedule: its history, characteristics, and validity. Arch Gen Psychiatry 38:381–389, 1981

Shaffer D, Gould MS, Brasic J, et al: A children's global assessment scale (C-GAS). Arch Gen Psychiatry 40:1228–1231, 1983

Spitzer R, Williams J, Gibbon M, et al: The Structured Clinical Review for DSM-III-R (SCID), I: history, rationale, and description. Arch Gen Psychiatry 49:624–629, 1992

Strober M, Morrell W, Burroughs J, et al: A family study of bipolar I in adolescence: early onset of symptoms linked to increased familial loading and lithium resistance. J Affect Disord 15:255–268, 1988

Tanguay PE: Mania in children with pervasive developmental disorder (discussion). J Am Acad Child Adolesc Psychiatry 36:1559–1560, 1997

Todd RD, Neuman R, Geller B, et al: Genetic studies of affective disorders: should we be starting with childhood onset disorders? J Am Acad Child Adolesc Psychiatry 32:1164–1171, 1993

Tohen M, Goodwin FK: Epidemiology of bipolar disorder, in Textbook in Psychiatric Epidemiology. Edited by Tsuang MT, Tohen M, Zahner GEP. New York, Wiley–Liss, 1995, pp 301–316

Towbin K, Dykens EM, Pearson GS, et al: Conceptualizing "borderline syndrome of childhood" and "childhood schizophrenia as a developmental disorder." J Am Acad Child Adolesc Psychiatry 32:775–782, 1993

Wozniak J, Biederman J, Kiely K, et al: Mania-like symptoms suggestive of childhood onset bipolar disorder clinically referred children. J Am Acad Child Adolesc Psychiatry 34:867–876, 1995

Early Prevention of Adult Psychiatric Disorders

Prevention of Mental Disorders and the Study of Developmental Psychopathology: A Natural Alliance

William R. Beardslee, M.D.

The design and evaluation of preventive interventions provide a natural complement to longitudinal studies of the development of psychopathology and should be considered in the conceptualization, design, and conduct of such studies. Historically, the study of the prevention of mental illness has received much less attention than the examination of the natural course, outcome, or treatment of psychiatric disorders. Recently, there has been significant progress in the science of prevention, particularly because of the application of investigative strategies closely related to those used in studies of the development of psychopathology. This chapter addresses the need for a greater focus on prevention by 1) reviewing the findings of one of the most recent comprehensive evaluations of preventive intervention, that of the Institute of Medicine (1994), and 2) describing the development and evaluation of a preventive intervention strategy for depressed parents.

One fundamental reason for the study of prevention is scientific; namely, as Dr. Felton Earls suggested (Earls 1989), the second phase of epidemiology should be the exploration of mechanisms for transmission of disorder through the initiation of interventions (i.e., a mechanism is fully understood only when the effects of that mechanism can be modified through intervention). Preventive intervention trials aim to change causal pathways enough to prevent the emergence of disorder in populations at risk and/or to significantly reduce the risk factors for the emergence of disorder. A second fundamental reason is that prevention can potentially alleviate the large burden of illness of those afflicted and thus have great benefit to both individuals and society.

Two factors that in the past have led prevention to not be fully considered are 1) concern about the degree of the methodological rigor with which trials have been conducted, and 2) the lack of substantive findings about the effects of preventive interventions. Over the last 10 years, increasingly rigorous designs have been employed, and a large body of well-conducted empirical trials has accumulated. These trials offer substantial evidence of the reduction of risk factors for mental disorders, with some studies actually demonstrating the prevention of disorders as well. Reports from a variety of different national committees have emphasized this (Coie et al. 1993; Institute of Medicine 1994; National Institute of Mental Health 1993, 1998). These reviews have employed rigorous methodological standards similar to those used in current, well-conducted longitudinal studies in psychopathology, such as appear in this volume:

- Full assessment with standardized measures prior to enrollment
- Testing of clearly specified, theory-driven hypotheses
- Randomization of subjects to well-defined, manualized conditions with appropriate evaluations of fidelity of intervention delivery
- Well-specified, objectively rated empirical outcomes
- Follow-up evaluations over long intervals

These standards, in combination with sophisticated data analytic techniques (i.e., growth curve modeling and logistic regression), have substantially improved the science of the study of prevention. Although there has been some confusion about definitions within the field, the characterization of prevention endeavors in the Institute of Medicine (1994) report provides the best organizing framework: "Preventive inter-

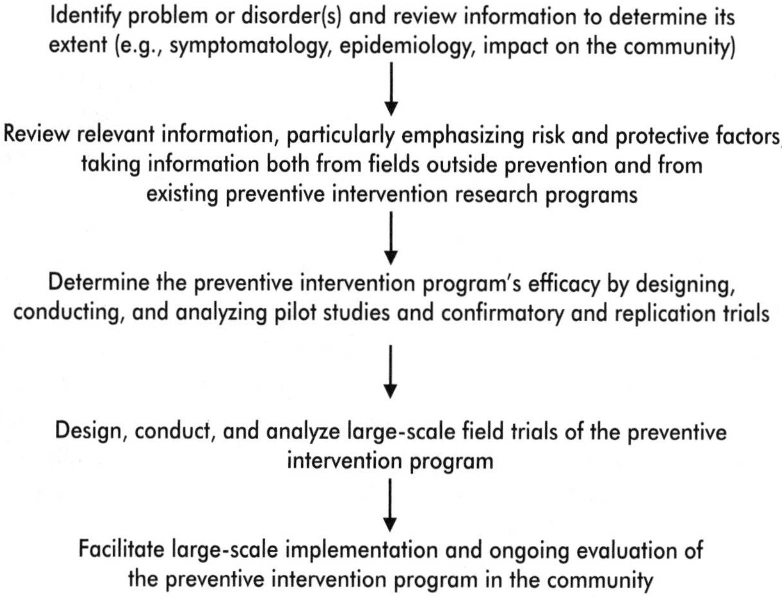

Identify problem or disorder(s) and review information to determine its
extent (e.g., symptomatology, epidemiology, impact on the community)

↓

Review relevant information, particularly emphasizing risk and protective factors;
taking information both from fields outside prevention and from
existing preventive intervention research programs

↓

Determine the preventive intervention program's efficacy by designing,
conducting, and analyzing pilot studies and confirmatory and replication trials

↓

Design, conduct, and analyze large-scale field trials of the preventive
intervention program

↓

Facilitate large-scale implementation and ongoing evaluation of
the preventive intervention program in the community

FIGURE 14–1. *The preventive intervention research cycle.*
Source. Adapted from Institute of Medicine: *Reducing Risks for Mental Disorders: Frontiers for Preventive Intervention Research.* Edited by Mrazek PJ, Haggerty RJ. Washington, DC, National Academy Press, 1994.

ventions for specific disorders are typically developed through a series of phases, each building on its predecessor, each supporting its successor" (p. 45). Figure 14–1 presents this characterization graphically.

The Institute of Medicine's framework is compatible with the study of developmental psychopathology. The model is made up of five categories, or stages. In fact, the first and second stages of the model, *identifying risk factors* and *describing the relative contributions of different factors to the disorder,* are in the domain of developmental psychology. The third stage of the model involves *applying strategies developed in pilot studies and completing efficacy trials to evaluate the overall effectiveness of these approaches.* The fourth stage, *carrying out effectiveness trials,* involves the examination of such strategies in multiple sites in large-scale investigations under non-ideal, real-world conditions. The final stage of the model consists of *implementing such strategies in large-scale public health campaigns.*

When this stage-sequential approach is used, the natural affinity between preventive intervention and the study of the development of psychopathology becomes clear. Questions asked concerning preventive intervention are similar to those asked in developmental psychopathology. Specifically, the questions asked in preventive intervention are, What are the risk factors for disorders? and How do they interact over time? It is also asked, Which of those factors are potentially responsive to intervention (biochemically, genetically, or psychosocially)? and, hence, How much of the variance is potentially amenable to change? It is then possible to estimate how much of the variance could be affected by a particular intervention strategy. These questions can be answered only with an understanding of the mechanisms of causation and the natural history of the course of disorder.

Preventive intervention is inherently a longitudinal endeavor. By definition, one cannot prevent illness in those already in the acute stage of that illness. On the other hand, in conducting preventive intervention experiments, the enrollment and follow-up of large samples over a considerable length of time are needed because only a few individuals in any short period of time will develop an episode of the disorder. Such an approach necessitates following a considerable number of individuals who will not become ill. Moreover, prevention involves understanding the broad effects of risk factors on outcomes (i.e., those who do not become ill are as important as those who do).

The prevention of disorder requires the use of more complex theoretical models and experimental designs than those in investigations of treatment strategies in which the effects are expected immediately after the delivery of the intervention. In this regard, the techniques used to study longitudinal outcome in developmental psychopathology are particularly relevant. In treatment research, the usual strategy is to select subjects who already have a specified acute condition, deliver an intervention targeted to changing that specific condition, and measure symptoms right after the intervention, usually no longer than 1–2 months later. In prevention trials with large samples followed over long time intervals, investigators must take into account the other intervening variables that may influence outcome—for example, the continued operation of the risk factors such as a parental illness, or developmental changes in subjects such as onset of puberty. They must understand the natural course of disorder and what influences it in order to attempt to show change in that natural course through the effect of the preventive intervention. The models for how to do this are those used in studies of the development of psychopathology over time.

The Institute of Medicine Report: Prevention of Mental Disorders

A brief review of some of the major approaches described in the Institute of Medicine (1994) report can serve as an overview of the kinds of preventive endeavors currently being studied. The intervention strategies described were grouped by the developmental age of subjects. A major emphasis in the Institute of Medicine report is that early in life, insults to the child's developing nervous system are potent risk factors for later mental disorders, be they the result of chemical factors (i.e., cocaine or alcohol) or prenatal factors (i.e., low birth weight or deprivation of nurturing). For infants and children, the Institute of Medicine emphasized the preventive value of large-scale epidemiological programs such as interventions to prevent low birth weight, immunizations against infectious disease, support for parenting (e.g., nursing home visitation) (Olds et al. 1986), high-quality day care (Schweinhart and Weikart 1992; Weikart et al. 1986), and Head Start (Kotelchuck and Richmond 1987). Emphasis on these programs for preventing mental disorder has historically been neglected in the mental health community.

For school-age children, social skills training and academic enhancement, such as increasing reading achievement, have been identified as important factors leading to later positive outcomes (Kellam and Rebok 1992; Shure and Spivack 1980, 1982). Also of demonstrated value are specific targeted interventions for youth at high risk of developing psychopathology because of diverse behaviors such as shyness, aggression, and substance abuse. For adolescents, in addition to interventions targeted at school, there has been an emphasis on community-based programs to control tobacco and alcohol use as well as programs focused on antisocial behavior, such as those described by Dr. David Offord in Chapter 16 of this volume.

In adulthood, for example, some interventions have focused on individuals under stress. In particular, the area of depression prevention has been emphasized. Programs involving rapid response to those undergoing job loss (Price et al. 1992), bereavement, and divorce (Bloom et al. 1985) have shown promising results. Programs later in life designed to reduce social isolation among the elderly and support their caregivers, as well as to provide adequate cognitive stimulation, are also prime examples of depression prevention programs.

The Institute of Medicine (1994) emphasized, in its report, the overlap between physical illness and mental illness. Investigations of the prevention of physical illness provide important conceptual models that are applicable to the prevention of mental illness. Three important strategies from the prevention of physical illness were reviewed. The first of these was based on the attempt to decrease risk factors associated with cardiovascular disease through large-scale, community-wide public education campaigns. These investigations took place under the direction of Dr. John Farquhar and associates, based at Stanford University. The project was initiated in the early 1970s. The attempt was made to change the entire community's habits through a combination of large-scale mass media approaches and work with practitioners, schools, and community education programs. Dr. Farquhar and colleagues based their approach on social learning and communication theories that emphasized the use of multiple domains of message delivery. This approach led to a series of interventions that could be delivered simultaneously. Farquhar's work demonstrated significant effects on risk factors for cardiovascular disease (Farquhar et al. 1990).

The second major area reviewed was that of smoking. Although a variety of factors have contributed to a reduction of smoking, there was, as Thomas Glynn (1991) pointed out, a lack of organization and integration of various approaches into an overall plan. In 1982, the National Cancer Institute launched the Smoking Tobacco and Cancer Program. A major aim of the project was to coordinate prevention trials and developing large-scale community prevention programs. In addition, the project identified and integrated the most effective programs. Over the subsequent 10 years, this approach proved effective. It is also important to note that although the connection between smoking and poor health had been established at the time the program was begun, there were very few data on the effects of various kinds of intervention. Coordinating the resources, integrating the approaches, and designing and implementing comprehensive programs centrally made possible the extraordinary gains in the prevention of smoking.

The third major area reviewed in the Institute of Medicine (1994) report was that of accident prevention. The emphasis in this approach is on a time-honored prevention strategy that changes the physical environment of individuals by limiting access to dangerous devices and diminishes the risk for potentially dangerous situations. One example is the pioneering work of William Hadden at the National Highway Traffic Safety Administration. He initiated a variety of programs aimed at prevention of morbidity and mortality from automobile accidents, such as programs focusing on seatbelts and better automobile design, at a time when few were concerned about those issues. Overall, such prevention campaigns are estimated to have had a significant effect on traffic fatalities, with approximately 30% fewer fatalities than would have occurred had such programs not been implemented (U.S. National Highway Traffic Safety Administration 1991). These investigators have used a strategy that might be termed "attacking the weakest link first," that is, the point at which a large impact may be achieved with a relatively small investment. For the most part, this meant changing the environment—namely, promoting the use of seatbelts or preventing childhood accidents through the design of playground structures or even household utilities in ways that will ensure that children are less likely to be harmed.

Preventive Intervention in Practice: Longitudinal Study of Families With Affective Disorders

The review of the Institute of Medicine (1994) report in the previous section provided a broad overview of the kinds of approaches that were considered to reflect the best in preventive intervention research. Clearly, many of these fall within the domains of public health and community intervention. In this section, based on our own work, the development and evaluation of a program for children of parents with affective disorders is described in order to show how, in one specific situation, the application of findings from a longitudinal risk study based on developmental principles can inform the development of a preventive intervention approach.

Our work has followed the sequence outlined in the Institute of Medicine report. We begin by describing the risks to children of parents with affective disorders and understanding the mechanism involved in the transmission of disorder from parent to child, as well as understanding the key construct of resilience. Our work is unique in that we have had the opportunity to go from conducting an initial risk study and gaining an understanding of resilience to designing standardized interventions that eventually could be widely used in public health settings and then to conducting a large-scale longitudinal efficacy trial in an area that had not been previously addressed—the prevention of depression in families.

Because our work is the first family-based cognitive psychoeducational preventive intervention trial, we have had the opportunity both to devise a highly specific, replicable set of interventions for prevention of childhood depression and, using that specific investigation, to explore how to develop a model for family-based preventive interventions in general. It is this dual focus of our work that has been particularly exciting. Our work has conclusively demonstrated both that families receive substantial benefits from preventive intervention and, conceptually, that such family-based approaches in general are possible, feasible, and safe and, indeed, should be much more widely considered. Moreover, although not the subject of this chapter, substantial opportunities are available for using clinical approaches for preventive intervention that have largely been neglected and should also be more fully considered (see Beardslee 1998).

Specifically, on the basis of the evidence that childhood depression is a severe and impairing disorder and that those at highest risk could be identified (Beardslee et al. 1999), we developed two preventive intervention strategies: delivery of psychoeducational material in a clinician-facilitated or a lecture format. We have been examining the effects of these interventions on families over time in a long-term efficacy trial. Although positive outcomes have been observed in both conditions, greater levels of benefit and change have been observed in families participating in the clinician-facilitated intervention.

A number of principles have guided our work:

1. Targeting of a mental illness that was quite prevalent
2. Selection of intervention strategies that could be widely used in public health models
3. Detailed understanding of the unfolding risk and resilience in the population targeted for intervention
4. Use of a standard longitudinal risk study design with the addition of randomly assigned prevention strategies for families
5. Examination of the role of core theoretical constructs in enhancing the family's ability to deal with depression

We chose to focus on depression in parents for a number of reasons. First, depression is common; according to Kessler (see Kessler et al. 1994), close to 20% of adults in the United States will meet the criteria for an episode of depression sometime during their lifetime. Evidence has accumulated that depression is a severe, impairing condition comparable to chronic medical illness in terms of cost. Moreover, depression remains one of the most treatable of the major mental illnesses, with clear evidence of the effectiveness of treatment in adults in terms of both psychopharmacological approaches and manual-based psychotherapeutic approaches (Gabbard 1995). In designing a preventive intervention for children, particularly one to effect psychosocial influences, we believed adequate treatment of the parents' mental illness was essential. Despite its treatability, depression remains largely undertreated (Keller et al. 1992), a fact that represented an important factor in our design, since we believe that the treatment of all those with acute illness is a necessary part of the prevention of mental illness. Depression profoundly impairs interpersonal functioning and, as accumulating evidence has shown, functioning within families and hence, in our opinion, needs to be viewed not only as an interpersonal illness but as a family illness as well. Thus, we employed a family approach.

Risk Factors for Development of Affective Illness

Youngsters growing up in homes where severe parental psychiatric disorder is present are at higher risk of receiving a psychiatric diagnosis (Beardslee et al. 1998; Downey and Coyne 1990). In most studies, the rates of diagnosis of depression are four to six times higher in children of parents with affective disorders than in children of parents with no disorders. The former are also at risk for difficulties in terms of general functioning (Forehand and McCombs 1988), guilt (Zahn-Waxler et al. 1990), and attachment difficulties (Teti et al. 1995). The risk to youngsters whose parents are depressed is significant, and consequently a number of experts have identified these children as a group to target for preventive intervention (Institute of Medicine 1994; National Institute of Mental Health 1993).

A number of investigators, including Dr. Myrna Weissman and her colleagues (see Chapter 11, this volume), have longitudinally followed the children of parents with affective disorders. The longitudinal evidence makes even more serious the concern for this population. Over a 10-year period, Dr. Weissman found higher rates of diagnosable disorders—in particular, major depression and anxiety—in the offspring of depressed parents, as did Hammen and Beardslee (Beardslee et al. 1993a; Hammen et al. 1990; Weissman et al. 1997).

Although there is undoubtedly a genetic influence in affective disorders, as evidenced by the data from family studies (Tsuang and Faraone 1990), there is also a strong psychosocial influence. Within the domain of psychosocial influence (Rutter 1990), poor marital relationships (Fendrich et al. 1990) and family cohesion/parenting problems (Billings and Moos 1983; Rutter and Quinton 1984) are associated with the transmission of affective illness from parent to child. High rates of marital conflict, separation, and divorce have been found in couples with a depressed spouse (Coyne et al. 1987; Hautzinger et al. 1982). Children in families with parental affective disorder who are exposed to marital conflict are significantly more likely to experience some form of psychopathology (including major depression) during their lifetime than are children in families with parental affective illness but no marital conflict (Fendrich et al. 1990). In addition, misunderstanding contributes to both interference with parenting and marital discord.

Moreover, it is clear that depression serves as an identifier of a constellation of risk factors that are linked to the poorest outcomes, just as indices of adversity have been found to be the most powerful predictors of poor outcome in epidemiological studies (Rutter 1986) and in developmental studies of young children (Sameroff et al. 1987). This is also in line with a major emphasis in the Institute of Medicine (1994) report, which is that there are common risk factors (i.e., severe marital discord and divorce, lack of attention to parenting, or abuse) that lead to a variety of negative outcomes in youngsters, rather than only one specific diagnosis.

In our own work, we identified predictors for the onset of affective disorder over a 4-year interval in a sample of subjects recruited from an HMO. Outcome was best predicted by three factors: 1) duration of parental affective disorder, 2) the number of parental nonaffective diagnoses, and 3) presence of all prior child diagnoses. The presence of these three factors together accounted for 50% of new onsets of depression over the 4-year interval, whereas only 7% of new onsets occurred when none of these factors were present. Clearly, impairment in the child and nonaffective illness in the parents represent common risk factors for later poor outcome.

Resilience

Central to our own work has been the attempt to incorporate a developmental transactional paradigm in understanding the connection between parental disorder and child outcome. Drs. Dante Cicchetti and Karen Schneider-Rosen (1986) have suggested that depression is best viewed as a consequence of various factors that together cause poor outcome. It is the balance of risk factors that change at different developmental stages and dynamically influence one another that determines outcome. Thus, ours is not a study of a clinical intervention, but an attempt to place an intervention in a developmental context that takes into account the balance of different factors.

In this regard, perhaps the most important finding from a wide number of risk studies, including in our own work with a sample of children of parents with affective disorder, is that pertaining to resilience. Compared with clinical approaches, our work was unusual in focusing on the enhancement of resilience rather than the removal of psychopathology. Moreover, our work had as its conceptual base a developmental framework rather than a framework based on more static studies of psychopathology as defined by disorders with which patients present in clinical centers. Understanding the concept of resilience was essential both in framing the intervention with families and in understanding the dynamic transactions among different factors leading to the emergence of disorder in children. The existence of resilience emphasizes the importance of developmental plasticity. The characteristics of resilient children offer examples of strengths and attributes whose development can, and in our view should, be encouraged in all youngsters at risk.

In examining resilience, we identified 18 young men and women from a much larger pool of subjects whom we had studied whose parents had experienced affective disorder. The individuals in the subsample were identified on the basis of high levels of adaptive functioning scores when they were first assessed and were interviewed with a combination of structured and open-ended formats some years later. These youngsters had two observable behavioral characteristics: 1) they were deeply involved in extracurricular and school activities and were very much activists and doers, and 2) they were deeply involved in and committed to interpersonal relationships.

A third major characteristic, self-understanding, was described by them as vital to their being able to cope with their parents' having severe illness (Beardslee and Podorefsky 1988). Implicit in the emphasis on this quality is that they knew that there was something physically wrong with their parents and that they were not to blame for the situation and, indeed, were free to go on with their own lives. Such recognition, they felt, was essential to their being able to go forward. Other investigators have emphasized the importance of intimate and supportive relationships (Garmezy 1985; Rutter 1987; Werner and Smith 1982) and the capacity to work. Cicchetti and Rogosch (1997) noted, when working with children who had been maltreated, the importance of self-confidence and self-reliance. A common fear of affectively ill parents was that they had irrevocably damaged their children and that nothing could be done. The existence of resilience—the example that many children fared well despite adverse life circumstances—provides a necessary and important corrective to this attitude and offers a legitimate basis for hope.

Preventive Interventions

The four main hypothesized mechanisms of our intervention program are presented in Table 14–1. In terms of our theoretical model, the

TABLE 14–1. *Hypothesized mechanisms targeted by intervention*

1. Increasing family understanding of affective disorders
2. Fostering prompter parental response to youngsters' needs
3. Promoting resilient traits in children
4. Lessening risk factors associated with parental affective illness (e.g., poor marital communication, parenting, and misunderstanding)

psychosocial interventions were designed to increase family communication and understanding, provide information about treatments when needed, diminish discord, and, above all, enhance parenting. The interventions had to be compatible with a variety of orientations, given that the majority or individuals, if they are treated at all, are treated by general practitioners. We developed manualized standardized versions of both interventions and then formulated an experimental design to test their relative efficacy. The design, too, was based on a set of developmental considerations. We chose to enroll youngsters aged 8–14 years and planned to follow them over the period when the risk for onset of childhood depression is the highest. Our basic approach was to use a risk study design—that is, to assess parents and children independently of one another serially over time at specified intervals. Assessment instruments derived from risk research (i.e., in-depth structured interviews for diagnoses and symptom levels) were utilized. Additional measures assessing dimensional functioning were also employed.

The interventions were different from one another by design. The lectures were standard, although time was allowed for group discussion. The clinician-facilitated intervention was slightly longer in total duration (6–8 sessions vs. 2 lectures) and involved sessions with parents, with children, and, eventually, with the family.

We hypothesized that within families many shared experiences regarding parental illness had gone undiscussed. This, we believed, was related to a general misunderstanding and stigma associated with mental illness. In the clinician intervention, in addition to transmitting information and teaching about resilience, we asked the parents to join us in running a family meeting in which depression was explained to their youngsters. Through this process, the cognitive information presented in the intervention sessions was linked directly to the shared life experience of the family. This approach proved to be an extremely potent way to help families both to make sense of the illness and to change their behavior—one that we happened on only because we were theoretically interested in changing families' behavior and empirically comparing outcomes.

Our empirical evaluation has proceeded in a standard step-by-step fashion. Initially, we established the safety of the intervention systematically. Since the interventions were new and involved approaching families of youngsters who were not ill, the possibility existed of stirring up parents' concerns needlessly. The interventions were demonstrated to be safe, feasible, and well tolerated by the families (Beardslee et al. 1992). In an initial pilot study comparing the two forms of intervention, we demonstrated that both forms resulted in changes. Greater levels of change, however, were observed in the families that participated in the clinician-facilitated intervention (Beardslee et al. 1993b). The follow-up of these families over several years has demonstrated sustained family effects. New changes have emerged in the families over time, with much greater and sustained change being observed in the clinician-facilitated group. In our most recent set of analyses, which has involved approximately half of the sample we will eventually enroll, we specifically looked at the effects of the interviews on parents and children over time, separately. We demonstrated that directly after intervention there were significant differences between the two groups and that these differences remained whether the unit of analysis was the mother or the father (Beardslee et al. 1997a). We also demonstrated that the differences between the families were sustained for 18 months and that youngsters, as well as adults, reported benefits (Beardslee et al. 1997b). Most importantly, we found that families that reported changes in psychosocial problem-solving strategies 1 month after intervention participation have youngsters who changed more in terms of either increased adaptive functioning or decreased depressive symptoms, as measured by Children's Depression Inventory scores, 18 months after enrollment in the study (Beardslee et al. 1997b).

Our basic theoretical model for prevention, derived from risk research, is presented in Figure 14–2. In this model, the mediating variable *family problem-solving strategy* is assessed after intervention, whereas child outcomes are assessed later. The mediating variable

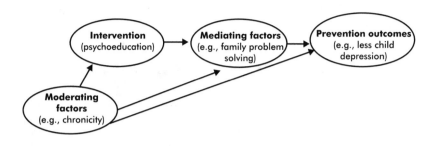

FIGURE **14–2.** *Overall prevention model of effects.*

change in family functioning (i.e., depressive symptoms) predicts success in later child outcomes. Moderating effects from factors such as chronicity of parental illness, which may be either genetic or psychosocial, operate at all levels—that is, they may affect both how the intervention is received and how the family members respond to family change. They may also have a direct effect on outcome. These effects were correlated with family change attributed to intervention participation at the prior assessment 1 year earlier—a finding that confirmed the validity of our model. Our long-term plan is to follow 100 families with youngsters in early adolescence to late adolescence and to look at the effects of not only the interventions but also specific risk factors such as illness in both parents and marital discord (moderating variable over time).

We have shown the compatibility of these approaches with a variety of different theoretical frameworks, including those of pediatrics, psychoanalytic practice, and family practice (Beardslee and MacMillan 1993a, 1993b). We have been repeatedly impressed with the need for family understanding in the face of a disorder, parental depression, that has largely been poorly understood and not discussed. We have found that depression profoundly disrupts the capacity of the family to have a coherent narrative and that our intervention helps restore the balance, enabling the families to take concrete actions and, indeed, to make sense of the illness (Focht and Beardslee 1996; Beardslee et al. 1996, 1999). Moreover, through this work, we have been able to address the fundamental public health question of how tightly tied to the individual life experience of the family the presentation of cognitive information needs to be in order to bring about change. In our work, a close linkage and the involvement of the entire family bring about far more change than intervention with less linkage.

Preventive Intervention Research: General Issues

It is essential that prevention strategies be considered from the onset when naturalistic studies of psychopathology risk factors are being designed. The questions asked by investigators concerned with prevention are relevant to, but slightly different from, those asked by investigators involved in naturalistic course and outcome studies. Specifically, the questions are from a developmental point of view across a given epoch: At what points are interventions capable of being mounted (i.e., choice of system—family, school, or community), and at what points, given a choice, are they most likely to have an effect (i.e., earlier in the course or at a developmental transition such as entering school or leaving home).

Longitudinal studies should include prevention questions in at least three areas. First, it is vital to understand resilience. Those variables in the lives of resilient individuals that are amenable to intervention offer particular opportunities for preventive intervention and, hence, need careful description. It is perhaps even more important to characterize the mechanisms underlying the emergence of resilience. As one example, the presence of mentors in crucial developmental points is generally regarded as helpful for youngsters at high risk who do well. In our own work, we found that the presence of a non-ill parent, an intact older sibling, a teacher, or a friend contributed significantly to positive outcome. Other studies have emphasized the positive impact of high-quality schools (Rutter 1994) or other opportunities within the environment, such as employment or the military (Werner and Smith 1982). The more these experiences are described as they occur in the context of naturalistic developmental studies, the greater the possibility that they can eventually be incorporated into preventive intervention trials. Second, it is important to have an awareness of the possibility of prevention when thinking about the range and depth of possible intervention strategies. Those concerned with the onset of psychopathology in adulthood may not think that high-quality day care or nursing home visitations are important interventions unless they are attuned to the considerable long-term effects of these types of programs in preventive intervention. At the least, characterization of naturally occurring interventions is important. Third, it is crucially important to understand the connection between risk factors and poor outcomes and to document ways in which risk factors may be potentially amenable to change.

It should be emphasized that all illnesses are not amenable to preventive interventions, and it is important to consider the reasons why developmental psychopathologists may not fully consider prevention. One factor in the hesitancy to consider prevention is the lack of effect of treatment in many naturalistic studies of the course and outcome of psychopathology. In a variety of large longitudinal studies, the effects of treatment do not appear to substantially alter outcome. This was true in the collaborative study of the psychobiology of depression (Rice et al. 1989), and it has proved true in the study of alcoholism (Vaillant 1993).

In light of the debate about preventive interventions, it is important to emphasize that only certain mental disorders are candidates for prevention trials. Many disorders are relatively rare and are only now coming to be understood fully, for example, childhood schizophrenia (see Chapter 8, this volume). These illnesses are unlikely to be candidates for successful prevention trials in part because they are so rare, and very large samples followed over long periods of time would be necessary to show the effects of a prevention approach in even 10%–20% of the cases. On the other hand, certain mental disorders are quite common, such as antisocial behavior (see Chapter 16, this volume) and depression, and therefore may be amenable to both preventive intervention and the adequate assessment of effects.

Recent studies have emphasized the difference between the study of clinical outcomes and research in standard practice (Weisz 1998). Interventions delivered in research settings tend to have much stronger effects than those delivered in clinical settings. Factors that account for these differences include sample differences (i.e., research participants are motivated, consent to treatment, and often are enrolled not in crisis or without serious comorbidity). In addition, treatments in research settings tend to be standardized and well supervised, and every emphasis

is made to include fidelity to well-defined standards. Treatment in longitudinal studies tends to represent the usual standard of care rather than
a specifically mounted preventive intervention. Moreover, in longitudinal studies, treatment is often being described years or even decades
earlier than the time of assessment. Finally, treatments when delivered
in naturalistic studies may be low in dose (i.e., medication). Certainly
in the areas of alcoholism and depression there have been dramatic
advances in the use of well-validated manual-based treatments. Thus,
the lack of effects of treatment in naturalistic studies should not be a
deterrent in considering the prevention of illness.

In the design of prevention programs, it is well to consider three
principles from the Institute of Medicine's (1994) report:

1. "Preventive intervention should be based on well-established theoretical frameworks" (p. 47). It is important that the testing of theoretical models, in terms of both causation and intervention pathways, will lead to far better data than simple assumptions about
   what might work.
2. "Preventive interventions need not always wait for complete scientific knowledge about etiology and treatment of disorder to be initiated" (p. 46). Since the days of the prevention of cholera there have
   been forward-thinking public health and social activists who have
   attempted preventive interventions without fully knowing all of the
   mechanisms in the causation of the disorder but while knowing
   the fundamental risk connection. For example, halting the spread
   of infectious disease, including recently AIDS, or reducing infant
   mortality is absolutely valid. Such approaches are justified when
   enough information can be gathered empirically to show that an
   intervention does in fact change a causal pathway. It may well be
   that the current epidemic of violence in this country can lead to
   such an approach—that is, prevention of violence may prevent a
   host of poor outcomes even though the mechanism by which those
   outcomes occur is not fully understood.
3. "Preventive interventions typically are most effective when they
   consider multiple domains of intervention" (p. 47). The point here
   is that trying to change behaviors over the long term in multiple
   domains involves a synergy and appears to have a much greater

effect than using different approaches singly in sequence. The corollary of this is the need to focus on the community for the implementation, because this has proved essential in a variety of different areas (Farquhar et al. 1990).

Conclusion

Given the advancements in the science of prevention and the natural affinities among the investigative techniques, awareness of and inquiries about the kind and positioning of preventive interventions should be a natural part of longitudinal investigations of psychopathology. In this regard, understanding resilience and the factors that contribute to it is particularly important. Enhancing the factors that encourage resilience provides natural guidelines of how to design interventions. Correspondingly, understanding who is at highest risk and what combination of factors leads to the poorest outcomes helps to define the targets for those individuals most in need of intervention. Finally, it is important to emphasize that the two fundamental principles of prevention — testing and understanding of causal mechanisms and provision of substantial help to families in great distress through prevention of disorder — offer considerable promise.

References

Beardslee WR: Prevention and the clinical encounter: implications from the development and evaluation of a preventive intervention for depression in families. Am J Orthopsychiatry 68:521–533, 1998

Beardslee WR, MacMillan HL: Preventive intervention with the children of depressed parents: a case study. Psychoanal Study Child 48:249–276, 1993a

Beardslee WR, MacMillan HL: Psychosocial preventive intervention for families with parental mood disorder: strategies for the clinician. J Dev Behav Pediatr 14:271–276, 1993b

Beardslee WR, Podorefsky D: Resilient adolescents whose parents have serious affective and other psychiatric disorders: the importance of self-understanding and relationships. Am J Psychiatry 145:63–69, 1988

Beardslee WR, Hoke L, Wheelock I, et al: Initial findings on preventive intervention for families with parental affective disorders. Am J Psychiatry 149:1335–1340, 1992

Beardslee WR, Keller MB, Lavori PW, et al: The impact of parental affective disorder on depression in offspring: a longitudinal follow-up in a nonreferred sample. J Am Acad Child Adolesc Psychiatry 32:723–730, 1993a

Beardslee WR, Salt P, Porterfield K, et al: Comparison of preventive interventions for families with parental affective disorder. J Am Acad Child Adolesc Psychiatry 32:254–263, 1993b

Beardslee WR, Wright E, Rothberg PC, et al: Response of families to two preventive intervention strategies: long-term differences in behavior and attitude change. J Am Acad Child Adolesc Psychiatry 35:774–782, 1996

Beardslee WR, Versage EM, Wright E, et al: Examination of preventive interventions for families with depression: evidence of change. Development and Psychopathology 9:109–130, 1997a

Beardslee WR, Wright E, Salt P, et al: Examination of children's responses to two preventive intervention strategies over time. J Am Acad Child Adolesc Psychiatry 36:196–204, 1997b

Beardslee WR, Versage EM, Gladstone TRG: Children of affectively ill parents: a review of the past ten years. J Am Acad Child Adolesc Psychiatry 37:1134–1141, 1998

Beardslee WR, Versage EM, Salt P, et al: The development and evaluation of two preventive intervention strategies for children of depressed parents, in Developmental Approaches to Prevention and Intervention (Rochester Symposia on Developmental Psychopathology, Vol 9). Edited by Cicchetti D, Toth SL. Rochester, NY, University of Rochester Press, 1999, pp 111–151

Billings AG, Moos RH: Comparisons of children of depressed and nondepressed parents: a social-environmental perspective. J Abnorm Child Psychol 11:463–486, 1983

Bloom BL, Hodges WF, Kern MB, et al: A preventive intervention program for the newly separated. Am J Orthopsychiatry 55:9–26, 1985

Cicchetti D, Rogosch FA: The role of self-organization in the promotion of resilience in maltreated children. Development and Psychopathology 9:799–817, 1997

Cicchetti D, Schneider-Rosen K: An organizational approach to childhood depression, in Depression in Young People: Developmental and Clinical Perspectives. Edited by Rutter M, Izard CE, Read PB. New York, Guilford, 1986, pp 71–134

Coie JD, Watt NF, West SG, et al: The science of prevention: a conceptual framework and some directions for a national research program. Am Psychol 48:1013–1022, 1993

Coyne JC, Kessler RC, Tal M, et al: Living with a depressed person. J Consult Clin Psychol 55:347–352, 1987

Downey G, Coyne JC: Children of depressed parents: an integrative review. Psychol Bull 108:50–76, 1990

Earls F: Epidemiology and child psychiatry: entering the second phase. Am J Orthopsychiatry 59:279–283, 1989

Farquhar JW, Fortmann SP, Flora JA, et al: Effects of community-wide education on cardiovascular disease risk factors: the Stanford Five-City Project. JAMA 264:359–365, 1990

Fendrich M, Warner V, Weissman MM: Family risk factors, parental depression, and psychopathology in offspring. Dev Psychol 26:40–50, 1990

Focht L, Beardslee WR: "Speech after long silence": The use of narrative therapy in a preventive intervention for children of parents with affective disorder. Fam Process 35:407–422, 1996

Forehand R, McCombs A: Unraveling the antecedent-consequence conditions in maternal depression and adolescent functioning. Behav Res Ther 26:399–405, 1988

Gabbard GO (editor-in-chief): Treatments of Psychiatric Disorders, 2nd Edition. Washington, DC, American Psychiatric Press, 1995

Garmezy N: Stress-resistant children: the search for protective factors, in Recent Research in Developmental Psychology (J Child Psychol Psychiatry Book Suppl No 4). Edited by Stevenson JE. Oxford, UK, Pergamon, 1985, pp 213–233

Glynn TJ: Comprehensive approaches to tobacco use control. Br J Addict 86:631–663, 1991

Hammen C, Burge D, Burney E, et al: Longitudinal study of diagnoses in children of women with unipolar and bipolar affective disorder. Arch Gen Psychiatry 47:1112–1117, 1990

Hautzinger M, Linden M, Hoffman N: Distressed couples with and without a depressed partner: an analysis of their verbal interaction. J Behav Ther Exp Psychiatry 13:307–314, 1982

Institute of Medicine: Reducing Risks for Mental Disorders: Frontiers for Preventive Intervention Research. Edited by Mrazek PJ, Haggerty RJ. Washington, DC, National Academy Press, 1994

Kellam SG, Rebok GW: Building developmental and etiological theory through epidemiologically based preventive intervention trials, in Preventing Antisocial Behavior: Interventions From Birth Through Adolescence. Edited by McCord J, Tremblay RE. New York, Guilford, 1992, pp 162–195

Keller MB, Lavori PW, Mueller TI, et al: Time to recovery, chronicity, and levels of psychopathology in major depression. Arch Gen Psychiatry 49:809–816, 1992

Kotelchuck M, Richmond JB: Head Start: evolution of a successful comprehensive child development program. Pediatrics 79:441–445, 1987

National Institute of Mental Health: The Prevention of Mental Disorders: A National Research Agenda. Bethesda, MD, National Institute of Mental Health, 1993

National Institute of Mental Health: Priorities for Prevention Research at NIMH. Bethesda, MD, National Institute of Mental Health, 1998

Olds DL, Henderson CR, Chamberlin RW, et al: Preventing child abuse and neglect: a randomized trial of nurse home visitation. Pediatrics 78:65–78, 1986

Price RH, van Ryn M, Vinokur A: Impact of a preventive job search intervention on the likelihood of depression among the unemployed. J Health Soc Behav 33:158–167, 1992

Rice J, Andreasen NC, Coryell W, et al: NIMH Collaborative Program on the Psychobiology of Depression: clinical. Genet Epidemiol 6:179–182, 1989

Rutter M: The developmental psychopathology of depression: issues and perspectives, in Depression in Young People: Developmental and Clinical Perspectives. Edited by Rutter M, Izard CE, Read PB. New York, Guilford, 1986

Rutter M: Psychosocial resilience and protective mechanism. Am J Orthopsychiatry 57:316–331, 1987

Rutter M: Commentary: some focus and process considerations regarding effects of parental depression on children. Dev Psychol 26:60–67, 1990

Rutter M: Fifteen Thousand Hours: Secondary Schools and Their Effects on Children. London, P Chapman, 1994

Rutter M, Quinton D: Parental psychiatric disorder: effects on children. Psychol Med 14:853–880, 1984

Sameroff AJ, Seifer R, Zax M, et al: Early indicators of developmental risk: Rochester Longitudinal Study. Schizophr Bull 13:383–394, 1987

Schweinhart LJ, Weikart DP: High/Scope Perry Preschool Program outcomes, in Preventing Antisocial Behavior: Interventions From Birth Through Adolescence. Edited by McCord J, Trembly RE. New York, Guilford, 1992, pp 67–86

Shure MB, Spivack G: Interpersonal problem solving as a mediator of behavioral adjustment in preschool and kindergarten children. J Appl Dev Psychol 1:29–44, 1980

Shure MB, Spivack G: Interpersonal problem-solving in young children: a cognitive approach to prevention. Am J Community Psychol 10:341–356, 1982

Teti DM, Gelfand DM, Messinger DS, et al: Maternal depression and the quality of early attachment: an examination of infants, preschoolers and their mothers. Dev Psychol 31:364–376, 1995

Tsuang MT, Faraone SV: The Genetics of Mood Disorders. Baltimore, MD, Johns Hopkins University Press, 1990

U.S. National Highway Traffic Safety Administration: Fatal Accident Reporting System: A Review of Information on Fatal Traffic Crashes in the United States in 1989 (Report No DOT-HS 807-693). Washington, DC, U.S. Department of Transportation, 1991

Vaillant GE: Is alcoholism more often the cause or the result of depression? Harv Rev Psychiatry 1:94–99, 1993

Weikart DP, Schweinhart LJ, Larner MB: A report on the High/Scope Preschool Curriculum Comparison Study: consequences of three preschool curriculum models through age 15. Early Childhood Research Quarterly 1:1–15,1986

Weissman MM, Warner V, Wickramarante P, et al: Offspring of depressed parents: ten years later. Arch Gen Psychiatry 54:932–940, 1997

Weisz J: Effects of psychopathology with children and adolescents: what we know and what we need to learn, in Developmental Approaches to Prevention and Intervention (Rochester Symposia on Developmental Psychopathology, Vol 9). Edited by Cicchetti D, Toth SL. Rochester, NY, University of Rochester Press, 1998

Werner EE, Smith RS: Vulnerable but Invincible: A Study of Resilient Children. New York, McGraw-Hill, 1982

Zahn-Waxler C, Kochanska G, Krupnick J, et al: Patterns of guilt in children of depressed and well mothers. Dev Psychol 26:51–59, 1990

CHAPTER 15

Prevention of Alcoholism: Reflections of a Naturalist

George E. Vaillant, M.D.

I f long-term follow-up often demolishes our fondest preconceptions, it also often supports our common sense. Two erroneous preconceptions regarding the etiology of alcoholism are the illusion of "psychiatric" causation and the illusion of single-gene causation. Prospective study of alcoholic individuals over several decades not only has dispelled these two illusions but also has arrived at the commonsensical conclusion that adequate prevention of alcoholism is most likely to come by supporting the cultural, social, and economic factors that contribute to moderate drinking.

Let me make these points one at a time. In so doing I will use data from the Study of Adult Development—a 50-year prospective study of 152 socially disadvantaged Core City and 52 college-educated alcoholic individuals (Vaillant 1995). However, the points that I shall make have also been confirmed by other studies.

This work is from the Division of Psychiatry, Department of Medicine, Brigham and Women's Hospital and the Study of Adult Development, Harvard University Health Services and is supported by research grants from the National Institute of Mental Health (MH-00364 and MH-42248).

Psychiatric Causation

Major stumbling blocks to the prevention and treatment of alcoholism are illusions about the etiology of alcoholism, especially illusions that suggest that psychiatric intervention will be particularly effective. Because alcoholism often occurs in individuals who had unhappy childhoods and in individuals with comorbid anxiety or depression or with antisocial disorders, these comorbid conditions are often credited with too much causal responsibility for the associated alcoholism.

In virtually all retrospective studies of alcoholic individuals (Barry 1974) and in two of the best prospective studies (McCord and McCord 1960; Robins 1966), unstable childhood seemed to predict future alcoholism. Broken homes, irresponsible fathers, marital discord, and inconsistent upbringing appear to be most often implicated. However, the subjects of both the McCords' and Robins's studies were drawn from cohorts of underprivileged youths known to be at high risk for delinquency. In addition, the hereditary contribution of parental alcoholism was not controlled. Haberman (1966) compared the children of alcoholic and nonalcoholic parents and noted that the former, if they lived with their parents, were more likely to stutter, wet the bed, misbehave, and manifest phobias. Is, then, the disturbed childhood environment of alcoholic individuals a cause of alcoholism or simply a manifestation of parental alcoholism that contributes to a child's subsequent alcoholism for hereditary rather than environmental reasons? Although the adult differences between social drinkers and alcohol-dependent individuals in the Study of Adult Development sample appear to be attributable to childhood environment, the prospective evidence suggests that the apparent differences between alcoholic subjects and matched control subjects can be attributed to alcoholism (Table 15–1). In childhood no differences could be discerned.

From studies of cross-fostered children, Goodwin (1976, 1979) has persuasively marshaled evidence that the observed increased rate of alcoholism in the descendants of alcoholic individuals appears to correlate with alcohol abuse in heredity, not in the environment. In a cross-fostering study of half-siblings, Schuckit et al. (1972) observed that in children with an alcoholic biological parent who were raised by nonal-

TABLE 15–1.   *Adult differences and childhood similarities between Core City men who never abused alcohol and those who became dependent on alcohol*

	Asymptomatic drinkers ($n = 260$),[a] %	Alcohol-dependent men ($n = 71$),[a] %
Differences in adulthood[b]		
10+ years unemployed	4	24
GAF score <70 (age 47)	24	51
Five or more sociopathic symptoms on Robins scale[c] (age 49)	0.4	30
Two or more times in jail (by age 42)	4	16
<10 grades of education	28	42
Social class V (age 47)	2	21
Similarities in childhood[d]		
IQ < 90	28	30
Parents in Social Class V	32	30
Multiproblem family	11	14
Warm relationship with mother	30	27
Inadequate maternal supervision	36	34
Emotional problems	32	30

Note. Core City sample from the Study of Adult Development (Vaillant 1995). GAF = Global Assessment of Functioning.
[a]Of the 456 men in the study, 71 could be classified at age 47 as alcohol-dependent and 260 as asymptomatic drinkers (one or no problems with alcohol). Of the remaining 125 men, 62 had two or three alcohol-related problems, 49 were classified as alcohol abusers but not as alcohol-dependent, and 14 were unclassified because of early death or lack of data.
[b]All comparisons (χ^2 test) significant, $P < 0.001$.
[c]Robins 1966.
[d]All comparisons (χ^2 test) not significant, $P > 0.05$.

coholic parents, the rate of alcohol abuse was three times higher than that in children without alcoholic parents who were raised by an alcoholic stepparent or surrogate.

Indeed, among the men in our study, the observed differences in childhood environmental weaknesses between future alcoholic individuals and social drinkers were no greater than could be accounted for by the presence of an alcoholic parent in the subject's family (Vaillant 1980, 1995). Put differently, of the 51 inner-city men who had been exposed to few childhood environmental weaknesses but did have an alcoholic parent, 27% became alcohol-dependent; of the 56 men from multiproblem families who did not have an alcoholic parent, only 5% developed alcohol dependence.

In addition to an unhappy childhood, three premorbid personality types have been repeatedly postulated to play an etiological role in alcoholism: the emotionally insecure, anxious, and dependent (Blane 1968; Simmel 1948); the depressed (Winokur et al. 1969); and the sociopathic and/or minimally brain-damaged (Robins 1966) (see Tarter 1981). Not until several prospective studies were available could we seriously entertain the hypothesis that these personality constellations might be secondary to the alcoholism and could we discard the popular illusion that alcoholism merely reflected one symptom of personality disorder.

First, alcoholic individuals are not more dependent premorbidly. Prospective studies by Jones (1968), Kammeier et al. (1973), and Vaillant (1980) concur that premorbid traits of dependency do not increase the risk of alcoholism.

The etiological link between anxiety disorder and alcoholism is less easy to dispel. As adults, the Core City men who developed alcohol dependence appeared twice as likely as those who never abused alcohol to manifest psychological dysfunction, and they were six times as likely to be chronically unemployed (Table 15–1). But as children, the men who became alcohol-dependent were only slightly more likely to come from multiproblem and welfare-dependent families, and they were no more likely to manifest childhood emotional problems.

Work by many investigators suggests that despite what alcoholic individuals tell us, objective observation in the laboratory reveals that chronic use of alcohol makes alcoholic subjects more withdrawn, less self-confident, and often more anxious (Logue et al. 1978; Nathan et al.

1970; Tamerin et al. 1970). Too often the "anxiety" that alcohol is most effective in relieving is not premorbid panic disorder but the tremulousness, fearfulness, and dysphoria produced by brief abstinence in an alcohol-dependent individual. Alcoholic individuals' verbal rationalizations for their behavior are highly noticeable, while the actual behavioral effects of the alcohol they consume often are ignored. Such misperception distorts our views regarding the etiology of alcohol abuse. For example, in an ingenious set of placebo-controlled experiments, Marlatt and Rohsenow (1980) assembled compelling evidence that the alleged relief of tension by alcohol has more to do with expectancy than with pharmacology. Prospective data from both the Core City and the college samples in the Study of Adult Development suggest that premorbidly anxious individuals are not at increased risk for alcoholism but that alcohol-dependent individuals are unusually anxious.

Brown and her colleagues (1991) studied the relationship between alcohol abuse and state and trait anxiety over time. For 4 months they repeatedly tested 171 hospitalized alcoholic men, 40% of whom reported significant state anxiety on admission. As would be expected these men reported themselves as chronically prone to anxiety and worry and perceived their drinking as a means of self-medicating anxiety. However, when they were administered the State-Trait Anxiety Inventory over time, a clear pattern emerged. After 2 weeks of abstinence, state anxiety levels, markedly elevated on admission, had returned to normal. At 3-month follow-up, among the men who had remained abstinent, both state and trait anxiety had declined still further. The men who, once in the community, had relapsed to alcohol abuse once again had elevated anxiety levels.

Finally, the family studies of Merikangas and Weissman (Merikangas et al. 1985; Weissman et al. 1984) show that patients with anxiety disorders without alcoholism do not have an increased number of alcoholic relatives compared with control subjects. In contrast, individuals manifesting both anxiety disorder and alcoholism do have more alcoholic relatives than do control subjects.

In conclusion, on the one hand, just as drugs like meprobamate and phenobarbital have rarely been more effective than placebo in treating chronic anxiety states, just so alcohol is probably not an effective means of self-medication for chronic anxiety. On the other hand, it seems clear that some facets of anxiety (e.g., guilt and muscle tension) are effectively relieved by low doses of alcohol, and in some individuals preexisting panic disorder may play an etiological role in the development of alcoholism.

The close association between depression and alcoholism has led some investigators to suggest that alcoholism is simply a forme fruste of major depressive disorder (Winokur et al. 1969). Although alcoholism and depression often occur in the same families, they do so for very complex reasons.

Numerous lines of evidence suggest that depression is a symptom caused by alcoholism far more often than the reverse.

1. Several laboratory studies have documented that alcohol ingestion increases, rather than reduces, depressive and suicidal ideation (Logue et al. 1978; Nathan et al. 1970; Tamerin et al. 1970).
2. There is very little evidence that the administration of either tricyclic antidepressants or lithium (pharmacological treatments that are effective in reducing the relapse rate for primary depression) alters the course of alcoholism (Dorus et al. 1989; Halikas 1983; Viamontes 1972). However, there is abundant evidence that abstinence from alcohol abuse alleviates depression (Brown et al. 1988; Pettinati et al. 1982).
3. Although Winokur et al. (1969) proposed genetic links between alcoholic and depressive disorders and documented that some cases of alcoholism may be variants of unipolar affective disorder, Morrison (1975) and Dunner et al. (1979) presented evidence that in family trees, alcoholism and bipolar affective illness are transmitted independently. Weissman and Merikangas (Merikangas and Gelernter 1990; Weissman et al. 1984) further clarified the fact that the family trees of alcoholism and major depressive disorder reflect quite separate lineages.
4. There is compelling prospective evidence that the prolonged abuse of alcohol causes, rather than alleviates, depression (Kammeier et al. 1973; McLellan et al. 1979).
5. The rate of alcohol dependence among patients with bipolar affective disorder does not seem to be greater than the rate of alcoholism among other psychiatric patients (Morrison 1974; Woodruff et al.

1973). It is true that many bipolar patients may drink excessively during a manic episode; but in an impressive 30-year follow-back study of the life course of more than 1,700 Scandinavian alcoholic individuals, Sundby (1967) determined that the occurrence of psychotic depression in this sample was, if anything, less than that observed for the general population.

The causal link between alcohol abuse and personality is less easy to dispel than the links between alcohol abuse and an unhappy childhood or comorbid anxiety or depression. Alcoholism is highly correlated with antisocial personality. Robins (1966) and the McCords (McCord and McCord 1960) found the antecedents of alcoholism and sociopathy to be very similar; but both of these prospective studies were limited by their focus on a relatively antisocial group of schoolchildren. In such studies, the interweaving of alcoholic heredity and environment with sociopathic heredity and environment could not be unraveled.

In the originally nondelinquent Core City sample, it remained difficult to disentangle alcoholism from sociopathy. Scales used to measure alcoholism correlated with scales used to measure sociopathy ($r = .6$). However, when multiple regression was performed, it was possible partially to tease apart the relationships between premorbid predictors and sociopathy and/or alcoholic outcome. On a univariate basis, all of the variables in Table 15–2 significantly ($P < 0.02$) predicted sociopathy, and all but boyhood competence, childhood environmental problems, and IQ predicted alcoholism. However, in a multivariate model, the predictors of alcohol abuse were quite different from those of sociopathy.

Our own data (Vaillant 1995), those of the McCords (McCord and McCord 1960), and those of the Gluecks (Glueck and Glueck 1950) all demonstrated that having criminal fathers and rejecting mothers correlate more highly with sociopathy than with alcoholism.

It was true that the 16 Core City men who by age 14 years were truant and exhibited school behavior problems were almost four times as likely as their peers to develop later alcohol dependence. And, since only 2 of these 16 men clearly abused alcohol before the age of 18, alcohol abuse could not be cited as the cause of their school misbehavior. Equally significant, however, from the viewpoint of etiology is that such serious truancy and school behavior problems were noted in only 9 of

TABLE 15–2.   *Childhood variables predicting alcoholism, mental health, and sociopathy in a sample of Core City men*

	Univariate Spearman rank correlation (ρ)[a]	
	Alcohol abuse[b] (1–3) ($n = 398$)	Sociopathy[c] (0–12) ($n = 430$)
Not significant in multivariate model		
Childhood emotional problems	0.02	0.15
IQ	0.00	–0.12
Sociopathy predictors		
Boyhood competence	–0.09	–0.24***
Multiproblem family	0.15	0.18**
Difficult infancy (maternal neglect) (yes/no)	0.12	0.13***
Alcoholism predictors		
Alcoholism in family	0.29***	0.20
Cultural background (1–3)[d]	–0.28***	–0.16

Note. Core City sample from the Study of Adult Development (Vaillant 1995).
[a]Significance based on controlling for all other variables by multiple regression.
[b]DSM-III (American Psychiatric Association 1980).
[c]Robins 1966.
[d]1 = Irish; 2 = Northern European, Canadian, American; 3 = Italian or other Mediterranean.
**$P < 0.01$, ***$P < 0.001$, Spearman's ρ.

the 71 Core City men who eventually became alcohol-dependent. In other words, many sociopathic individuals later abuse alcohol as part of their antisocial behavior; but most alcoholic individuals are not premorbidly sociopathic.

Genetic Factors

Considerable controversy exists as to whether the familial transmission of alcohol abuse is caused by environmental or genetic factors. Because of the seemingly intractable, involuntary nature of alcoholism, investigators have hypothesized that alcoholism is an inherited disease of disordered metabolism. Such studies have failed to fully appreciate that alcohol abuse may be as polygenic in etiology as height or IQ.

Although genetic factors do control the rate of the metabolism of alcohol (Seixas 1978; Vesell et al. 1971), alcohol elimination rates do not differ among the children of alcoholic and nonalcoholic parents (Utne et al. 1977). In other words, interindividual and interracial differences in alcohol metabolism exist, but these differences in metabolism do not seem to be powerfully related to risk of alcohol dependence.

In the past 10 years an increasingly convincing body of evidence has emerged suggesting that if alcoholism is not primarily caused by alcoholism in the child's environment, neither is it the result of a simple hereditary metabolic defect. In the Core City sample from the Study of Adult Development, a familial history of alcohol abuse was a potent predictor that the men themselves would abuse alcohol (Table 15–3). The presence of alcoholism in the parents also greatly increased the risk of alcoholism in their children. Of the 244 men who grew up in households where neither parent nor parent surrogate abused alcohol, 11% became alcohol-dependent. In contrast, 28% of the men with alcohol-abusing fathers and 36% of the men with alcohol-abusing mothers (many of whom were also married to alcohol-abusing husbands) developed alcohol dependence.

TABLE 15–3. *Relation of family history of alcohol abuse to alcohol abuse among a sample of Core City men*

	Proportion of sample with known alcohol-abusing relatives (%)	
	No relatives ($n = 155$)	Three or more relatives ($n = 80$)
No alcohol abuse ever	80	45***
Alcohol abuse ever[a]	13	20*
Alcohol dependence ever[a]	7	35***

Note. Core City sample from the Study of Adult Development (Vaillant 1995).
[a]DSM-III (American Psychiatric Association 1980).
*$P < 0.05$. ***$P < 0.001$.

In reviewing the relationship between alcoholism in probands and family history of alcohol abuse, Goodwin and others suggested that *familial* alcoholism may be different from *acquired* alcoholism (Cloninger et al. 1981; Goodwin 1979). The former is thought to have a poorer prognosis and to begin at an earlier age. Implicit in this view is the belief that familial alcoholism, analogous to early-onset diabetes or process schizophrenia, is a more malignant subtype. The data from the Core City sample of men did not support this point of view (Table 15–3). We compared the 155 men with no alcohol-abusing relatives with the 80 men who had three or more alcohol-abusing relatives. As a group, the alcohol-abusing men with many known alcoholic relatives were five times more likely to develop alcohol dependence, but the symptom pattern in the alcohol-abusing men with many alcoholic relatives did not seem very different from that in the alcohol-abusing men with no known alcoholic relatives (Valliant 1994).

Failure to separate heredity from environment has also led to what, I believe, is the misleading distinction between type 1 and type 2 alcoholism (Cloninger 1987b; Cloninger et al. 1988; von Knorring et al. 1985). Type 1 alcoholism is believed to affect both sexes and to have a relatively late onset (after age 25 years). The alcohol-related problems associated with this type of alcoholism are relatively mild and rarely involve antisocial activity. Persons with type 1 alcoholism are thought to demonstrate the personality trait of high harm avoidance; thus, they are cautious and more likely to worry and feel guilt over their alcoholism (Cloninger 1987b). It has been suggested that type 1 alcoholism is analogous to reactive schizophrenia and adult-onset diabetes.

Clinically, it is hypothesized, type 2 alcoholism affects males and has an early onset (prior to age 25 years). A person with type 2 alcoholism has many male alcoholic relatives and manifests a history of violence and illegal activities both with and without alcohol use. He is more often a polydrug abuser. The personality traits of low harm avoidance (i.e., little need for social approval and a lack of inhibition) and of high novelty seeking are hypothesized to be present (Cloninger 1987b). Thus, he uses alcohol for its euphoric effects and is more likely to develop alcohol dependence.

Before the hypothesized typology of alcoholism can be confirmed, however, it must be tested in a psychiatrically normal community sample. Then, the environmental effects of alcoholic parents must be distinguished from the genetic effects of alcoholic parents. Finally, individuals alleged to manifest type 1 and type 2 personalities must be contrasted at the same age. The personalities of most people, including alcoholic individuals, change between ages 16 and 46 years. By this I mean that many novelty-seeking, harm-ignoring adolescents grow up to become novelty- and harm-avoiding grandparents.

Early onset of problem drinking among the Core City alcoholic men was not associated with alcoholic heredity (Table 15–4). Men with no alcoholic relatives were as likely to develop alcohol abuse early as late. Men with many alcoholic relatives were as likely to develop alcoholism late as early. When the data were further analyzed, early onset of alcohol abuse among the Core City men appeared to be more closely associated with family breakdown and number of antisocial relatives than with number of alcoholic relatives.

At the present time, a commonsense view of the role of genetic factors in alcoholism seems appropriate. All of the investigations reviewed by Schuckit (1992) have demonstrated that after modest doses of alcohol, despite having identical blood alcohol concentrations, individuals with family histories of alcohol abuse have less intense subjective feelings of intoxication. Like cultural susceptibility, genetic susceptibility to alcoholism is but one of many risk factors and is most likely polygenic. The number of alcoholic relatives is an important predictor of *whether* an individual develops alcoholism, and an unstable childhood environment is an important predictor of *when* an individual develops alcoholism. Harm avoidance and novelty seeking in men may be affected as much by age as by genes.

Other Etiological Factors

Many other etiological factors besides genes and psychiatric causation affect the probability that an individual will develop alcohol dependence. The most important etiological factor in alcoholism, of course, is that alcohol use is addictive. However, the use—without abuse—of alcohol is endemic throughout much of the world. Thus, in the attempt to understand why alcohol use evolves into a disorder, appreciation of

TABLE 15–4. *Associations of "biological" and "environmental" factors with age at onset of alcoholism in a sample of Core City men*

		Age at onset of alcoholism (years)		
	n	9–21 (*n* = 40)	22–34 (*n* = 69)	35–57 (*n* = 40)
"Biological factors"				
No alcoholic relatives	43	12 (30%)	20 (29%)	11 (27%)
Two or more alcoholic relatives	95	21 (53%)	40 (58%)	24 (60%)
Alcohol dependence (ever)	77	22 (55%)	38 (55%)	17 (43%)
Stable abstinence (age 60)	47	13 (33%)	22 (32%)	12 (30%)
"Environmental" factors				
Multiproblem family	25	10 (25%)	11 (16%)	4 (10%)
Alcoholic caretaker	79	30 (75%)	32 (46%)	17 (43%)*
Abuse from alcoholic caretaker	38	15 (38%)	16 (23%)	7 (18%)*
Five or more sociopathic traits	27	15 (38%)	10 (14%)	2 (5%)**
Incarceration (ever)	26	10 (25%)	14 (20%)	2 (5%)*
School behavior problems	13	8 (20%)	4 (6%)	1 (3%)*
Multiple alcohol-related arrests	54	20 (50%)	28 (41%)	6 (15%)**

Note. Core City sample from the Study of Adult Development (Vaillant 1995). Number of individuals with each factor by age-at-onset group, along with proportion of the total number in that age group with that factor, is shown.
*$P < 0.05$. **$P < 0.01$.

host resistance to addiction is crucial. Most etiological factors that affect host resistance are sociocultural modulators of alcohol use. But with the exception of Moslem and Hindu countries, where social taboos against alcohol use have been successful, prohibition has rarely been an effective solution. In other words, *proscriptions* against alcohol use have rarely been as effective as social *prescriptions* for alcohol use.

At least eight environmental factors have been well documented that significantly affect host resistance to alcohol dependence, and none of them are primarily "psychiatric."

Rapidity of alcohol's effects on the brain. The rapidity with which alcohol reaches the brain affects resistance to alcohol dependence. Thus, social patterns that encourage consumption of low-proof alcoholic beverages or that direct that alcohol be drunk only with food that delays intestinal absorption of alcohol reduce the likelihood that an individual will develop dependence (Jellinek 1960). In contrast, drinking practices that encourage high-proof alcohol to be ingested in the absence of food (e.g., in inner-city bars and in the gin mills at the perimeter of Native American reservations) increase the likelihood of alcohol dependence.

Society's attitudes toward alcohol use. Cultures that teach children to drink responsibly and cultures that have ritualized when and where to drink tend to have lower rates of alcohol abuse than cultures that forbid children to drink and/or exert little social control over when and how adults are to drink. And, as Heath (1975) demonstrated, how a society socializes drunkenness is as important as how it socializes drinking. For example, both France and Italy inculcate in their children responsible drinking practices; but public drunkenness is far more socially acceptable in France than in Italy, and France experiences a higher rate of alcohol abuse.

By chance, the Study of Adult Development offered unique controls for many of the confounding variables. Virtually all of the Core City men lived in an urban environment (Boston) where alcohol was readily available and was the principal recreational drug of choice. The Core City men shared the same schools and legal system, and they shared the same ethnically diverse peer group. The Core City men differed from one another, however, in terms of the cultural background of their parents. Sixty-one percent of their parents were born in foreign countries. The prognostic power of classifying men according to the extent to which their culture sanctions childhood drinking and proscribes intoxication is underscored in Table 15–5. In the Core City sample, alcohol dependence developed seven times more frequently in those of Irish descent than in those of Mediterranean descent. The Italians provide children with a long education in moderate alcohol use and encourage drinking with family members. They inculcate drinking practices that diminish the alcohol "high"; these practices include using low-proof alcohol and drinking alcohol with food. In contrast, the Irish forbid children and adolescents from learning how to drink, but they tolerate—and covertly praise—the capacity of men to drink large amounts of alcohol. The Irish prefer drinking in pubs, where alcohol intake is carefully separated from the family dinnertable and often from food intake of any kind (Stivers 1976). (A little reflection will bring to mind that the drinking practices that occur on many of our Native American reservations are an exaggeration of the drinking practices in Ireland.)

TABLE 15–5.   *Relationship between the culture in which fathers were raised and the development of alcohol dependence in their sons*

	Fathers' culture		
Alcohol use[a]	Irish (n = 75)	Other[b] (n = 195)	Mediterranean (n = 128)
No alcohol abuse	59%	58%	86%[c]
Alcohol abuse without dependence	13%	19%	10%
Alcohol dependence	28%	23%	4%

Note. Core City sample from the Study of Adult Development (Vaillant 1995).
[a]DSM-III (American Psychiatric Association 1980). The proportion of men from each parental background with the specified pattern of alcohol use is presented.
[b]Canadian, American, and Northern European.
[c]$P < 0.001$ (χ^2).

Occupation.   Occupation is an important contributing factor in the development of alcohol dependence (Plant 1979), especially occupations that break down the time-dependent rituals that help to protect "social" drinkers from persons who engage in round-the-clock alcohol consumption. Occupations like bartending and the diplomatic service put an individual in close contact with alcohol throughout the day. Similarly, unemployment and occupations, such as writing and journalism, that deprive an individual of the structure of the workday and therefore facilitate drinking at odd times are associated with increased rates of alcoholism.

Drinking patterns of the immediate social group.   The drinking habits of an individual's immediate social group powerfully affect how the individual uses or abuses alcohol (Bacon 1957; Cahalan and Room 1972; Jessor and Jessor 1975). It has been consistently shown that the heavy-drinking adolescent can be distinguished from his or her more abstemious peers by social extroversion, dependence on peer-group pressure, independence from parental or religious-group pressure, and social involvement in heavy-drinking peer groups (Fillmore et al. 1979; Jessor and Jessor 1975; Margulies et al. 1977). The drinking habits of one's marital partner also significantly affects the risk of alcoholism. A common reason for the young men in the Core City group to shift from a pattern of heavy, prealcoholic drinking to "social" drinking was marriage and a concomitant shift in social network.

Availability. The success of legal prohibition of alcohol seen in Moslem countries is supported not only by social mores concerning the use of mood-altering drugs but also by agricultural and climatic patterns that inhibit production of crops from which alcohol may be cheaply produced. In contrast, the greatest lesson of prohibition in the United States was that in the absence of cultural support and alternative "recreation of drugs," the legal proscription of alcohol per se will be an ineffective remedy. Age limits for legal drinking and time and location of alcohol sales also affect rates of alcohol abuse.

Cost. The extent of alcohol abuse appears to be directly related to the per capita consumption of alcohol (de Lint and Schmidt 1968; Schmidt and Popham 1975). Thus, to the extent that social policy and price structure affect alcohol consumption, these factors will also influence risk of alcohol abuse. At the present time, the evidence that the consumption of distilled spirits is affected by price relative to disposable income appears incontrovertible (Bruun et al. 1975; Lau 1975; Ornstein 1980; Special Committee of the Royal College of Psychiatrists 1979). In the laboratory, Mello et al. (1968) observed experimentally that when alcoholic subjects were working for alcohol on an operant apparatus, the blood alcohol level of the alcoholic subjects was directly related to the number of responses (the behavioral "cost") necessary to produce a reinforcement of beverage alcohol. In terms of prevention of alcohol abuse, two melancholy facts deserve attention. Fifty percent of all alcohol sold is consumed by alcoholic individuals, and the advertising budget of the beer, wine, and spirits industry is 10 times the budget of the National Institute on Alcohol Abuse and Alcoholism.

Social instability. Another etiological factor in alcoholism is social instability (Leighton et al. 1963; Pittman and Snyder 1962). As already pointed out, alcohol is an addictive substance, and to some degree all alcohol users are at risk for dependence. When societies are stable and have evolved rituals for social drinking, rates of alcohol abuse are lower; when societies break down and individuals become demoralized and societal control over alcohol ingestion is diminished, rates of alcohol abuse are higher. Alcohol abuse is often a concomitant of the destabilization that accompanies the impact of a modern industrial society on a society less industrialized. According to Edwards et al. (1974), ritualized controlled social drinking will break down when any of three conditions are met: 1) when the culture itself is changing and loosening its control over individual members, 2) when the sudden introduction of a substance with high dependence-inducing properties imposes a particular threat to an unprepared society, or 3) when individuals are unresponsive to cultural influences and use addictive drugs.

Gender. Because alcoholism occurs less often in women than in men, many have speculated that alcoholism in women may be different (Schuckit et al. 1969; Winokur et al. 1971). At least until very recently, American social mores tolerated drunkenness in men but not in women. In American movies male drunks are hilarious, but female drunks are pathetic. As a result, among women who abuse alcohol, more etiological risk factors are usually present and in greater severity (Hesselbrock 1981). Alcohol metabolism is also affected by sex differences (Camberwell Council on Alcoholism 1980; Frezza et al. 1990). However, several recent studies suggest that in most respects female alcohol abusers do not differ from their male counterparts (Kagle 1987; Vaillant 1995; Wilsnack and Beckman 1989).

Conclusion

In this chapter I have suggested that alcohol abuse and/or social drinking are predicted by a set of variables depending on social, economic, and genetic factors that are quite different from the variables predicting other mental illnesses and sociopathy. We must stop trying to treat alcoholism as if it were merely a symptom of underlying psychic distress. Instead, we must learn to heed an old Japanese proverb: "First, the man takes a drink, then the drink takes a drink, then the drink takes the man." Thus, the treatment of alcohol abuse must depend more on social structure and behavior modification than on relief of psychopathology (Vaillant 1995).

A second conclusion is that if culture does play such an important role in the genesis of alcoholism, we must try to uncover ways of socializing adolescents in healthy drinking practices so that the use of alcohol will remain for a lifetime under the individual's conscious choice. Introducing children to the ceremonial and sanctioned use of low-proof alcoholic beverages taken with meals in the presence of others, coupled with social sanctions against drunkenness and against drinking at unspecified times, would appear to provide the best protection against future alcohol abuse. Within reason, altering price structure can sometimes affect alcohol use; governments should experiment with ways of reducing overall consumption, especially of high-proof alcohol, by price manipulation and education. The covert advertising by the alcohol industry, which serves to promote the likelihood of addiction, must be economically combated as the covert advertising by the tobacco industry has been by antismoking groups. Society must learn to recognize the health consequences and to appreciate the long-range dangers of providing cheap alcohol as a fringe benefit. Finally, if genetic factors play an important etiological role in alcoholism—and I believe that they do—individuals with many alcoholic relatives should be alerted to learn safe drinking habits (i.e., never consume more than 30 grams, or 2 drinks, of alcohol in a 24-hour period).

Finally, the prevention of alcoholism appears to be different from preventing heroin addiction and Alzheimer's disease. In preventing heroin addiction and and cigarette smoking, prohibition is useful. In preventing Alzheimer's disease and bipolar illness, genetic breakthroughs may become terribly important. However, in order to prevent alcoholism, the same principles must be applied as in the prevention of heart disease and most forms of obesity, namely, moderation in all things.

References

American Psychiatric Association: Diagnostic and Statistical Manual of Mental Disorders, 3rd Edition. Washington, DC, American Psychiatric Association, 1980

Bacon SD: Social settings conducive to alcoholism. JAMA 164:177–181, 1957

Barry HB III: Psychological factors in alcoholism, in The Biology of Alcoholism, Vol 3: Clinical Pathology. Edited by Kissin B, Begleiter H. New York, Plenum, 1974, pp 53–107

Blane HT: The Personality of the Alcoholic: Guises of Dependency. New York, Harper & Row, 1968

Brown SA, Irwin M, Schuckit MA: Changes in depression among abstinent alcoholics. J Stud Alcohol 49:412–417, 1988

Brown SA, Irwin M, Schuckit MA: Changes in anxiety among abstinent male alcoholics. J Stud Alcohol 52:55–61, 1991

Bruun K, Edwards G, Lumio M, et al: Alcohol Control Policies in Public Health Perspective. Helsinki, Finnish Foundation for Alcohol Studies, 1975

Cahalan D, Room R: Problem drinking among men aged 21–59. Am J Public Health 62:1472–1482, 1972

Camberwell Council on Alcoholism: Women and Alcohol. London, Tavistock, 1980

Cloninger CR: A systematic method for clinical description and classification of personality variants: a proposal. Arch Gen Psychiatry 44:573–588, 1987b

Cloninger CR, Bohman M, Sigvardsson S: Inheritance of alcohol abuse: cross-fostering analysis of adopted men. Arch Gen Psychiatry 38:861–868, 1981

Cloninger CR, Sigvardsson S, Bohman M: Childhood personality predicts alcohol abuse in young adults. Alcohol Clin Exp Res 12:494–505, 1988

de Lint J, Schmidt W: The distribution of alcohol consumption in Ontario. Q J Alcohol Stud 29:968–973, 1968

Dorus W, Ostrow DG, Anton R, et al: Lithium treatment of depressed and nondepressed alcoholics. JAMA 162:1646–1652, 1989

Dunner DL, Hensel BM, Fieve RR: Bipolar illness: factors in drinking behavior. Am J Psychiatry 136:583–585, 1979

Edwards G, Kyle E, Nicholls P: A study of alcoholics admitted to four hospitals, I: social class and the interaction of the alcoholics with the treatment system. Quarterly Journal of Studies on Alcohol 35:499–522, 1974

Fillmore KM, Bacon SD, Hyman M: The 27-Year Longitudinal Panel Study of Drinking by Students in College, 1949–1976. Final Report to the National Institute on Alcohol Abuse and Alcoholism. Contract No ADM 281-76-0015, 1979

Frezza M, di Padova, Pozzato G, et al: High blood alcohol levels in women: the role of decreased gastric alcohol dehydrogenase activity and first-pass metabolism. N Engl J Med 322:92–95, 1990 [Published errata appear in N Engl J Med 322:1540, 1990 and N Engl J Med 323:553, 1990]

Glueck S, Glueck E: Unravelling Juvenile Delinquency. New York, The Commonwealth Fund, 1950

Goodwin DW: Is Alcoholism Hereditary? New York, Oxford University Press, 1976

Goodwin DW: Alcoholism and heredity. Arch Gen Psychiatry 36:57–61, 1979

Haberman PW: Childhood symptoms in children of alcoholics and comparison group parents. Journal of Marriage and the Family 28:152–154, 1966

Halikas JA: Psychotropic medication used in the treatment of alcoholism. Hospital and Community Psychiatry 34:1035–1039, 1983

Heath DB: A critical review of ethnographic studies of alcohol use, in Research Advances in Alcohol and Drug Problems, Vol 2. Edited by Gibbins RJ, Israel Y, Kalant H, et al. New York, Wiley, 1975, pp 1–92

Hesselbrock MN: Women alcoholics: a comparison of the natural history of alcoholism between men and women, in Evaluation of the Alcoholic: Implications for Research, Theory and Treatment. Edited by Myer RR, et al. Washington, DC, National Institute on Alcohol Abuse and Alcoholism, 1981

Jellinek EM: The Disease Concept of Alcoholism. New Haven, CT, Hillhouse Press, 1960

Jessor R, Jessor SL: Adolescent development and the onset of drinking. J Stud Alcohol 36:27–51, 1975

Jones MC: Personality correlates and antecedents of drinking patterns in adult males. J Consult Clin Psychol 32:2–12, 1968

Kagle J: Women who drink: changing ages, changing realities. Social Work Education 3:21–28, 1987

Kammeier ML, Hoffmann H, Loper RG: Personality characteristics of alcoholics as college freshmen and at time of treatment. Quarterly Journal of Studies on Alcohol 34:390–399, 1973

Lau H: Cost of alcoholic beverages as a determinant of alcohol consumption, in Research Advances in Alcohol and Drug Problems, Vol 2. Edited by Gibbins RJ, Israel Y, Kalant H, et al. New York, Wiley, 1975, pp 211–246

Leighton DC, Harding JS, Macklin DB, et al: Psychiatric findings of the Stirling County Study. Am J Psychiatry 119:1021–1026, 1963

Logue PE, Gentry WD, Linnoila M, et al: Effect of alcohol consumption on state anxiety changes in male and female nonalcoholics. Am J Psychiatry 135:1079–1081, 1978

Margulies RZ, Kessler RC, Kandel DB: A longitudinal study of onset of drinking among high school students. J Stud Alcohol 38:897–912, 1977

Marlatt GA, Rohsenow DJ: Cognitive processes in alcohol use: expectancy and the balanced placebo design, in Advances in Substance Abuse: Behavioral and Biological Research. Edited by Marlow NK. Greenwich, CT, JAI Press, 1980, pp 159–200

McLellan AT, Woody GE, O'Brien CP: Development of psychiatric illness in drug abusers: possible role of drug preferences. N Engl J Med 301:1310–1314, 1979

McCord W, McCord J: Origins of Alcoholism. Stanford, CA, Stanford University Press, 1960

Mello NK, McNamee HB, Mendelson JH: Drinking patterns of chronic alcoholics: gambling and motivations for alcohol. Psychiatric Research Reports 24:83–118, 1968

Merikangas KR, Leckman JR, Prusoff BA, et al: Familial transmission of depression and alcoholism. Arch Gen Psychiatry 42:367–372, 1985

Merikangas KR, Gelernter CS: Comorbidity for alcoholism and depression. Psychiatr Clin North Am 13:613–632, 1990

Morrison JR: Bipolar affective disorder and alcoholism. Am J Psychiatry 131:1130–1133, 1974

Morrison JR: The family histories of manic depressive patients with and without alcoholism. J Nerv Ment Dis 160:227–229, 1975

Nathan PE, Titler NA, Lowenstein LM, et al: Behavioral analysis of chronic alcoholism. Arch Gen Psychiatry 22:419–430, 1970

Ornstein S: Control of alcohol consumption through price increases. Quarterly Journal of Studies on Alcohol 4:807–818, 1980

Pettinati HM, Sugerman AA, Maurer HS: Four year MMPI changes in abstinent and drinking alcoholics. Alcohol Clin Exp Res 6:487–494, 1982

Pittman DJ, Snyder CR: Society, Culture and Drinking Patterns. New York, Wiley, 1962

Plant ML: Drinking Careers. London, Tavistock, 1979

Robins LN: Deviant Children Grown Up: A Sociological and Psychiatric Study of Sociopathic Personality. Baltimore, MD, Williams & Wilkins, 1966

Schmidt W, Popham RE: Heavy alcohol consumption and physical health problems: a review of the epidemiological evidence. Drug Alcohol Depend 1:27–50, 1975

Schuckit MA: Advances to understanding the vulnerability to alcoholism, in Addictive States. Edited by O'Brien CP, Jaffe JH. London, Raven, 1992, pp 93–108

Schuckit MA, Pitts FN, Reich T, et al: Alcoholism, I: two types of alcoholism in women. Arch Environ Health 18:301–306, 1969

Schuckit MA, Goodwin DW, Winokur G: A half-sibling study of alcoholism. Am J Psychiatry 128:1132–1136, 1972

Seixas R: Racial difference in alcohol metabolism: introduction. Alcohol Clin Exp Res 2:59, 1978

Simmel E: Alcoholism and addiction. Psychoanal Q 17:6–31, 1948

Special Committee of the Royal College of Psychiatrists: Alcohol and Alcoholism. London, Tavistock, 1979

Stivers R: A Hair of the Dog. University Park, PA, Pennsylvania State University Press, 1976

Sundby P: Alcoholism and Mortality. Oslo, Universitets Forlaget, 1967

Tamerin JS, Weiner S, Mendelson JH: Alcoholics expectancies and recall of experiences during intoxication. Am J Psychiatry 126:1697–1704, 1970

Tarter RE: Minimal brain dysfunction as an etiological predisposition to alcoholism, in Evaluation of the Alcoholic: Implications for Research, Theory and Treatment. Edited by Meyer RE, et al. Washington, DC, National Institute on Alcohol Abuse and Alcoholism, 1981

Utne HE, Vallo Hansen F, Winkler K, et al: Alcohol elimination rates in adoptees with and without alcoholic parents. Quarterly Journal of Studies on Alcohol 38:1219–1223, 1977

Vaillant GE: Natural history of male psychological health, VIII: antecedent of alcoholism and orality. Am J Psychiatry 137:181–186, 1980

Vaillant GE: Evidence that the type 1/type 2 dichotomy in alcoholism must be re-examined. Addiction 89:1049–1057, 1994

Vaillant GE: Natural History of Alcoholism Revisited. Cambridge, MA, Harvard University Press, 1995

Vesell ES, Page JF, Passananti GT: Genetic and environmental factors affecting ethanol metabolism in man. Clin Pharmacol Ther 12:192–201, 1971

Viamontes JA: Review of drug effectiveness in the treatment of alcoholism. Am J Psychiatry 128:1570–1571, 1972

von Knorring AL, Bohman M, von Knorring L, et al: Platelet MAO activity is a biological marker in subgroups of alcoholism. Acta Psychiatr Scand 72:51–58, 1985

Weissman MM, Gershon ES, Kidd KK, et al: Psychiatric disorders in the relatives of probands with affective disorders. Arch Gen Psychiatry 41:13–21, 1984

Wilsnack SC, Beckman LJ (eds): Alcohol Problems in Women. New York, Guilford, 1989

Winokur G, Clayton DJ, Reich T: Manic Depressive Illness. St Louis, MO, CV Mosby, 1969

Winokur G, Rimmer J, Reich T: Alcoholism, IV: is there more than one type of alcoholism? Br J Psychiatry 118:525–531, 1971

Woodruff RA, Guze SB, Clayton PJ, et al: Alcoholism and depression. Arch Gen Psychiatry 28:97–100, 1973

CHAPTER 16

Prevention of Antisocial Personality Disorder

David R. Offord, M.D.

Antisocial personality disorder begins in childhood and extends into adult life (American Psychiatric Association 1994; Robins et al. 1991). To qualify for the diagnosis, the person must show evidence of onset of conduct disorder before age 15 years. In adult life, after the age of 15, the individual must exhibit three or more behaviors that indicate "a pervasive pattern of disregard for and violation of the rights of others" (American Psychiatric Association 1994, p. 649). Antisocial personality disorder is a relatively rare disorder, with an estimated 4% of the U.S. population having ever warranted this diagnosis (Robins et al. 1991). The focus of this chapter is broader than consideration of the prevention of antisocial personality disorder per se. The chapter addresses the prevention of serious antisocial behavior throughout the life cycle regardless of whether, in the case of adults, the affected individual qualifies for a diagnosis of antisocial personality disorder.

The Case for Prevention

The prevention of antisocial behavior is attractive not only because of the general disadvantages of the treatment of mental disorders but also because of special features of antisocial behavior in general and antisocial personality disorder in specific.

Clinical programs that focus on the treatment of mental disorders in childhood and adolescence have serious limitations (Offord et al. 1998). It is difficult to provide adequate coverage for those with clinically important emotional and behavioral problems, and compliance is a vexatious issue. For example, among families who begin treatment because of a child's having emotional or behavior problems, 40%–60% withdraw from treatment prematurely (Kazdin 1996). Further, the possible stigmatization of having one's behavior labeled antisocial can itself lead to an increase in the behavior (Farrington 1977). Moreover, treatment is expensive, and by the time the child and the family have entered treatment, they have suffered a good deal and the disorder and associated dysfunction may be well entrenched. All of these disadvantages make prevention attractive for mental disorders in children and adolescents.

In addition, certain features of antisocial behavior make prevention especially appealing. First, the condition is associated with a heavy burden of suffering (Reid and Eddy 1997), and because of the high prevalence of the condition, even if effective treatments were available, the number of children and young adolescents with clinically important levels of antisocial behavior (e.g., conduct disorder) would far exceed the resources available to treat them. Second, the results of treatment of antisocial behavior have been discouraging (Kazdin 1997; Offord and Bennett 1994). Third, in most instances, serious antisocial behavior—whether occurring in the developmental years or in adulthood—has recognizable antecedents, usually consisting of the milder forms of antisocial behavior (Loeber and Farrington 1997). Thus, identifying groups of individuals at increased risk for serious antisocial behavior is at least plausible. The advantages of preventing antisocial behavior before it gathers momentum and becomes established are overwhelming. The question is, How can it be done?

The Need for a Developmental Model

Prevention efforts focused on antisocial behavior must be guided by a developmental model. The model should have several characteristics.

First, it should differentiate clearly among correlates, risk factors, markers, and causal risk factors for antisocial behavior (Kraemer et al. 1997). For example, markers can serve to identify a high-risk population for prevention initiatives, but causal risk factors, not correlates or noncausal risk factors, should be the focus of the intervention. Second, the causal risk factor or factors on which the intervention program is centered must have been shown to have high *attributable risk*. This measure indicates the proportion of new cases of a disorder or condition, such as antisocial behavior, that would be prevented if the causal effects of the risk factor could be eliminated (Kleinbaum et al. 1982, p. 160). If risk factors with low attributable risk are the focus of interventions, the expected reduction in the level of antisocial behavior will be modest even if the intervention program is effective. Third, the model should indicate that the nature of the intervention will differ depending on the stage of development at which the intervention takes place (Reid and Eddy 1997). For example, interventions in the prenatal period will, by necessity, focus on the mother. In contrast, interventions in middle childhood will have multiple foci, including the child, the parents, teachers, and peers. Fourth, the elements of the intervention should be clearly described, and evidence of the effectiveness of the proposed elements of the intervention in reducing the risk factors themselves or in altering the mechanisms by which the risk factors have their effects should be presented. Lastly, the model should indicate what proximal effects of the intervention should be evaluated along with more distal outcomes. If, for example, a parent management program is one of the elements of the intervention, a proximal outcome that should be assessed is the extent to which parenting behaviors have improved. The evaluation of distal outcomes alone is unwise and fails to monitor the short-term benefits of particular elements of the intervention.

Overall Approach to the Prevention of Antisocial Behavior

The prevention of antisocial behavior cannot be accomplished by a one-step intervention program. It instead requires both universal and targeted programs set in the context of a civic community.

Civic Community

Robert Putnam, in his seminal work *Making Democracy Work: Civic Traditions in Modern Italy* (Putnam 1993a), traces the development in different parts of Italy of regional governments set up in 1970. Over the succeeding 20 years, large regional differences in the performance of these governments were noted; the regional governments in the north did much better than those in the south. A major explanatory factor was that in northern Italy, the communities were far more "civic" than in southern Italy. A civic community is a community in which there is civic engagement. Citizenship in a civic community is marked, first, by active participation in public affairs (Putnam 1993a, 1993b); there is solidarity, trust, and tolerance among the citizens. Citizens are helpful and trustful of one another, even when they have different views on important matters. They set up community activities such as athletic teams and choral societies, and there is a sense of collective responsibility for children in the community. The presence of both a high degree of *collective efficacy*, defined as social cohesion among neighbors as well as a willingness to intercede on behalf of the common good (Sampson et al. 1997), and strong horizontal ties in the community ensures that social capital (Coleman 1988) will be present in impressive amounts.

Prevention programs for antisocial behavior, whether universal or targeted, have little chance of success if the context in which they are placed is a disorganized, uncivic community. These programs are fragile, and a necessary prerequisite for their success is a modicum of civicness in the setting in which they exist. For example, an intervention program in the schools, either universal or targeted, requires that the schools be adequately staffed and organized if the program is to have a chance of success. The effects of a disorganized, uncivic community on the development of antisocial behavior cannot be "cured" by placing a universal or targeted program in that community.

Universal Programs

Advantages and Disadvantages

In universal programs, all residents in a geographic area or setting (e.g., a school) receive the intervention. The individuals do not seek help, and no one is singled out for the intervention. The universal approach has many advantages and disadvantages (Table 16–1). One major advantage is that there is no labeling or stigmatization of individuals, since the intervention is offered to the entire population of interest. Another advantage is that the members of the middle class will be involved in the program, and they tend to demand that the program be well run. Economically disadvantaged parents, for example, may be less likely than middle-class parents to find fault with a program and complain about its deficiencies. Yet another advantage is that a universal program, though not expected to have large effects on individuals, can have a sizable cumulative effect on the population. Suppose, for example, that a universal intervention raises the IQ scores an average of 1 or 2 points for all individuals in the population; although the improvements are slight for individuals, the gains can be considerable for the population as a whole.

TABLE 16–1.   *Selected advantages and disadvantages of universal programs for the prevention of antisocial behavior*

Advantages	Disadvantages
Involves no labeling or stigmatization	Hard to convince public and politicians of widespread usefulness of program
Is accompanied by demand from the middle class that the program be well run	Has small benefit to the individual
Has large potential for the population	Is hard to detect an overall effect
Has potential for focus on community-wide contextual factors	May have the greatest effect on those at lowest risk, thus increasing inequality
Is behaviorally appropriate	Is unnecessarily expensive
Sensitizes the setting ("tills the soil") for targeted interventions	Denies the non-high-risk population the opportunity of doing good
	May undermine community initiatives
	May be perceived by the low-risk population as having little benefit for their children

Some further advantages of a universal approach are in areas in which the targeted approach has distinct disadvantages. A universal program can contain elements that are directed at community-wide factors, whereas a targeted program focuses on variables that differentiate the high-risk group from the low-risk group (Rose 1985). Suppose, for example, that community A has high rates of conduct disorder compared with community B. A targeted preventive approach would look for variables within the children in community A that distinguish the children at high risk for conduct disorder from those at low risk for that condition. However, suppose that in community A there is a community-wide factor — for example, a paucity of well-run day care centers — that contributes significantly to increased rates of conduct disorder overall in that community compared with community B. The latter community has a plethora of well-run day care centers and thus much lower rates of conduct disorder. A universal intervention would focus on a community-wide contextual element, such as increasing the number of effective day care centers, whereas a targeted intervention would not consider this community-wide factor in developing its potential elements.

Yet another advantage of the universal approach is that by not singling out children for the intervention, specific children are not being asked to change their behavior in a context in which all children are behaving in a similar, though not as severe, manner. It is difficult, for example, to expect specific children with behavior disorders to lessen their troublesome behavior in a context in which most children are behaving in a similar fashion.

One further advantage of the universal approach is that it "tills the soil" for a targeted program. If a universal program is in place in a setting such as a school, the milieu is one that is accustomed to the presence of the program. If a targeted program is then implemented, it is more likely to be widely embraced, and the identified children are less likely to feel labeled and stigmatized.

The disadvantages of universal programs are several. First, it is hard to convince the public and politicians of the widespread usefulness of such programs. These programs do not deal with dramatic clinical cases and can raise concerns about social engineering or about interfering with personal freedoms or intruding in family business. Second, there is only a small benefit to the individual. Third, in terms of evaluating program effectiveness, since the effect sizes are small, it is difficult to ascertain reliably whether the intervention has been effective. Fourth, although universal programs are put in place in many instances to reduce the inequality among groups of children in a population, they may have the opposite effect. There is the concern, for example, that universal programs aimed at reducing antisocial behavior in a population may have their greatest effect on those children with low levels of antisocial behavior. They will in effect make "nice kids even nicer" but will have little or no beneficial effect on children with troublesome antisocial behavior. Thus, inequality, in terms of levels of antisocial behavior, will be increased in the population. In a similar fashion, universal programs aimed at benefiting poor children and their families end up benefiting the middle class to a greater extent (Howe and Longman 1992; Jones 1994). Fifth, a universal program may be unnecessarily expensive. The majority of children receiving the program may not need it. If a universal program has as its goal, for example, the prevention of clinically important antisocial behavior, the at-risk group may constitute no more than 20% of the population, and thus 8 out of 10 children do not need the universal intervention.

The last three disadvantages of universal programs center on the reactions of the non-high-risk group. With a universal program in place, members of the non-high-risk group may feel that the efforts they would make, under ordinary circumstances, to help out the more disadvantaged members of the population are no longer needed. The universal program is in fact fulfilling that need. In a similar vein, a universal program may undermine a community initiative. The initiative is perceived by the residents as not needed anymore because of the presence of the universal program. Lastly, it may be that the low-risk population will view a universal program unenthusiastically because, for example, the parents of the low-risk children know that the program is not needed for their children. They may feel that the unstated purpose of the universal program is to serve the high-risk population, and it can be irritating to them that this is done under the guise of providing a program for all children.

Tri-Ministry Study and
Other Universal Programs

Our group at the Centre for Studies of Children at Risk in Hamilton, Ontario, has recently completed a large-scale prevention project, the Tri-Ministry Study. This initiative is a school-based trial aimed at reducing or preventing problem behavior, including antisocial behavior, among children in the primary division (kindergarten to grade 3) of Ontario schools. The trial was carried out between 1991 and 1995, and the elements of the intervention were a parent management training program, a classwide social skills training program, and a partner reading program. These three elements, plus selected combinations, were evaluated for their effectiveness during the trial. Sixty schools were selected by the 11 participating school boards and randomly assigned to one of the intervention programs throughout the course of the study. The evaluation database consisted of detailed follow-up assessments (observations, ratings, and standard tests) on 2,439 children. Assessments of school climate variables were furnished annually by more than 500 teachers. Three-level growth trajectory models were used to evaluate program effects.

Preliminary results indicate that there were significant gains on children's positive playground behavior and significant reductions in children's inappropriate classroom behavior among children in schools receiving the classwide social skills training program either alone or in combination with the partner reading program. The source of data used in the evaluation of these gains was independent observation by trained observers. Further, it was found that the combined social skills training and partner reading program produced gains in children's reading achievement, as indicated by scores on the Wide Range Achievement Test, and in teacher ratings of children's externalizing problems. No significant effects for any interventions were found on measures of parent-rated externalizing problems and on ratings by teachers or parents of social competence. Lastly, it should be noted that although the positive results reported here were statistically significant, the effect sizes (see Cohen 1988) were in the moderate range (0.17–0.44) and diminished over time.

In addition to the Tri-Ministry Study, there are six universal programs focusing on a nonclinic community sample of children in which the intervention was initiated in the school setting for groups of children, most of whom were in kindergarten to grade 3. Available outcome data included a measure of externalizing behavior, and results have been reported since 1987 (Cunningham et al. 1998; Garaigordobil and Echebarria 1995; Grossman et al. 1997; Kellam et al. 1994; O'Donnell et al. 1995; Sharpe et al. 1995).

As would be expected, the results were mixed, but most studies found some improvement in externalizing behavior. A common thread was that none of the results had a large effect size. There are a number of reasons why it would not be expected that the results from the Tri-Ministry Study and similar universal interventions would be stronger than were demonstrated.

Selection of schools.   Schools that volunteer for participation in a study may be on positive trajectories for a reduction in behavior problems. In addition, the selection of a school for study itself, regardless of whether the school is receiving the intervention or not, may stimulate positive changes that reduce behavior problems. Similarly, the fact that repeated measures are being taken on children's behavior, classroom and school atmosphere, and teacher satisfaction may in itself induce positive changes in a school, even if the school is not receiving the intervention. Monitoring may prompt a school to introduce changes it is already contemplating. One or more of these mechanisms may account for the striking finding in the Tri-Ministry Study of marked positive trajectories in outcome measures for children in both the nonintervention (control) schools and the experimental schools. Thus, the trajectories in the outcomes in the intervention schools, if the intervention is to be deemed effective, would have to be more markedly positive than the trajectories in the outcomes in the control schools.

Design.   A randomized controlled trial has the advantage of being the strongest design with which to evaluate the effectiveness of an intervention program. However, when the unit of assignment and analysis is a school, two potential limitations arise immediately. First, there may be large differences among the schools—at the outset of the study and throughout the study—on variables measured cross-sectionally or longitudinally that are highly relevant to the measured outcomes. In short, the differences between schools may be so great that they dwarf changes that could be expected between schools because of the intervention. In the Tri-Ministry Study, there were sizeable differences among the schools at the beginning of the study on relevant prognostic variables. Second, when the unit of randomization is the school, there will be marked limitations on the sample size in the study. If the unit of randomization is the individual, a large sample involving hundreds of subjects randomized to the experimental and control groups could be expected to deal adequately with the differences among individuals. It would be far more likely that the experimental and control groups, because of randomization, would be equivalent on relevant prognostic variables.

A second aspect of the role of design deserves mention. The follow-up period of 42 months in the Tri-Ministry Study is not adequate to evaluate the possibility that the effects of the interventions may grow over time or that there may be long-term effects (so-called sleeper effects). Such patterns have been reported elsewhere in intervention studies with children (e.g., Tremblay et al. 1996).

Lastly, in a randomized controlled trial, it is expected that the experimental group will receive the intervention and the control group will not. However, by the time a commitment is made to evaluate a universal program, it is likely that the elements of the program are already being widely implemented (e.g., Winkleby et al. 1987). Thus, it is very difficult to select comparison sites where the program element to be tested in the intervention sites is not present in some form. For example, in year 1 of the Tri-Ministry Study, 36% of the control schools had social skills programs in place, and by year 4 the proportion of control schools having such programs increased to 51% in the first cohort of children. This increase during the study of social skills programs in the control schools may have been stimulated by knowledge of the systematic social skills program under way in the experimental sites.

Interventions.   First, the duration of the intervention may affect the magnitude of the outcome. The small effect of the size of the positive results in the Tri-Ministry Study can be accounted for in part by the short duration of the interventions (typically 1 year). The short duration of the intervention programs may be responsible for the finding of a diminution in the magnitude of the positive intervention effects over the 42-month time period.

Second, interventions may have to be of enough intensity before they can be expected to produce a sizeable population effect on the outcomes of interests. The intervention in the Tri-Ministry study may not have been intense enough to effect such outcomes.

Third, it may be that some elements of the intervention implemented over the course of the project are not appropriate ones for providing large effect sizes in the outcome variables. In the Tri-Ministry Study, for example, the absence of an intervention element focusing on changing parenting behaviors could be seen as a major deficit in a program aimed at preventing antisocial behavior in young children. A parent training program was part of the original intervention package in the Tri-Ministry Study. However, this element was dropped at the end of year 2 because attendance levels were too low (14.3%) for a population effect to be demonstrated.

Fourth, the interventions themselves may not be delivered as planned by a sufficient number of teachers and facilitators. The information available on this issue in the Tri-Ministry Study suggests that the program components were implemented quite well. The data on the fidelity of program implementation do not, however, have reliability estimates and are not objective.

Lastly, the high rates of mobility of teachers, principals, and students make it impossible to have continuity of the intervention program in terms of either the deliverers of the program or its recipients. Over the 5 years of the Tri-Ministry Study, on average, 21% of the teachers, 16% of the principals, and 35% of the students moved each year.

Measures. The measures of the outcomes of interest may not be sensitive enough to pick up changes in the outcomes of the magnitudes that could be expected from a study such as the Tri-Ministry Study.

Universal strategy. A universal program cannot be expected to have large effects on the population as a whole. Even if the program were of acceptable duration, the elements were appropriate, the delivery was as planned, and mobility was not a problem, the intervention would not be expected to have large effects. The absence of a large effect is the consistent finding from universal intervention programs, regardless of whether they focus on changing children's antisocial behavior or adults' health practices (e.g., Winkleby et al. 1987). There are two reasons for this. First, most members of the population of interest will not have the behavior that is to be prevented, or at least will not exhibit very much of it. Thus, they cannot show improvement at all in this domain or can show only a small amount. For example, in the case of antisocial behavior in young children, which is a major focus of the Tri-Ministry Study, most young children will have minimal levels of antisocial behavior, if they have any at all. Second, since the intensity of the program is limited because it has to be delivered to so many individuals, the program cannot be expected to produce marked positive results in that small proportion of the population that has high and severe levels of the behavior of interest.

An intervention program to prevent antisocial behavior delivered universally to a population of children cannot be expected to have marked positive effects on those children at highest risk of developing antisocial behavior or with the highest level and severity of the behavior. Universal programs can be expected to have their beneficial effect on that relatively small group of children in a population who have mild forms of the behavior of interest. Even if programs are highly effective with this subgroup, the overall population effects of the program cannot be expected to be marked.

In summary, there are a number of reasons why the positive results of the Tri-Ministry Study were not more widespread and of greater magnitude. Universal programs will have some positive effects and, as noted previously, will sensitize the setting to interventions and evaluations that make it further receptive to more intense, targeted programs.

Targeted Interventions

In targeted interventions, the recipients—for example, children and their families—do not seek help, but rather individual children are singled out for the intervention. The children are identified as in need of the intervention because they are thought to be at high risk for developing a disorder (e.g., conduct disorder). Children can be identified as being at increased risk on the basis of either identifying characteristics that lie outside the child (e.g., family on social assistance) or distinguishing features of the child himself or herself (e.g., mild antisocial behavior). In the book on prevention by the Institute of Medicine (1994), these two types of targeted prevention programs are termed *selective preventive interventions* and *indicated preventive interventions*, respectively, and in the past, the term *secondary prevention* was used for these endeavors.

Selected advantages and disadvantages of targeted programs are presented in Table 16–2. Advantages of targeted programs include the possibility that such programs are potentially efficient and that they can address problems early on before they become severe. These possibilities can be realized only if the high-risk group can be targeted accurately.

Targeted programs have several disadvantages. One disadvantage is that labeling and stigmatization can be a problem, particularly if children in, for example, the high-risk group are incorrectly identified.

TABLE 16–2.   *Selected advantages and disadvantages of targeted programs for the prevention of antisocial behavior*

Advantages	Disadvantages
Is potentially efficient	Can lead to labeling and stigmatization
Can address problems early on	Involves issues regarding difficulties with screening
	Cost and commitment
	Uptake least among those at greatest risk
	Boundary problem
	Risk status unstable
	Difficulty targeting accurately
	Has limited potential for individuals and populations
	Power to predict future disorder usually very weak
	More cases of disease possibly attributable to the large number of people at small risk than to the small number at high risk
	Tends to ignore the social context as a focus of intervention
	Is behaviorally inappropriate

A second disadvantage of a targeted program is that the necessity of screening, in itself, raises a number of issues. The cost and commitment to carry out the screening year after year must be considered. Further, noncompliance with the screen can be expected to be highest among those at increased risk (Rose 1985; Rutter et al. 1970). The issue of where one sets the threshold for including children in the targeted group is also a factor. This issue becomes even more problematic if the risk status is unstable and repeated screenings are necessary—a situation that emphasizes the advantage of using a stable marker to indicate the high-risk group. Lastly, it can be difficult to target a population accurately. Lipman et al. (1998), using data from the Ontario Child Health Study (a large, provincewide community survey of the mental health of children aged 4–16 years), showed that of children identified as antisocial at ages 4 and 5 years, a maximum of 50% would still be antisocial 4 years later (i.e., positive predictive value = 50%). Further, of those children who were antisocial at ages 8 and 9 years, a maximum of 50% would have been identified 4 years earlier on a screen as being antisocial at ages 8 or 9 (i.e., sensitivity = 50%). It should be kept in mind that clinicians are concerned primarily with the positive predictive value: How likely is it that the patient they are seeing will have the current disturbed behavior down the road? Public health officials, on the other hand, are concerned not just with positive predictive value but with sensitivity as well: What proportion of individuals with the behavior at issue would have been identified by a screen administered some years before? The answers to these questions bring up the relative importance of false positives and false negatives. These issues, the discussion of which is outside the scope of this chapter, have been covered elsewhere (Offord et al. 1998).

A third disadvantage of the targeted program is that it has limited potential for individuals and populations (Rose 1985). The power to predict future disorder is usually very weak (e.g., White et al. 1990). Further, although members of a high-risk group can be expected to have a greater proportion of individuals who will eventually qualify for the disorder of interest if effective intervention does not occur, the vast majority of the cases will come from the low-risk group. For example, data from the Ontario Child Health Study reveals that, as expected, children living in families with an annual income level under Can$10,000 are at high risk for developing one or more psychiatric disorders, with more than one-third of them (36.3%) having conditions that qualify as cases. However, only 7.3% of children in Ontario are from families in this income category. Thus, economically disadvantaged children account for only 14.5% of the population with psychiatric disorder in the province. However, children who live in families that are more well off financially (annual income of Can$25,000 or more) account for more than one-half (59%) of the children with psychiatric disorder. The risk for disorder is much lower in the relatively well-off population of children than in the economically disadvantaged population, but the large number of these children means that their contribution to the population of children with disorder is far greater than that of the poor children. An implication of this finding is that one targeted program, even if successful, cannot be expected to have marked effects at the population level.

Two further disadvantages of targeted programs — namely, that such programs tend to ignore the social context as a focus of intervention and that they can be behaviorally inappropriate — have been alluded to previously in the discussion of the advantages of universal programs.

Four targeted programs in the literature focusing on interventions with children in early elementary school have produced improvement in externalizing behavior during the intervention or at post-test on at least one measure or for at least one intervention group (Bierman et al. 1997; Bloomquist et al. 1991; Conduct Problems Prevention Research Group 1992, 1997; Prinz et al. 1994). Evidence for delayed positive effects was found for a fifth targeted program (Tremblay et al. 1996).

Tremblay and Craig (1995) did an extensive review of targeted programs aimed at preventing antisocial behavior and delinquency. The intervention programs focused on three risk factors: socially disruptive behavior, cognitive deficits, and poor parenting. The authors noted that experiments with juvenile delinquency as an outcome demonstrated that positive results were more likely when the interventions were implemented before adolescence, focused on more than one risk factor, and lasted for a relatively long time. Early childhood interventions focusing on the three aforementioned risk factors were reported to have generally positive results. The authors concluded by pointing out that the majority of studies were of small scale and that the next step was to test the effectiveness of large-scale efforts.

Prevention of Antisocial Behavior

The prevention of antisocial behavior will require a combination of strategies. Clearly, methods must be found and efforts must be put forth to enable communities to have the necessary infrastructure, the civicness if you like, to support programs aimed at reducing the incidence of antisocial behavior. There is no substitute for this first step. Given a community with civic characteristics, the most promising approach is to have a combination of universal and targeted programs. The universal program will accomplish two major goals: it will lead to some reduction in antisocial behavior, and it will increase the community's motivation to implement a series of targeted programs for children who were not helped sufficiently by the universal programs in such a way that labeling and stigmatization are minimized. There are examples in the literature of combined universal and targeted programs in which a classwide social skills curriculum is used in combination with a targeted intervention (Bloomquist et al. 1991; Conduct Problems Prevention Research Group 1997).

It could be argued that universal programs, such as the teaching of social skills in elementary schools, should be an integrated part of the curriculum and be explicit and systematized. The results of the program could be continuously monitored, and, indeed, schools should be centrally involved in monitoring the health and well-being of their children.

Two other issues deserve mention. The first involves finding ways to ensure that successful programs in one setting can be disseminated to and maintained in other settings. Barriers to dissemination, discussed elsewhere (Offord 1997), include the following:

- There is insufficient information on the costs of the program, or the costs are prohibitive.
- The program is not feasible and acceptable to either the deliverers of the program or the target population.
- The program was imposed on the setting by people or organizations from the outside.
- The program has a high reliance on exceptional people who cannot easily be duplicated.

A second issue has to do with the allotment of limited research funds. Difficult decisions will have to be made between funding descriptive longitudinal studies and funding experimental studies (Robins 1978), and between funding small-scale efficacy studies (Will the intervention do more good than harm under ideal conditions?) and funding larger-scale effectiveness studies (Will the intervention do more good than harm when carried out in real-world conditions?). It would appear not only that each of these endeavors needs support but also that, to reduce the burden of suffering of antisocial behavior, work must proceed on discovering effective interventions—universal, targeted, and clinical.

The enterprise of preventing antisocial behavior, although difficult, remains so attractive because, as Lee Robins has noted (Robins 1974), if we could discover how to prevent antisocial behavior successfully in childhood and adolescence, we could reduce antisocial behavior and antisocial personality disorder markedly within one generation.

References

American Psychiatric Association: Diagnostic and Statistical Manual of Mental Disorders, 4th Edition. Washington, DC, American Psychiatric Association, 1994

Bierman KL, Miller CL, Stabb SD: Improving the social behavior and peer acceptance of rejected boys: effects of social skills training with instructions and prohibitions. J Consult Clin Psychol 55:194–200, 1987

Bloomquist ML, August GJ, Ostrander R: Effects of a school-based cognitive-behavioral intervention for ADHD children. J Abnorm Child Psychol 19:591–605, 1991

Cohen J: Statistical Power Analysis for the Behavioral Sciences, 2nd Edition. Hillsdale, NJ, Lawrence Erlbaum, 1988

Coleman JS: Social capital in the creation of human capital. American Journal of Sociology 94(suppl):S95–S120, 1988

Conduct Problems Prevention Research Group: A developmental and clinical model for the prevention of conduct disorder: the FAST Track Program. Dev Psychopathol 4:509–527, 1992

Conduct Problems Prevention Research Group: Prevention of antisocial behavior: initial findings from the FAST Track Program. Symposium at the biennial meeting of the Society for Research in Child Development, Washington, DC, April 1997

Cunningham CE, Cunningham LJ, Martorelli V, et al: The effects of primary division, student-mediated conflict resolution programs on playground aggression. J Child Psychol Psychiatry 39:653–662, 1998

Farrington DP: The effects of public labelling. British Journal of Criminology 17:112–125, 1977

Garaigordobil M, Echebarria A: Assessment of peer-helping game program on children's development. Journal of Research in Childhood Education 10:63–69, 1995

Grossman DC, Neckerman HJ, Koepsell TD, et al: Effectiveness of a violence prevention curriculum among children in elementary school. JAMA 277:1605–1611, 1997

Howe N, Longman P: The next New Deal. Atlantic Monthly, June 1992, pp 88–99

Institute of Medicine: Reducing Risk for Mental Disorders: Frontiers for Preventive Intervention Research. Edited by Mrazek PJ, Haggerty RJ. Washington, DC, National Academy Press, 1994

Jones MB: Undoing the effects of poverty in children: non-economic initiatives, in Improving the Life Quality of Children: Options and Evidence (Post-Symposium Working Papers). Hamilton, Ontario, Centre for Studies of Children at Risk, 1994

Kazdin AE: Dropping out of child psychotherapy: issues for research and implications for practice. Clin Child Psychol Psychiatry 1:133–156, 1996

Kazdin AE: Practitioner review: psychosocial treatments for conduct disorder in children. J Child Psychol Psychiatry 38:161–178, 1997

Kellam SG, Rebok GW, Ialongo N, et al: The course and malleability of aggressive behavior from early first grade into middle school: results of a developmental epidemiologically-based preventive trial. J Child Psychol Psychiatry 35:259–281, 1994

Kleinbaum DG, Kupper LL, Morgenstern H: Epidemiologic Research: Principles and Quantitative Methods. New York, Van Nostrand Reinhold, 1982

Kraemer HC, Kazdin AE, Offord DR, et al: Coming to terms with the terms of risk. Arch Gen Psychiatry 54:337–373, 1997

Lipman EL, Bennett KJ, Racine YA, et al: What does early antisocial behavior predict: a follow-up of 4- and 5-year-olds from the Ontario Health Study. Can J Psychiatry 43:605–613, 1998

Loeber R, Farrington DP: Strategies and yields of longitudinal studies on antisocial behavior, in Handbook of Antisocial Behavior. Edited by Stoff DM, Breiling J, Maser JD. New York, Wiley, 1997, pp 125–139

O'Donnell J, Hawkins JD, Catalano RF, et al: Preventing school failure, drug use, and delinquency among low-income children: long-term intervention in elementary schools. Am J Orthopsychiatry 65:87–100, 1995

Offord DR: Bridging development, prevention, and policy, in Handbook of Antisocial Behavior. Edited by Stoff DM, Breiling J, Maser JD. New York, Wiley, 1997, pp 357–364

Offord DR, Bennett KJ: Long-term outcome of conduct disorder and interventions and their effects. J Am Acad Child Adolesc Psychiatry 33:1069–1078, 1994

Offord DR, Kraemer HC, Kazdin AE, et al: Lowering the burden of suffering from child psychiatric disorder: trade-offs among clinical, targeted, and universal interventions. J Am Acad Child Adolesc Psychiatry 37:686–694, 1998

Prinz RJ, Blechman EA, Dumas JE: An evaluation of peer-coping skills training for childhood aggression. J Clin Psychol 23:193–203, 1994

Putnam RD: Making Democracy Work: Civic Traditions in Modern Italy. Princeton, NJ, Princeton University Press, 1993a

Putnam RD: The prosperous community: social capital and public life. The American Prospect, Spring 1993b, pp 35–42

Reid JB, Eddy JM: The prevention of antisocial behavior: some considerations in the search for effective interventions, in Handbook of Antisocial Behavior. Edited by Stoff DM, Breiling J, Maser JD. New York, Wiley, 1997, pp 343–356

Robins LN: Antisocial behavior disturbances in childhood: prevalence, prognosis and prospects, in The Child in His Family: Children at Psychiatric Risk. Edited by Anthony EJ, Koupernick C. New York, Wiley, 1974, pp 447–460

Robins LN: Psychiatric epidemiology. Arch Gen Psychiatry 35:697–702, 1978

Robins LN, Tipp J, Przybeck T: Antisocial personality, in Psychiatric Disorders in America: The Epidemiologic Catchment Area Study. Edited by Robins LN, Regier DA. New York, Free Press, 1991, pp 258–290

Rose G: Sick individuals and sick populations. Int J Epidemiol 14:32–38, 1985

Rutter M, Tizard J, Whitmore K: Education, Health and Behaviour. London, Longman, 1970

Sampson RJ, Raudenbush SW, Earls F: Neighborhoods and violent crime: a multilevel study of collective efficacy. Science 277:918–924, 1997

Sharpe T, Brown M, Crider K: The effects of a sportsmanship curriculum intervention on generalized positive social behavior of urban elementary school students. J Appl Behav Anal 28:401–416, 1995

Tremblay RE, Craig WM: Developmental crime prevention, in Building a Safer Society: Strategic Approaches to Crime Prevention, Vol 19. Edited by Tonry M, Farrington DP. Chicago, IL, University of Chicago Press, 1995, pp 151–236

Tremblay RE, Masse LC, Pagani L, et al: From childhood aggression to adolescent maladjustment: the Montreal Prevention Experiment, in Preventing Childhood Disorders, Substance Abuse, and Delinquency. Edited by Peter RD, McMahon RJ. Thousand Oaks, CA, Sage, 1996, pp 268–298

White JL, Moffit TE, Earls F, et al: How early can we tell? Predictors of child conduct disorder and adolescent delinquency. Criminology 28:507–533, 1990

Winkleby MA, Miller CL, Stabb SD: Improving the social behavior and peer acceptance of rejected boys: effects of social skills training with instructions and prohibitions. J Consult Clin Psychol 55:194–200, 1987

Index

Page numbers printed in *boldface* type refer to tables or figures.